T5-BBU-994

CLINICAL CARE
in the Rheumatic Diseases

STEPHEN T. WEGENER, PhD, EDITOR

BASIA L. BELZA, PhD, RN, ASSOCIATE EDITOR

ERIC P. GALL, MD, CONSULTING EDITOR

Published by the American College of Rheumatology
60 Executive Park South
Suite 150
Atlanta, Georgia 30329

Library of Congress Cataloging-in-Publication Data

Clinical care in the rheumatic diseases / Stephen T. Wegener, editor:
  Basia L. Belza, associate editor; Eric P. Gall, consulting editor.
      p.   cm.
    Includes bibliographical references and index.
    ISBN 0-9654316-0-6 (pbk.)
    1. Rheumatism—Patients—Care.   2. Rheumatism—Patients—
Rehabilitation.   I. Wegener, Stephen T., 1952–   .   II. Belza, Basia
L., 1954–   .   III. Gall, Eric P. (Eric Papineau), 1940–   .
    [DNLM: 1. Arthritis—therapy.   2. Arthritis—diagnosis.
    3. Rheumatic Diseases—therapy.   4. Rheumatic Diseases—
diagnosis. WE 344 C6403 1996]
RC927.C528   1996
616.7'23—dc20
DNLM/DLC
for Library of Congress   96-41776
                                                                        CIP

Managing Editor: Cynthia M. Kahn
Editorial/Publication Assistant: Angela M. Wiens
Executive Director, Association of Rheumatology Health Professionals: Julie Epps
ISBN 0-9654316-0-6

Authors

Saralynn Allaire, ScD, RN, CRC
Health Services/Epidemiology Research Unit
Boston University Arthritis Center
Boston, MA

Thomas D. Beardmore, MD, FACP, FACR
University of Southern California
Rancho Los Amigos Medical Center
Downey, CA

Basia L. Belza, PhD, RN
University of Washington
Seattle, WA

Michele Boutaugh, BSN, MPH
The Arthritis Foundation
Atlanta, GA

Laurence A. Bradley, PhD
University of Alabama at Birmingham
Birmingham, AL

Teresa J. Brady, PhD
Chronic Disease Services
Fairview Health Systems
Minneapolis, MN

Kenneth D. Brandt, MD
Indiana University Multipurpose Arthritis
and Musculoskeletal Diseases Center
Indiana University School of Medicine
Indianapolis, IN

David S. Caldwell, MD
Duke University Medical Center
Durham, NC

Leigh F. Callahan, PhD
Thurston Arthritis Research Center
University of North Carolina at Chapel Hill
Chapel Hill, NC

A. Betts Carpenter, MD, PhD
Marshall University School of Medicine
Huntington, WV

Bruce M. Clark, RPT
The Mary Pack Arthritis Center
BC and Yukon Division, The Arthritis
Society
Vancouver, BC, Canada

Sharon R. Clark, PhD, RN-C, FNP
Oregon Health Sciences University
Portland, OR

Diane Erlandson, RN, MS, MPH
Hingham Visiting Nurse and Community
Service, Inc.
Hingham, MA

Judith A. Falconer, PhD, MPH, OTR
Programs in Physical Therapy
Northwestern University Medical School
Chicago, IL

Robert G. Frank, PhD
College of Health Professions
University of Florida Health Science
Center
Gainesville, FL

Victoria Gall, PT, MEd
Brigham and Women's Hospital
Boston, MA

Sandy B. Ganz, PT, MSCHE
Amsterdam Nursing Home Corp.
The Hospital for Special Surgery
New York, NY

Marie R. Griffin, MD, MPH
Vanderbilt University
Nashville, TN

Nortin M. Hadler, MD, FACP, FACR
School of Medicine
University of North Carolina at
Chapel Hill
Chapel Hill, NC

Kristofer J. Hagglund, PhD
School of Medicine
University of Missouri-Columbia
Columbia, MO

Pamela B. Harrell, OTR, CHT
Arthritis and Osteoporosis Care Center
Baptist Hospital
Nashville, TN

Donna J. Hawley, EdD, RN
Professor School of Nursing
Wichita State University
Wichita, KS

Karen W. Hayes, PhD, PT
Programs in Physical Therapy
Northwestern University Medical School
Chicago, IL

Francis J. Keefe, PhD
Duke University Medical Center
Durham, NC

John H. Klippel, MD
National Institute of Arthritis and
Musculoskeletal and Skin Diseases
Bethesda, MD

Kate R. Lorig, DrPH
Stanford Arthritis Center
Stanford University School of Medicine
Stanford, CA

Christopher D. Lorish, PhD
University of Alabama at Birmingham
School of Health Related Professions
Birmingham, AL

Michael J. Maricic, MD
University of Arizona Health Sciences Center
Tucson, Arizona

Donald R. Miller, PharmD
College of Pharmacy
North Dakota State University
Fargo, ND

Marian A. Minor, PhD, PT
School of Health Related Professions
University of Missouri
Columbia, MO

Carolee Moncur, PhD, PT
University of Utah
Salt Lake City, UT

Lisa A. Nichols, MSN, RN, FNP-C
The University of Texas
Southwestern Medical Center at Dallas
Dallas, TX

Jill A. Noaker, OTR/L, CHT
St. Margaret Memorial Hospital
Pittsburgh, PA

Richard S. Panush, MD
St. Barnabas Medical Center
University of Medicine and Dentistry of
New Jersey-New Jersey Medical School
Livingston, NJ

Jerry C. Parker, PhD
Harry S. Truman Memorial Veteran's
Hospital
University of Missouri-Columbia School of
Medicine
Columbia, MO

Theodore Pincus, MD
Vanderbilt University School of Medicine
Nashville, TN

Michael Rapoff, PhD
University of Kansas Medical Center
Kansas City, KS

Laura Robbins, DSW, MSW
Hospital for Special Surgery
Cornell Multipurpose Arthritis and
Musculoskeletal Disease Center
Cornell University Medical College
New York, NY

Kathleen M. Schiaffino, PhD
Fordham University
Bronx, NY

H. Ralph Schumacher, Jr., MD
University of Pennsylvania School of
Medicine
Veterans Affairs Medical Center
Hospital of the University of Pennsylvania
Philadelphia, PA

C. Michael Stein, MBCHD, MRCP
Vanderbilt University School of Medicine
Nashville, TN

Gigi Viellion, RN, ONC
Beth Israel Medical Center-North Division
New York, NY

Stephen T. Wegener, PhD
Johns Hopkins University
Baltimore, MD

Gail E. Wright, PhD
Harry S. Truman Memorial Veteran's
Hospital
University of Missouri-Columbia School of
Medicine
Columbia, MO

Contributors

The following individuals made publication of *Clinical Care in the Rheumatic Diseases* possible by participating in project development, the editorial process, or serving as chapter reviewers. Contributors of illustrations are identified in figure legends.

John P. Allegrante, PhD
Karen O. Anderson, PhD
Judith C. Bautch, PhD, RN, CS
Susan Belanger, MS
Cynthia Belar, PhD
Coleen Bertsch, RN, MSN
Mary J. Bridle, MA, OTR
Melanie Brown, MD
Danuta I. Bujak, MSN, CFNP
John L. Chase, MSN, RN, FNP
Mary P. Clapper, MSc, PT
Michael R. Clark, MD
Timothy Dillingham, MD
David Felson, MD, MPH
Judith Fifield, RN, PhD
Gloria Furst, OTR, MPH
Gregory Gardner, MD
Lynn Gerber, MD
Kathleen Haralson, PT, MLA
Scott M. Hasson, PT
Marc C. Hochberg, MD, MPH
Gaye M. Koenning, MS, RD
Amye L. Leong, MBA

Matthew H. Liang, MD, MPH
Martha K. Logigian, MS, OTR
Daniel Lovell, MD, MPH
Richard Maisiak, PhD, MPH
Diane Miller, RN
Gerri Neuberger, RN, EdD
Perry M. Nicassio, PhD
Nancy Olson, MD
Helen Ornstein, MS, RN, FNP
Alison J. Partridge, LICSW
Janice S. Pigg, BSN, RN, MS
Janet Poole, PhD, OTR
Marilyn K. Sanford, PT, PhD
Judy R. Sotosky, MEd, PT
Timothy M. Spiegel, MD, MPH
Barbara Stokes, PT
Annette M. Swezey, MSPH
Steven A. Stuchin, MD
Robert Willkens, MD
H. James Williams, MD
Lynn Yasuda, MSEd, OTR
Edward Yelin, PhD
Kathryn Zavadak, BS, PT

Table of Contents

FOREWARD

The publication of *Clinical Care in the Rheumatic Diseases* marks the culmination of a number of years of hard work and devotion on the part of the volunteers and staff of the Association of Rheumatology Health Professionals (ARHP). The ARHP, a division of the American College of Rheumatology, is a professional membership society composed of individuals from a variety of disciplines such as nursing, physical therapy, occupational therapy, social work, and other health professions. It is the only organization that brings together an interdisciplinary group of caregivers, educators, and researchers focused solely on rheumatic diseases.

Clinical Care in the Rheumatic Diseases is the ARHP's response to a perceived need in the rheumatology community for a text that addresses a focused approach to the continuum of care for people with rheumatic diseases. Until now, there has been no central source of clinical information to serve as a reference for health care providers involved in the diagnosis, treatment, and management of people with rheumatic disease.

The Association of Rheumatology Health Professionals is proud to offer this text as a cornerstone of our mission for all health care practitioners and providers who care for patients with rheumatic disease. *Clinical Care in the Rheumatic Diseases* is an excellent example of how ARHP's members view their commitment as premier providers of care in rheumatic diseases. This text now takes its place alongside the other important educational benefits (such as *Arthritis Care and Research*, national scientific meetings, workshops, and the ARHP Slide Collection) that ARHP currently provides.

In keeping with ARHP's dedication to serving the needs of its members and the greater rheumatology community, this text will be regularly updated and revised to provide the most up-to-date information on clinical care. We hope that, by providing this volume of information, we can contribute to the quality of care of individuals with rheumatic diseases. I commend the 44 volunteer authors, the staff, and most especially, Editor Stephen Wegener and Associate Editors Basia Belza and Eric Gall for their significant role in this contribution to the field.

Diana Anderson, RN, MSN
President
Association of Rheumatology Health Professionals

The American College of Rheumatology (ACR) is an organization of physicians, health professionals, and scientists that serves its members through programs of education, research, and advocacy that foster excellence in the care of people with arthritis, rheumatic, and musculoskeletal complaints. This first edition of *Clinical Care in the Rheumatic Diseases* effectively meets the long-term goals of the organization. The text represents another major educational endeavor by the ACR and the Association of Rheumatology Health Professionals. It emphasizes the interdependence of biological, sociological, and psychological factors in determining rheumatic disease onset, course, severity, and outcomes.

The six sections within the book outline the role of the specialist, the societal impact of rheumatic diseases, the use of cost effective diagnostic testing, appropriate treatment, and the importance of coordinated longitudinal multidisciplinary care. Critically important topics such as the psychosocial aspects of rheumatic disease, health status assessments, social and cultural aspects of rheumatic disease, physical therapy modalities, occupational therapy adaptive and assistive devices, management of fatigue and sleep disorders, work disability, public health aspects of rheumatic disease, evaluation of outcomes data, and determinations of cost effectiveness are discussed in detail.

The rheumatic diseases have a profound effect on the function, productivity, and quality of life of the individual, and they have a major economic impact on society. This volume of *Clinical Care in the Rheumatic Diseases* will be of immense value to the rheumatologists, rheumatology health professionals, and primary care providers who care for the millions of patients with these disorders.

Arthur L. Weaver, MD, FACP, FACR
President
American College of Rheumatology

INTRODUCTION

Clinical Care in the Rheumatic Diseases was conceived and developed to fill a need for a single, concise source of information on the treatment of persons with rheumatic diseases for an inter-disciplinary audience. The cover art was chosen to convey the fundamental message of this volume: the text is a blueprint for building the structure of care for persons with rheumatic diseases. Blueprints are only two-dimensional; the finished structure requires the art and attention of each clinician to shape the blueprint to the needs of each patient.

Clinical Care in the Rheumatic Diseases differs from existing rheumatology texts. First, and in contrast to texts grounded solely in the medical model, *Clinical Care* is based on the biopsychosocial model of health care (1). While the medical model continues to guide advances in modern medicine, rheumatic disease researchers have added to the growing body of knowledge on the interdependence of biological, psychological, and sociological factors in determining the course and outcome of disease. Based on this philosophy and ongoing research, the structure and content of the text were carefully developed.

Second, this volume emphasizes clinical information. Chapter topics were selected based on the needs of clinicians; authors were chosen based on their clinical expertise. Over 40 experts in rheumatology — in the fields of medicine, nursing, physical therapy, occupational therapy, pharmacy, and the behavioral sciences — have collaborated on this text, which attempts to address the more commonly encountered clinical problems associated with the treatment of the rheumatic diseases.

Third, *Clinical Care in the Rheumatic Diseases* is designed to be a basic text for both health care professionals who provide clinical care to persons with rheumatic diseases and for students in these disciplines. This audience includes primary care providers such as family practice, pediatric, and internal medicine physicians, nurse practitioners, physician assistants, and students and post-graduate trainees in medicine, nursing, physical therapy, occupational therapy, and social sciences. While specialists in rheumatic disease care may be familiar with the base of knowledge within their discipline, this volume can serve as a source of information regarding other disciplines. In addition to being of value to clinicians, this volume is appropriate for educators teaching students in their own disciplines about rheumatic disease care, as well as educating students regarding the role various health professionals play in rheumatic disease care and comprehensive patient education.

The text is divided into six sections, each addressing a broad area of clinical care. The first section, Clinical Foundations, includes chapters on the musculoskeletal system, immunology and inflammation, and psychosocial aspects of rheumatic disease across the life span. The second section, Assessment and Evaluation, encompasses the components of a comprehensive patient evaluation: history and physical examination, health status assessment, diagnostic tests, psychological assessment, and social and cultural assessment. The third section, Clinical Interventions, consists of 10 chapters outlining the various options available to clinicians in the management of the rheumatic diseases, including patient education, cognitive behavioral interventions, pharmacologic interventions, rest and exercise, physical modalities, splinting, functional ability, management and ambulation of foot problems, surgical management, and interventions of questionable efficacy.

The fourth section, Problem-Focused Management, contains chapters on the clinical management of common problems such as pain, fatigue, sleep disturbance, mood disorders, deconditioning, adherence, and work disability. Each chapter in the fifth section, Common Rheumatic Diseases, provides a review of the etiology, pathogenesis, incidence diagnosis, clinical course, and treatment associated with the more frequently seen rheumatic diseases. The sixth and final section covers two increasingly important topics related to the clinical management of rheumatic disease — public health aspects of rheumatic disease and evaluation of treatment efficacy and cost effectiveness.

Clinical Care in the Rheumatic Diseases has been several years in development and is a tangible result of the new relationship between the Association of Rheumatology Health Professions (ARHP) and the American College of Rheumatology (ACR). Numerous members and staff of these organizations have played key roles in bringing the volume to fruition. The associate editor, Basia L. Belza, PhD, RN, provided enthusiasm and innovation, and the consulting editor, Eric Gall, MD, provided perspective and guidance; both contributed clinical expertise critical to the success of this project. Authors and reviewers generously volunteered their knowledge and their time.

Ruth Martin, previous ARHP Executive Director, saw the project through the difficult early stages. Julie Epps and the other ARHP and ACR staff saw it through to publication. Special thanks to Cynthia Kahn, managing editor, and Angela Wiens, editorial/publication assistant. The staff and faculty at The Johns Hopkins Department of Physical Medicine and Rehabilitation also provided support, making my contribution possible. As in rheumatic disease care, this outcome of our efforts would not have been successful except for the collaboration of this team.

The publication of this first edition of *Clinical Care in the Rheumatic Diseases* is not an end unto itself. Like a blueprint, it may — and indeed should — be altered in succeeding editions to reflect new data and new treatments. Until then, our goal will be met if this volume leads to an improvement in care and quality of life for the nearly 40 million persons with rheumatic disease.

Stephen T. Wegener, PhD, Editor
Baltimore, MD

1. Engel GL: The need for a new medical model: a challenge for biomedicine. Science 196:129-136, 1977

SECTION A: CLINICAL FOUNDATIONS

CHAPTER 1

The Musculoskeletal System

CAROLEE MONCUR, PhD, PT

To appreciate the impact of rheumatic disease on the musculoskeletal system, it is important to have some understanding of the anatomic characteristics and biomechanical responses of the tissues at risk for developing arthritis. Muscles, bones, cartilage, tendons, ligaments, aponeuroses, and fascia are all dynamic tissues important to the integrity, stability, and mobility of the musculoskeletal system. This chapter presents a brief overview of these structures.

JOINTS

Joints are concerned with differential growth (1), with the transmission of tensile, shear, compressive, and torsion forces (2), and with movement (3). The dominant function at any given time depends on the location of the joint and the age of the individual (4). The scientific study of the functional topography and unique anatomy of each joint is called *arthrology.*

Classification schemes for joints range from simple to more complex systems; the more complex are used by specialists in the intricacies of human movement. For this review, joints can be assigned to one of two categories: synarthroses or diarthroses. Synarthrodial joints are solid, non-synovial joints. They are grouped either as fibrous joints or cartilaginous joints, depending on their mode of ossification. Synarthroses are found in the cranial junctions, epiphyseal plates, and various midline joints of the body such as the symphysis pubis (4).

Diarthrodial or Synovial Joints

Diarthrodial or synovial joints are of primary interest in joint pathology. Each articular surface is composed of specialized hyaline cartilage strongly adherent to the underlying subchondral bone. On the outer surface, the cartilage is macroscopically smooth and free to be lubricated. This provides a near frictionless surface over which to move in concert with another articular surface. A classification scheme for diarthrodial joints is presented in Figure 1.

A typical example of the knee synovial joint is shown in Figure 2. Characteristic structures include two bones linked by a fibrous capsule that may have intrinsic ligamentous thickenings to support the joint, a layer of synovial membrane deep to the fibrous capsule, an articular disc and/or meniscus not covered by the synovial membrane, a fibrocartilage labrum (as

in the case of the hip), fat pads, and a vascular, neural, and lymphatic supply.

Joint Capsule. The joint capsule ensheathes the two ends of the bone. Because the fibrous layer of the joint capsule blends with the periosteum of the bones, meeting some distance away from the articulating ends, it does not impede movement. The fibrous layer is composed of relatively inelastic sheets of white collagen fibers, which contributes to joint stability. Blood vessels and nerves perforate the layer, and occasionally gaps are present.

Ligaments of the joint represent cord-like thickenings of parallel collagen bundles formed intrinsically in the fibrous layer of the capsule. They may be separated from the capsule by bursae formed from outpouchings of the synovial lining. Ligaments are pliant and structured to resist excessive or abnormal movements of the joints, yielding very little to tension. Reflex neural mechanisms protect the ligament from excessive tension and stretch (5). In some joints, such as the knee, the intrinsic ligamentous properties are critical to the arthrokinematics of the joint.

Synovial Membrane. The synovial membrane or *synovium* lines the joint everywhere, with the exception of the articular cartilage. The inner surface of the membrane is usually smooth and glistening, and it may be folded into numerous processes called *villi.* Synovium is abundantly supplied with blood vessels, nerves, and lymphatics (4). Synovial tissues are capable of rapid and complete repair when injured or surgically removed (6,7).

Blood Vessels and Lymphatics. Synovial joints have a relatively rich blood supply. The branches of arteries to a joint commonly supply three structures: the epiphysis, the joint capsule, and the synovium. Arteriovenous anastomoses are formed in these joints, but their significance has not yet been determined. Due to the enriched vasculature of the synovial membrane, injury to the joint may allow blood to escape into the joint space and mix with the synovial fluid (4,7).

Nerve Supply. Hilton's law (8) continues to be the fundamental statement regarding the nerve supply to joints. This law postulates that the nerve trunks supplying joint musculature furnish innervation to skin over the muscle and to the tissues of the joint. An array of afferent receptors are found in and near the articular capsule. These provide information regarding the position, movement, and stresses that act on the joint. At least four types of receptors have been identified (9). Type I endings (Ruffini type) are found in the superficial layers of the fibrous capsule and are slowly adapting mechanoreceptors. They pro-

1

Surface Shape	Surface Topology
plane = gliding joints spheroid = ball and socket or enarthrosis ellipsoid = condyloid ginglymus = hinge bicondylar = double condyloid trochoid = pivot sellar = saddle joint	simple (concave and convex surfaces) compound (concave and convex surfaces) sellar (concave and convex surfaces)
Axes of Movement	**Joint Mechanics**
uniaxial biaxial triaxial polyaxial	Movements are related to the concept of the mechanical axis of a bone. Movements are all resolvable as rotations around one, two or three orthogonal axes, i.e., possessing 1-3 degrees of freedom of motion.
Types of Movement	**Types of Movement**
Translation Angulation Rotation Circumduction Examples: flexion/extension abduction/adduction pronation/supination elevation/depression protraction/retraction isometric (neuromuscular) stabilizing (mechanical: close-packing)	Terms refer to one mobile articular surface moving relative to its fixed partner: **Spin**: pure rotation of a surface around its mechanical axis. Two varieties of spin: pure and impure. **Roll**: tips of mechanical axis move end over end. **Slide**: tips of mechanical axis trace an translatory path (like ice on ice).
Fundamental Joint Positions	
Loose Packed: controlled free mobility Close Packed: position of functional rigidity	

Figure 1. Classification of diarthrodial joints (4).

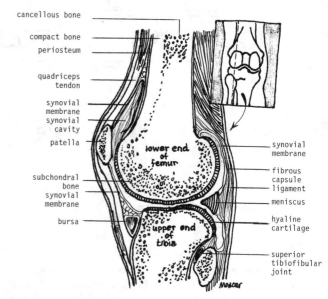

Figure 2. Characteristics of a diarthrodial joint as depicted by the knee joint.

vide awareness of joint position and movement, particularly in terms of postural control. Type II endings (Pacinian type) occur in small groups in the deeper structures of the joint capsule. They are rapidly adapting, low-threshold mechanoreceptors that are sensitive to movement and pressure changes within the joint capsule. Type III endings (Golgi type) are identical to neurotendinous organs in structure and function and are found in the articular ligaments of the joint. They appear to be high-threshold, slowly adapting receptors that prevent excessive tension and stress on the joint by reflex inhibition of the adjacent musculature. Type IV endings are free terminals of myelinated and non-myelinated fibers located in the articular capsule, the adjacent fat pads, and around the blood vessels of the synovial layer. These endings are high-threshold, slowly adapting receptors that appear to respond to excessive motion or injury. They may provide a basis for articular pain (9).

Articular Cartilage. Healthy hyaline cartilage is a specialized connective tissue characterized by considerable extracellular matrix. The matrix is composed mainly of proteoglycans, collagen, glycoproteins, other proteins (such as chondronectin and anchorin CII) and water. Chondrocytes are responsible for the homeostasis of the cartilage matrix. Located at a distance from blood vessels, chondrocytes receive their nutrition via diffusion or convection through the matrix. This arrangement has led to the common understanding that hyaline cartilage is avascular and receives nutrients from the synovial fluid during the movement and loading of the joint. Hyaline cartilage is also aneural. Collagen, proteoglycans, other proteins, and glycoproteins represent about 20% of the tissue wet weight; water and inorganic salts constitute the remainder. Maintenance of the water content is critical to maintaining the resilience and function of the cartilage in terms of joint nutrition and lubrication (4,7,10,11).

Synovial Fluid and Lubrication. Synovial fluid is produced by the cells lining the intima of the synovia and is found in the joint space, within bursae, and in tendon sheaths. It provides a liquid environment for joint surfaces; nutrition for articular cartilage, articular discs, and menisci; and lubrication and reduction of erosion of the joint surfaces and structures. Because the synovium has a rich vascular supply that is fenestrated (has openings), diffusion between the plasma and interstitial spaces can occur. A delicate balance exists between the exchange rate of plasma and synovial fluid particularly in the medical and rehabilitation treatment of the inflammatory arthritides. Severe impairment of this process can create ischemia, effusion, and increased intra-articular temperature (12).

The joint lubrication is an intricate process. Proposed models have followed engineering physics and attempted to equate the human joint with a hydrodynamic function. Considerable data have shown that the human joint is more remarkable than any hydrodynamic system, and that the coefficient of friction is very low in a healthy joint (13). The coefficient of friction is defined as a measure of the energy required to move the joint in proportion to the energy available to do the work of moving the joint. That synovial joints possess a highly effective lubrication system is widely appreciated; however, the mechanics are less well understood. Current descriptions include a component called *boundary layer lubrication* and a second component referred to as *hydrodynamic lubrication* (11,14–16).

Boundary layer lubrication occurs as a result of a proposed small glycoprotein called lubricin. This substance appears to bind to the weight-bearing surface and facilitate the intrinsic arthrokinematics of the joint, while providing protection against wear. Lubricin is a synovium-derived molecule that binds to articular cartilage and retains molecules of water. These properties not only contribute to lubrication of the joint but also to joint stability (16).

Hydrodynamic lubrication seems to contribute to the low friction of the joint during motion. The theory is that load-induced compression of hyaline cartilage will force interstitial fluid to flow laterally to an unloaded surface where it exudes over the surface of the cartilage, thus generating a cushioning layer of fluid when the joint is further loaded. This may reduce the shearing stresses and friction between the joint surfaces (11,14–16).

Intra-articular Menisci. Not all diarthrodial joints have menisci; however, when present and during embryonic development, menisci differentiate into fibrocartilage. Menisci may have a free inner border (as in the knee joint) or they may traverse the joint, dividing it into two separate synovial cavities (as in the sternoclavicular joint). The function of intra-articular fibrocartilage may include absorbing shock, improving fit between articulating surfaces, improving the mechanics of movement, checking translatory motions of joints, deploying weight over a large surface, and helping dissipate the synovial fluid throughout the joint space (4).

Surface Shape and Topology. Some synovial joints have two articulating surfaces forming simple articulations. In this case, one surface is convex and the other is concave, as in the metacarpophalangeal (MCP) joint. Joints such as the elbow are compound articulations, because there are two convex surfaces (capitulum and trochlea) that articulate with two concave surfaces (radius and ulna). Furthermore, in the elbow the circumference of the convex radial head articulates with the concave radial notch of the ulna. Joints such as the knee, which contain an intracapsular disc or meniscus, are complex articulations (4).

The general shape of synovial joints has been classified into seven different categories (Figure 1). *Plane or gliding joints* are articulations between almost flat surfaces, such as between the carpal or tarsal bones. *Ginglymi or hinge joints* resemble a hinge and are restricted to one plane of motion, as demonstrated by the phalanges. *Trochoid or pivot joints* are also uniaxial; however, these rotate around a longitudinal axis, as in the case of the radial head and ulnar notch, or the atlas around the dens of the axis. *Bicondylar joints* such as the knee have two convex condyles that articulate with two concave surfaces. *Ellipsoid joints* are oval and convex. They articulate with an elliptical concave surface, as in the radiocarpal or MCP joints. *Sellar or saddle joints* are concavoconvex surfaces, meaning that both a convex and a concave surface are found on the articulating surfaces. The carpometacarpal joint of the thumb is an example of a sellar joint. *Spheroidal or ball and socket joints* are formed by a spherical surface directed into a cup-like articulating surface, as seen in the hip and shoulder joints (3,4).

TENDONS, LIGAMENTS, APONEUROSES, AND FASCIA

Tendons

Tendons, which are largely composed of collagen fibers, are somewhat flexible and resistant to over-stretching. They are white, due to the low density of vascular supply. The anatomic sites where tendons attach to bone are called *entheses*. At these locations the collagen fibers of the tendon have undergone a transition to fibrocartilage and become continuous with the Sharpey's fibers of the bone. Sharpey's fibers serve as anchorage for tendons, ligaments, and the periodontal membranes of the teeth by becoming buried in bones (7). Entheses can become inflamed in the spondylarthropathies.

The blood supply to tendons is sparsely provided by small arterioles that run parallel to the adjacent musculature and intercommunicate freely. These arterioles are accompanied by vena communicantes and lymphatic vessels. Although the metabolism of tendinous tissue is low, it increases in reaction to an injury or insult. Repair is almost exclusively due to proliferation of fibroblasts associated with collagen fibers (4,7). Tendons severed in accidents heal very well with proper surgical management and rehabilitation.

The nerve supply to tendons appears to be mostly afferents, and there is no clear evidence of vasomotor control. Specialized neurotendinous endings called Golgi tendon organs exist in tendons, particularly at the myotendonous junction.

Bursae are present where tendons are deflected around bones or pass under a retinaculum near a joint. The bursa is a simple, flattened sac of synovial membrane supported by dense regular connective tissue. It decreases friction by allowing complete freedom of movement over a limited range. Each bursa contains a lubricating film of synovial fluid. The majority of bursae occur between tendon and bone, tendons and ligaments, or between tendons.

Tendon synovial sheaths occur where tendons would otherwise rub against bone or other friction-generating surfaces. They are arranged in a closed double-walled cylinder, separated by a thin film of synovial fluid. The inner sheath attaches to and encloses the tendon. The external layer attaches to the neighboring connective tissue structures, allowing surfaces to glide easily past one another in healthy tissues.

The tendon's primary function is to attach muscle to bone and to transmit tensile loads from muscle to bone during joint movement. The tendon guides the muscle belly to maintain optimal distance from the joint center during movement. Tendons have viscoelastic properties that give them a tensile strength that is greater than necessary during normal movement. The tensile strength of tendon is similar to that of bone, which is about one-half that of steel. A tendon of 1 cm^2 cross-sectional area can support 600–1,000 kg of weight. During muscle contraction, tendons become elastic and can have considerable contractile energy transferred to them during movement (17).

During normal activity, a tendon is subjected to less than one-fourth of its ultimate capacity to handle tension (18). Factors that can affect the ability of both tendons and ligaments to accomplish their tensile responsibilities include aging, disease, trauma, medications, mobilization, immobilization, or pregnancy.

Ligaments

Ligaments attach one bone to another and are often thickenings of the joint capsule. Like tendons, ligaments are dense, regular connective tissue of parallel arranged collagenous tissue that are sparsely vascularized. Ligaments also undergo transition into fibrocartilage and attach to the bone, forming an enthesis.

The collagen arrangement in ligaments is aligned parallel and straight, therefore restricting elongation. This lends to the stability and protection of the joint from abnormal motion or force. A minor amount of elasticity is present in the collagen fibers of ligaments, which allows some deformation and then return of the fiber to the original position. Excessive or prolonged elongation may impair the ability of the ligament to return to its original position, thus compromising joint stability.

Aponeuroses

Aponeuroses are flat sheets of densely arranged collagen fibers showing a surface iridescence when newly exposed. Aponeuroses usually consist of several layers, with the fasciculi of fibers arranged parallel within one layer but inclined in a different direction in subsequent layers. Typical examples are the aponeurosis forming the sheath of the rectus abdominis muscle and the iliotibial band of the thigh. Smaller aponeuroses are found in the palm of the hand and on the plantar surface of the foot. The aponeurosis of the rectus sheath houses the muscle and serves as a midline attachment for the other abdominal musculature. The iliotibial band lends support laterally to the integrity of the hip and the knee. The palmar aponeurosis is important to the arches of the hand; similarly, the plantar aponeurosis is important to the bony arches of the foot.

Fascia

Fascia can describe a variety of connective tissues large enough to be seen with the unaided eye. Typically, fascia forms the enveloping fibers of muscles, nerves, and tendons, and the sheaths between whole muscles, viscera, and skin. Superficial fascia is found deep to the dermis and serves as an insulator. It also connects the skin to deeper structures. It sometimes contains muscle fibers, for example, the muscles of facial expression. It is distinct and of variable thickness over the anterior abdominal wall, the limbs, and the perineum. Fascia tends to be thinnest over the hands and feet, the side of the neck, around the anus, and especially over the penis and scrotum. It is particularly dense in the scalp, the palms, and the soles.

Deep fascia forms intermuscular septa that separate muscles or groups of muscles while connecting extensively to bone. The crural fascia of the leg is an example. Sometimes the deep fascia becomes specialized into localized transverse thickenings and is attached at both ends to local bony prominences. An example is the wrist flexor retinaculum, which helps form the carpal tunnel.

BONE

The skeletal system provides a rigid framework for support and weightbearing by the body. In addition, it forms a lever system to which muscles attach and provides smooth, polished surfaces for joints. Other functions include protection for vulnerable viscera; formation of hematopoietic tissue for production of erythrocytes, granular leukocytes, and platelets; and storage of calcium, phosphorus, magnesium, and sodium.

Cells and the Intercellular Substance of Bone

In order to appreciate how bone develops, it is important to understand the duties and functions of the cells and intercellular substance of bone. Bone is a living tissue. Modeling and remodeling occurs in healthy bone and requires healthy cells and a healthy environment. Osteogenic (bone-producing) cells lie on the deep layers of the periosteum and endosteum of bone. The periosteal membrane covers the outer surface of the bone, except where there is hyaline cartilage. Comprised of an outer fibrous coat and an inner cellular coat of osteogenic cells, this membrane is highly vascularized with vessels that enter and leave the nutrient foramen of the bone. There are myelinated and non-myelinated neural fibers accompanying the arteries, some of which are nociceptors.

The endosteum lines the inner spaces of the marrow cavity, spaces of cancellous bone, and the canals of compact bone. Large, multinucleated cells called *osteoclasts* are scattered along the inner layer of these membranes and function to resorb bone. During growth, the osteoclasts of the endosteum widen the marrow cavity. After growth, the endosteum becomes a resting membrane unless a fracture or change in hormonal levels occur, requiring an increase of osteoclast production.

Osteoblasts, derived from osteogenic cells, synthesize and secrete the organic matrix of bone around their cell processes to form canaliculi and future osteons of bone. When mature, they become osteocytes that reside in the lacunae of bone and maintain bone metabolism. Their cell junctions with other osteocytes appear to maintain the integrity of the bone matrix. The matrix or intercellular substance of bone is composed of collagen fibers and amorphous ground substance containing water, glycoproteins, and inorganic materials of calcium, phosphate, fluoride, magnesium, and sodium (4,7).

Bone Remodeling and Healing

Remodeling of bone occurs in response to change in type or amount of physical stresses (or to the lack of them), healing fractures, or rheumatic disease. The phenomenon of bone deposited in sites subjected to stress and reabsorbed in sites where there is little stress is known as Wolff's law. This is exemplified by marked cortical thickening on the concave side of a curved bone. The trabeculae align along the lines of weight-bearing stress in the internal architecture of the bone.

Bone healing consists of several phases that occur concurrently: inflammation, soft callus formation, hard callus formation, and remodeling. Soft and hard callus formation are equivalent to the proliferative phase of wound healing. *Soft callus* is the term given to soft, collagenous, revascularizing, osteogenic tissue that unites bone fragments and from which bone regenerates. In primary bone healing, new Haversian systems or osteons are regenerated across the site of the fracture. Osteoclasts assemble at ends of the Haversian canals near the fracture site forming spearheads or cutting cones, which advance at a rate of 50 to 80 μm/day across the fracture, enlarging the canals as they advance. These are closely followed by osteoblasts, which form new Haversian systems in the enlarged canals and cross the fracture site to link bone fragments. The entire process takes about 5 or 6 weeks; however, any major surgical intervention increases the trauma to the tissues and may prolong the healing process (4,7). Excessive motion at the site or an infection may also prolong healing.

Comparison of Cartilage and Bone

Like cartilage, bone consists of cells and an organic intercellular matrix, which in turn consists of collagen fibers embedded in an amorphous component. The osteocytes of bone, like the chondrocytes of cartilage, live in lacunae within a matrix. Just as a cartilage structure is covered with *perichondrium,* the outer surface of a bone is covered with a membrane called *periosteum*. Finally, bone tissue, like cartilage, develops from a mesenchymal model (4).

Unlike cartilage, bone is a highly vascular, living, constantly changing, mineralized connective tissue. It is remarkable for its hardness, resilience, characteristic growth mechanisms, regenerative capacity and its stone-like resistance to bending during weight-bearing. While all bone consists of cells embedded in an amorphous and fibrous organic matrix permeated by inorganic bone salts, its fine structure varies widely with age, site, and natural history. Thus, bone may develop by direct transformation of condensed mesenchyme, or it may be preceded by a cartilaginous model which is later replaced by bone. The inorganic matrix may exist as irregular, dense masses with scattered bone cells, or it may be arranged as a series of thin sheets (lamellae) in a variety of more or less precise patterns, with intervening rows of bone cells. Both lamellar and non-lamellar bone often develops as minute rough cylindrical masses or *osteons*, each with a central vascular canal.

Bone nutrition differs from that of cartilage. If the organic matrix of bone in which osteocytes live were solidly calcified, no diffusion of nutrients could occur. The osteocytes would die just as chrondrocytes die if the matrix surrounding them becomes calcified. Ground bone sections show that osteocytes in calcified bone are connected both to each other and to a canal, or to some other surface where there is tissue fluid, by what appears as fine lines. These lines, called *canaliculi*, are tiny tubular passageways through the calcified matrix. They contain tissue fluid and hair-like cytoplasmic processes of osteocytes that connect osteocytes together. Canaliculi provide the means for nutrients to reach osteocytes, thus keeping them alive within a calcified matrix (7).

SKELETAL MUSCLE

Muscle fibers are the cellular units of skeletal muscle and are bound by a plasma membrane called the *sarcolemma*. This membrane encloses numerous nuclei and a large amount of cytoplasm, called *sarcoplasm*. Groupings of muscle fibers (fasciculi) can vary in size and pattern depending on the individual muscle. Connective tissue sheaths surround different components of the muscle, including the delicate network between muscle fibers termed the endomysium; a stronger perimysium ensheathing individual fascicles of muscle fibers; and epimysium, which encases the entire muscle and is continuous with the perimysium and the external connective tissue.

Skeletal muscles vary considerably in size, shape, fascicular architecture, type of fiber, and attachment to bone. Each muscle is composed of numerous longitudinal cylindrical myofibrils. These are contrived to provide range, direction, velocity, and force of action appropriate to the particular joint. Myofilaments of actin and myosin are located on the myofibrils, forming serial units called *sarcomeres* that are visible only with an electron microscope. Sarcomeres can be considered the functional unit of skeletal muscle.

Contraction and Relaxation

Much has been written on the contraction of skeletal muscle. Individual muscle fibers demonstrate differences in their rates of contraction, development of tension, and suscepti-

bility to fatigue. All of these are characteristics that classify muscle fibers according to the type of metabolic and contractile properties they display (19–21). Three fiber types have been identified: type I, slow-twitch oxidative fibers; type IIA, fast-twitch oxidative-glycolytic fibers; and type IIB, fast-twitch glycolytic fibers. Type I fibers are characterized by a relatively slow contraction time and have a high potential for aerobic activity. Very difficult to fatigue, type I fibers are capable of prolonged, low intensity work. The myoglobin content is high in type I fibers, giving the muscle a distinct red color.

Type IIA muscle fibers have a fast contraction time, providing a moderately well developed capacity to do both aerobic and anaerobic work. Possessing a well-developed blood supply, they can maintain contractile activity for relatively long periods providing the rate of activity does not exceed the ability of the fiber to utilize adenosine triphosphate (ATP). Once exceeded, the muscle will fatigue. Myoglobin content is fairly high in this muscle type; therefore, it is often classified as red muscle.

Type IIB fibers contain very little myoglobin and are often referred to as white muscle. These fibers rely primarily on glycolytic (anaerobic) activity for ATP production. Very few capillaries appear in the vicinity of these fibers. While type IIB fibers are able to produce energy rapidly, they fatigue very quickly as their high rate of ATP utilization depletes the glycogen needed for metabolism. These large muscles can produce considerable tension for a short period of time before they fatigue (19–21).

Researchers have demonstrated that the innervation to the muscle fiber determines the type it will become; thus, each motor unit innervates a single type of muscle fiber (19). The fiber composition of a muscle depends on the function of that muscle. The soleus muscle of the calf is an example of a muscle with a high percentage of type I fibers, which are necessary in a postural muscle. Muscles that perform both endurance and strength activities are generally composed of a mixture of the three fiber types. There is a controversy in the literature whether fiber types are genetically determined.

The most widely held theory of muscle contraction is the sliding filament theory proposed by Huxley et al (22) and refined by others (23,24). As proposed, muscle contraction requires the sarcomere to actively shorten due to the relative movement of the actin and myosin filaments past one another in response to a variety of stimuli. Wilkie (25) described the activity of the actin and myosin to be "similar to a man pulling on a rope hand over hand."

Once the motor neuron has initiated an action potential along the sarcolemma, an orderly sequence of events occurs to proliferate fiber contraction. From the sarcolemma, the action potential proceeds through the T-tubule system to the sarcoplasmic reticulum, resulting in the release of calcium into the sarcoplasm. Calcium concentrations increase, causing release of actin. This allows actin and myosin cross-linkages or bridges to proceed, leading to shortening of the myofilaments. Shortening continues until the calcium source is actively pumped back into the sarcoplasmic reticulum, breaking the cross-linkages between actin and myosin and allowing the muscle to relax. Both contraction and relaxation of the muscle are active processes.

Energy Metabolism

Energy for the cross-linkage between actin and myosin is provided in the form of hydrolysis of ATP to diphosphate $(ADP+P_1)$ by an ATPase. The splitting of ATP releases energy for the mechanical work of moving the actin filaments along the myosin filaments. Once ATP is hydrolyzed, the remaining ADP and free phosphate leave the binding site on the myosin. The energy required to release a contraction of the myofilaments is provided by ATP. The muscle relaxes when new ATP is bound to the myosin, promptly disassociating actin from myosin by breaking the cross-linkage. Absence of ATP would result in permanent bonding between actin and myosin, as seen in rigor mortis.

JOINT MECHANICS AND MOVEMENT

A classification scheme for the shape of synovial joints is depicted in Figure 1. Movement of the joints is often taken for granted, and the complexity for accomplishing movement is not consciously considered. Kinesiology and biomechanics have become intricate and complex sciences, made more intriguing when a joint has been affected by rheumatic disease. The study of the structure, function, and movement of joints is called *arthrokinesiology.*

Fundamental Joint Positions

Joint surfaces are capable of becoming fully congruent with each other at some point in the range of motion. At this juncture, the soft tissues around the joint become elongated, tense, and slightly stretched. One example of this occurs during full extension of the knee and is called the *close-packed position* of the knee. No further intrinsic motion can occur and an excessive external force applied to the knee may disrupt tissues. Close packing is the terminal limiting position of the joint; any further attempt to increase motion will be resisted by reflex protective contraction of the associated muscles around the joint. Excessive close packing can cause deformation of the ligaments and joint structures, including articular cartilage.

When the joint capsule is lax and the articular surfaces are not congruent, the joint is said to be in the *loose-packed position.* In mid-position of the range of motion, capsules are lax enough that an external force to the knee may allow separation of the bony surfaces. This concept is the basis for using mobilization techniques to increase the motion of a joint following knee surgery, for example. Furthermore, the loose-packed position allows normal movement to occur in joints. Thus, loose-packed positions are important for joint mobility, while close-packed position are necessary for joint stability (3,4).

Kinematics

The study of the motion within the joint or between bones is called kinematics, without regard for the force that caused the motion. *Osteokinematics* is a subcategory of kinematics that describes the motion of a rotating bone around an axis of rotation oriented perpendicular to the path of the moving bone. An example of osteokinematics would be a description of the relationship between the femur and the tibia when the knee is flexed or extended. Another way of describing the osteokinematics of bone is by linkages. An open kinematic chain describes the relationship of a moving distal bone to a proximal stable bone (foot and tibia moving on a stable femur). A closed kinematic chain describes the relationship of a proximal moving bone to a distal stable bone (foot and tibia fixed on the floor and femur moving).

Arthrokinematics describes the motions occurring within the joint or between joint surfaces. In the case of the knee, the femoral condyles, tibial plateaus, and patella are related to each other during these motions. Because the femoral condyles are smooth and rounded, while the tibial plateaus are more flattened with a meniscus on each, the arthrokinematics of the motions of flexion and extension requires the bones to slide, spin, and roll to accomplish the movements. These intricate movements require the joint to be in loose-packed position.

Kinetics

Kinetics comprises the unique science of biomechanics and describes the forces and torques necessary to cause the joint to move. Active forces are generally produced by muscle contraction. Passive forces may be generated by the intrinsic structures of the joint such as the joint capsule, ligaments, or other connective tissues. When evaluating joint motion kinetically, consideration must be given to the ability of the muscle to produce force, integrity of the bone and joint structures, amount of work the muscle can generate, the power or rate the muscle can perform the work, and external forces such as gravity, body weight, and general health of the person.

Types of Movement

There are many descriptions of the movement of joints (Figure 1); however, most joint movement could be considered to be translation, angulation, rotation, and circumduction. Translation (gliding) is sliding without rotation or angulation of the bone. It is a common arthrokinematic motion, which is frequently combined with other motions, such as a spin or rolling on the joint surfaces. Angulation describes an osteokinematic movement of bones as seen in flexion/extension or abduction/adduction. Rotation is used to describe movement around the longitudinal axis of a bone, as seen in pronation/supination of forearm or internal/external rotation of the glenohumeral joint. Circumduction is commonly ascribed to ball and socket joints, which circumscribe their movements in the shape of a cone, thus combining all of the above motions (3,4).

Axes of Movement

The axes of movement are dictated by the type and shape of the synovial joint. Axes of movement are usually perpendicular to the moving bone. However, bones have a mechanical axis that runs perpendicular to the articular center and allows the bone to rotate or spin in such movements as supination and pronation. Uniaxial joints commonly move in one plane of motion (sagittal, frontal, horizontal) such as flexion and extension; biaxial joints move in two planes such as flexion/extension and abduction/adduction; triaxial joints move in three planes of motion such as flexion/extension, abduction/adduction and internal/external rotation. Finally, multi- or polyaxial joints are capable of moving in all planes of motion, usually resulting in circumduction (4).

SUMMARY

Successful management of the joint impairment caused by rheumatic diseases can be enhanced if the health provider appreciates the intricate nature of the structures of the musculoskeletal system. Beyond the effects of rheumatic disease on the musculoskeletal system, considerations should also be given to the effects of age, medications, exercise history, and environment in which the person with arthritis must function. Understanding human movement involves integration of the knowledge of the anatomy, biomechanics, and arthrokinesiology of the musculoskeletal system; the attributes of the specific rheumatic disease and its impact on these structures; and an appreciation of the personal performance attributes and attitudes of the person with arthritis.

REFERENCES

1. Larsen WJ: Development of the limbs. In, Human Embryology. New York, Churchill-Livingstone, 1993, p. 289
2. Viidik A: Biomechanics and functional adaptation of tendons and joint ligaments. In, Studies on the Anatomy and Function of Bones and Joints. Edited by FG Evans. Berlin, Springer-Verlag, 1966, pp. 17–39
3. Norkin C, LeVange P: Biomechanics. In, Joint Structure and Function: A Comprehensive Analysis. Philadelphia, FA Davis, 1992, pp. 3–51
4. Williams PL, Warwick R, Dyson M, Bannister LH, editors: Arthrology. Gray's Anatomy. Thirty-seventh edition. Edinburgh, Churchill-Livingstone, 1989, pp. 460–485
5. Smith JW: Muscular control of the arches of the foot in standing: an electromyographic assessment. J Anat 88:152–163, 1954
6. Key JA: The reformation of synovial membrane in knees of rabbits after synovectomy. J Bone Joint Surg 7:793–813, 1925
7. Ham AW, Cormack DH: Histophysiology of Cartilage, Bone and Joints. Philadelphia, JB Lippincott, 1979, pp. 475–476
8. Hilton J: Lecture VII. In, On Rest and Pain: A Course of Lectures on the Influence of Mechanical and Physiological Rest in the Treatment of Accidents and Surgical Diseases, and the Diagnostic Value of Pain. Edited by WHA Jacobson. New York, William Wood & Co, 1879, p. 96
9. Wyke B: The neurology of joints: a review of general principles. Clin Rheum Dis 7:223–239, 1981
10. Myers ER, Mow VC: Biomechanics of cartilage and its response to biomechanical stimuli. In, Cartilage. I. Structure, Function and Biochemistry. Edited by BK Hall. New York, Academic Press, 1983, pp. 313–341
11. Mow VC, Proctor CS, Kelly MA: Biomechanics of articular cartilage. In, Basic Biomechanics of the Musculoskeletal System. Second edition. Edited by M Nordin, VH Frankel. Philadelphia, Lea & Febiger, 1989, pp. 5–8
12. Simkin PA: The musculoskeletal system: joints. In, Primer on the Rheumatic Diseases. Edited by HR Schumacher, JH Klippel, WF Koopman. Atlanta, Arthritis Foundation, 1993, pp. 5–8
13. Charnley J: The lubrication of animal joints. In, Proceedings of the Symposium on Biomechanics: London, 1959. London, Institution of Mechanical Engineers, 1959, pp. 12–19
14. McCutcheon CW: Boundary lubrication by synovial fluid: demonstration and possible osmotic explanation. Fed Proc 25:1061–1068, 1966
15. Swann DA, Radin EL, Hendrin RB: The lubrication of articular cartilage by synovial fluid glycoproteins (abstract). Arthritis Rheum 22:665–666, 1979
16. Swann DA, Silver FH, Slayter HS, et al: The molecular structure and lubricating activity of lubricin isolated from bovine and human synovial fluids. Biochem J 225:195–201, 1985
17. Carlstedt CA, Nordin M: Biomechanics of tendons and ligaments. In, Basic Biomechanics of the Musculoskeletal System. Second edition. Edited by M Nordin, VH Frankel. Philadelphia, Lea & Febiger, 1989, pp. 59–74
18. Kear M, Smith RN: A method for recording tendon strain in sheep during locomotion. Acta Orthop Scand 46:896–905, 1975
19. Astrand P-O, Rodahl K: Textbook of Work Physiology: Physiological Basis for Exercise. Second edition. New York, McGraw Hill, 1977, pp. 37–52
20. Engel WK: Fiber-type nomenclature of human skeletal muscle for histochemical purposes. Neurology 25:344–348, 1974
21. Huxley AF: Muscular contraction. J Physiol 243:1–43, 1974
22. Huxley AF, Huxley HE: Organizers of a discussion of the physical and chemical basis of muscular contraction. Proc R Soc Lond B Biol Sci 160:433–437, 1964
23. Huxley HE: The mechanism of muscular contraction. Science 164:1356–1366, 1969
24. Weber A, Murray JM: Molecular control mechanisms in muscular contraction. Physiol Rev 53:612–673, 1973
25. Wilkie DR: The mechanical properties of muscle. Br Med Bull 12:177–182, 1956

CHAPTER 2

Immunology and Inflammation

A. BETTS CARPENTER, MD, PhD

The immune system is a complex system crucial to our survival. The immune system provides our primary defense against foreign substances. Immunity may be thought of as either innate or acquired. Innate immunity does not require previous exposure and involves phagocytic cells, natural physical barriers, and a special group of lymphocytes, termed *natural killer* (NK) cells. Acquired immunity has great specificity, requiring previous exposure to foreign pathogens, and involves lymphocytes. When referring to the immune system, one is usually referring to acquired immunity, however in this review, components of both the innate and acquired immunity will be discussed. The specific immune system is divided into two parts, humoral and cellular, which relate to the response of distinct types of lymphocytes. *Humoral* responses are mediated by B lymphocytes, and they produce specific antibodies whose function is to neutralize foreign substances known as *antigens*. Antibody-mediated responses can be transferred from one individual to another by serum or plasma. Humoral immunity is predominately concerned with protection against bacterial pathogens. *Cellular* responses are mediated by T lymphocytes, which produce soluble factors for the immune response. Cellular responses are transferred via cells, and are mainly involved with immunity against fungi, parasites, and intracellular bacteria (1–3).

CELLS OF THE IMMUNE SYSTEM

B Lymphocytes

B lymphocytes make up a major cell population vital to the immune system (1–4). They respond to extracellular antigens of many different types: proteins, lipids, nucleic acids, and others. The major mediators are known as **B** lymphocytes, because they are a product of an organ in the chicken, the **B**ursa of Fabricius. This organ is unique to the chicken; however, the mammalian equivalent is the **B**one marrow. B lymphocytes are the sole producers of proteins called immunoglobulins, which are called *antibodies* when produced in response to a specific antigen. B lymphocytes have antigen-binding surface membrane receptors with the same specificity as the immunoglobulin they secrete.

There are five major classes of immunoglobulins produced: IgM, IgG, IgA, IgE, and IgD. All immunoglobulins consist of at least two heavy chains (with a molecular weight of 50,000–70,000) and two light chains (with a molecular weight of 23,000) which form a basic Y shape (Figure 1). Each chain is composed of a *constant region* in which the amino acids are relatively unchanged between different molecules, and a *variable region*, which is composed of different amino acids between different molecules. Within the variable region, there are areas with much variability of amino acids, the hypervariable region. These areas are responsible for the antigen-binding

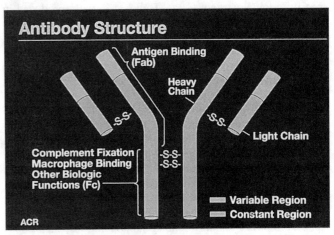

Figure 1. Antibody structure (reprinted from the Clinical Slide Collection on the Rheumatic Diseases, copyright 1995).

specificity of each immunoglobulin. The variable or "V" end of the molecule is where the antigen binding specificity is located; this area is alternatively termed the fragment antigen-binding (FaB) region. The straight end of the molecule is composed exclusively of the constant region and is involved in other activities of the immune system, such as binding of complement. It is termed the Fc region. Various inflammatory cells have Fc receptors that can bind immunoglobulin via their Fc end, and this can facilitate phagocytosis of foreign particles.

Each of the five classes of immunoglobulins have distinctive characteristics. IgM is the largest immunoglobulin, with five unit immunoglobulin molecules. Its primary task is to respond to antigen on initial exposure. IgG is the most prevalent immunoglobulin in the serum, and responds mostly to antigen on secondary exposure. IgA is predominately produced by lymphocytes that are present submucosally. This immunoglobulin provides protection at mucosal surfaces, and is highly concentrated in tears, saliva, bronchial secretions, breast milk, intestinal fluids, and other body fluids. IgE mainly responds to allergens and is also important in response to parasitic infections. IgD has the lowest concentration in the serum, is important mainly as a cell surface immunoglobulin, and has a role in differentiation of B cells.

Upon first exposure to an antigen, a resting B cell—with the help of T lymphocytes—responds by proliferating and differentiating into an activated B cell, which can produce antibodies to bind and neutralize specific antigens. With this first exposure (primary response), the major immunoglobulin produced is IgM; during subsequent responses, IgG is the predominant immunoglobulin secreted. At the initial antigen exposure, there are several paths of differentiation the B cell can take. It may become an activated B cell, which can go on to an end stage of development, the plasma cell. These cells are chiefly found in organ sites, where they represent constitutive producers of

9

antibodies. Alternatively, some B cells differentiate to form the memory cells that allow the immune system to remember and respond quickly to antigen upon repeat exposure. These cells are responsible for the long-term efficacy of vaccines.

T cells

T lymphocytes are the other major cell population of the specific immune system (1–4). They are initially produced in the bone marrow and then complete their development in the thymus, thus the term **T** cells. They are vital in defense against viruses, intracellular bacteria, fungi, protozoa, and tumor cells. In contrast to B cells, T cells can respond only to peptides, and only after they have been processed by antigen-presenting cells (APC). In addition, they are complexed with protein products of the major histocompatibility complex (MHC), a complex of genes important in the immune system (see below). The T cell expresses a protein expressed on its surface that can bind antigen (cell surface antigen receptor). This is similar to the cell surface antigen receptor also expressed on the B cell. B and T cells cannot be differentiated by microscopy. They must be identified by cell surface protein receptors, which in turn can be identified by their reactivity with monoclonal antibodies. To simplify the many cellular subpopulations, each population has been given a CD (cluster of differentiation) designation followed by a number. All mature T cells are CD3 antigen positive, thus T cells are alternatively referred to as CD3 cells. The major T cell subpopulations are helper cells (CD4) and cytotoxic/suppressor cells (CD8). CD4 cells are crucial in the body's defense against infectious agents. This is especially highlighted in acquired immunodeficiency syndrome, where depleted CD4 cells cause a profound immunodeficiency. CD8 cells are preferentially termed cytotoxic cells. In the past, these cells were termed suppressor cells; however, it is not universally accepted that suppressor cells are a distinct cellular entity. CD8 cells have an important role in the lysis of virally infected cells and in killing of tumor cells. T cells do not produce antibodies. They produce soluble mediators, termed *cytokines*, which are important mediators of these cells.

Phagocytic Cells

The major phagocytes are monocytes/macrophages, and neutrophils (2,5). Monocytes circulate in the peripheral blood, and once they home to the tissues, they are termed macrophages, or histiocytes. In the tissue, multiple histiocytes coalesce to become giant cells. Macrophages in different body sites have different designations: kuppfer cells (liver), alveolar macrophages (lung), glial cells (brain). Mononuclear phagocytes are involved in mediating cellular responses, especially pathogenic responses to intracellular organisms such as mycobacterium. They are also important phagocytic cells. Many microbes, such as encapsulated bacteria, do not readily bind to the surface of phagocytes for engulfment. However, upon coating with substances such as products of the complement system and immunoglobulins, the particles are recognized as foreign and can bind to the Fc portion of the immunoglobulin molecule and/or complement receptors on the macrophage cell surface. This process, called opsonization, facilitates the process of phagocytosis. Macrophages also function in cell-to-cell interactions as APCs. Along with the protein products of the MHC, they

process and express protein antigen to T lymphocytes. Macrophages also produce cytokines, which effect cell interactions and recruit inflammatory cells to sites of injury.

Neutrophils are the other major phagocytic cells (2,6). They comprise the major population of white cells in the peripheral blood (up to 80%). Neutrophils are formed in the bone marrow from myelocytic precursors. They are terminally differentiated, living only 1–2 days after reaching the peripheral blood. They have a multi-lobed nucleus and a variety of storage cytoplasmic granules, which contain digestive enzymes that act to break down particles that have been phagocytized. Neutrophils provide one of the first lines of defense against foreign invaders, and are one of the first cell populations present in tissues with an acute infection. They mediate their effects via phagocytosis or release of granules either intracellularly or extracellularly.

Natural Killer Cells

Natural killer cells are a population of cells distinct from T or B cells (7,8). They have large cytoplasmic granules, and are thus called large-granular lymphocytes. These cells are able to kill tumor cells and virally infected cells. In contrast to the tumor cell killing by cytotoxic CD8+ T cells, NK-cell mediated killing does not require previous exposure or products of the MHC. In addition, NK cells can interact with antibody-coated tumor cells and kill them in a process termed *antibody-dependent cellular cytotoxicity*. The exact role of NK cells in normal immunity has not been unequivocally established. Rare individuals with NK cell deficiency have been shown to develop severe viral infections.

SOLUBLE MEDIATORS OF THE IMMUNE SYSTEM

Cytokines are soluble mediators produced by a variety of cell types (1–3,9). Most of these substances are produced in very small amounts and act either on adjacent cells or the cell that produced them. However, some act on distant cells and tissues. Cytokines have a wide variety of effects on many cellular functions and cell populations. Their major roles include mediating effects induced by infectious agents, regulating lymphocyte growth, stimulating growth of precursor cell populations, and mediating inflammatory reactions. One major group of cytokines are the interleukins (IL) which are presently numbered IL1–12. Some additional cytokines include tumor necrosis factor (TNF), T cell transforming factor, and interferons Only some of the cytokines with special relevance to the rheumatic diseases will be discussed.

Interleukin-1 (IL-1) and TNF are two cytokines that differ structurally but have very similar physiological effects. Interleukin-1 can be produced by essentially all nucleated cells, but most predominately by macrophages and activated T cells. Both IL-1 and TNF are important co-stimulators in the antigen-induced activation of T cells. They are important mediators of inflammatory responses. In addition, they cause fever, thus they are endogenous pyrogens. Both of these cytokines act on hepatocytes to induce the synthesis of plasma proteins termed *acute phase reactants*, which are increased in infection, neoplasia, burns, and trauma. Multiple proteins can be increased in an acute phase reaction, including such proteins as the third component of complement (C3), C-reactive protein, serum amyloid protein, and haptoglobin. These proteins can be measured by laboratory tests to determine whether a patient is undergoing an inflammatory response. Interleukin-1 and TNF affect cells important in rheumatic disease. These two cytokines can induce bone resorption by osteoclasts, increase cartilage turnover by chondrocytes, and cause proliferation of fibroblasts and synovial cells (1–3). Studies have shown increased levels of IL-1 and TNF in joint fluid from patients with rheumatoid arthritis (RA). There has been interest in treating RA patients with inhibitors of these cytokines. One recent trial using an antibody against TNF in 20 patients with active RA showed that the treatment was safe and resulted in significant laboratory and clinical improvement (10).

Interleukin-2 is a crucial growth factor for T cells. Activated T cells produce IL-2, which then acts on the same cell that produced it to further stimulate its growth. It also stimulates the growth of nearby cells. Interleukin-2 has allowed the growth of T cells in the laboratory, furthering our knowledge of cellular interactions. It has also been used therapeutically in the treatment of some cancers.

Interleukin-6 is produced by monocytes/macrophages, endothelial cells, and fibroblasts in response to IL-1 and TNF, and it has two major effects. It stimulates hepatocytes to increase the production of fibrinogen, which causes red blood cells to stack. An increase in this protein is measured by the erythrocyte sedimentation rate (ESR) test, frequently used in rheumatology patients to assess inflammation and follow their disease course. In addition, IL-6 acts as a B cell growth factor.

THE COMPLEMENT SYSTEM

The complement system, a complex group of serum proteins, is important to both natural and acquired immunity (1,2,11). It is a cascade system of approximately 25 serum proteins, including the regulatory proteins, that are normally inactive. Upon activation, they sequentially mediate a number of biologic effects. The main actions of the complement system are as follows: 1) mediate lysis of antibody-coated targets, such as bacteria, viruses, cells, and others; 2) act as mediators of inflammation via recruitment of inflammatory cells and cellular products to the sites of inflammation; and 3) aid in removal of foreign pathogens through increasing the efficiency of phagocytosis through opsonization.

The complement system is divided into two pathways: the classical (discovered first) and the alternative. There are three key proteins that are unique to each pathway along with a number of proteins common to both. C3 is a crucial protein component in both pathways. The classical pathway only interacts with IgG and IgM when they are complexed with antigen to form an immune complex. The unique classical pathway components, C1, C2, and C4, are sequentially activated and then interact with C3 to form a complex that interacts with the common terminal components of the system (C5–C9). The classical complement pathway is a major effector mechanism of humoral immunity, because it allows the destruction of antibody-coated microbes and the recruitment of inflammatory cells to sites of inflammation. The alternative pathway is also important as part of the innate or natural immune system, allowing complement to interact directly on the surface of the

molecule without the requirement for antigen–antibody complexes. Proteins unique to the alternative pathway include factors B, D, H, I, and properdin. The end result of activation of either pathway is the formation of the membrane attack complex (MAC). This mediates cell lysis by intercalating into the lipid bilayer membrane and forming lytic pores, which allow the passage of water into the cell and cause subsequent cell lysis.

In addition to direct destruction of cell targets by the MAC, complement split products cause a variety of effects. C5a and C3a are anaphylatoxins that cause release of histamine from mast cells and smooth muscle contraction. In addition, C5a attracts and activates neutrophils. C3b bound to the surface of microorganisms binds to receptors on macrophages and neutrophils and promotes phagocytosis. Complement also enhances solubilization and clearance of immune complexes by interacting with the formation of immune complexes and enhancing clearance by phagocytic cells.

A deficiency of complement can lead to altered patterns of complement activation, causing either increased or decreased patterns of activation. There are a variety of genetic deficiencies of various complement components, commonly the early pathway proteins, C2 and C4. Over 50% of the patients with deficiencies of C2 and C4 have systemic lupus erythematosus (SLE). C2 and/or C4 deficiencies may lead to altered clearance of immune complexes and immune complex disease characteristic of SLE. In addition, in patients without an inherited complement deficiency, there can be alterations in the normal levels of complement. In the presence of activation by a persistent infection or an autoimmune disease such as SLE, there can be persistent activation of the complement system, resulting in low levels. Generally, the serum levels of C3 and C4 correlate with disease activity and they are followed in patients with SLE.

INFLAMMATION

Inflammation is the response of the body to injured tissues (1–3,12). It is characterized by the movement of vascular fluid and cells from the vessels into the extravascular spaces. The inflammatory response is a complex process initiated from a variety of foreign insults (microbes, altered cells, foreign particles), and involving a variety of cells and soluble inflammatory mediators. It can be acute or chronic. Acute inflammation often occurs as the initial response to highly virulent organisms and tissue injury, and it is characterized by a cellular infiltrate primarily of neutrophils. A chronic inflammatory response occurs later (usually as a response to a persistent and/or intracellular organism), and it is characterized by an infiltrate of primarily lymphocytes, plasma cells, and macrophages.

The local signs of inflammation were originally described by Celsus in the second century AD as: rubor (redness), calor (heat), tumor (swelling), and dolor (pain). In response to an inciting noxious agent that causes tissue injury, the capillary and postcapillary venules containing the inflammatory cells respond to the injury. There is a disruption of the endothelial cells lining the vessel walls, thus allowing movement of fluid and cells into the extravascular spaces and to the site of injury. The inflammatory cells (neutrophils, platelets, mast cells, eosinophils, basophils, and lymphocytes) release mediators with a myriad of effects, including an increase in vascular perme-

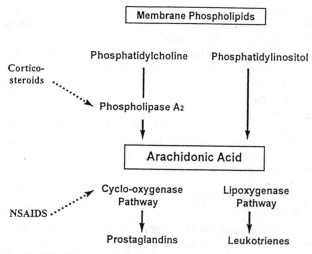

Figure 2. Arachidonic acid pathway.

Table 1. Association of human leukocyte antigens with rheumatic diseases (1–3, 13–14).

Disease*	HLA Antigen	Relative Risk
AS	HLA–B27	69–90
RS	HLA–B27	37
RA	HLA–DR4	2.7–6
SS	HLA–DR2	5.2–9.7
	HLA–DR3	3.6
SLE	HLA–DR2	2.3
	HLA–DR3	2.5–5.8

* AS-ankylosing spondylitis; RS-Reiter's syndrome; RA-rheumatoid arthritis; SS-Sjogren's syndrome; SLE-systemic lupus erythematosus.

ability, recruitment of additional cells, contraction of smooth muscle, and release of additional mediators. Thus, from the initial injurious stimuli, the body responds with a cascade of events.

The inflammatory response usually resolves the noxious assault and restores the tissues to normal physiologic integrity and functioning. However, in a number of pathological situations, tissue injury results from the inflammatory response. The inflammatory response may become chronic due to characteristics of the inciting agent (persistent, intracellular) or to factors in the host, or both.

A variety of inflammatory mediators are released from the infiltrating cells during the inflammatory response. Some are preformed and in cytoplasmic granules or are formed from the metabolism of membrane phospholipids, for example, prostaglandins and leukotrienes. In addition, cytokines are released from infiltrating macrophages or lymphocytes, and complement split products are produced from the activation of the complement system.

Arachidonic acid (AA) is a 20-carbon fatty acid that is the central compound in the generation of both prostaglandins and leukotrienes (Figure 2). It is created during the inflammatory process from membrane phospholipids in two ways. It can be generated from membrane phosphatidylinositol via cleavage by phospholipase C to diacylglycerol, followed by the generation of arachidonic acid from diacylglycerol by the action of diacylglycerol lipase. Alternatively, phosphatidylcholine is acted upon by phospholipase A2 to generate AA directly. From this point, AA can proceed either by the cyclo-oxygenase pathway to prostaglandins/thromboxanes or via the lipo-oxygenase pathway to leukotrienes. Prostaglandins and leukotrienes have diverse proinflammatory actions, including chemotaxis, smooth-muscle constriction, and vasoactive properties. Corticosteroids act as anti-inflammatory agents by inducing an inhibitor of phospholipase A2, thus inhibiting the formation of AA. Nonsteroidal anti-inflammatory agents (NSAIDs) directly inhibit the cyclo-oxygenase pathway, inhibiting the formation of prostaglandins and thromboxanes.

Inflammatory responses that result in tissue injury are termed *hypersensitivity reactions*. These include allergic reactions, antigen–antibody reactions that are cytotoxic, immune complex reactions, and cell-mediated responses. The most relevant to rheumatic disease is the immune complex reaction, which involves immune complexes that deposit in the tissue. Complement is activated and neutrophils are attracted to the site of deposition, causing local damage. Tissue injury occurs primarily from the resultant inflammatory reaction. The antigen may be exogenous or endogenous (an autoantigen). This immune mechanism is responsible for much of the tissue destruction seen in SLE.

HUMAN HISTOCOMPATIBILITY COMPLEX

The human MHC is a group of closely related genes on human chromosome 6, which encodes proteins important in the immune system (13,14). The protein products of these loci are called human leukocyte antigens (HLA). The gene products are highly polymorphic, meaning that there are many alleles or forms of the genes in different individuals. This system was first discovered in graft rejection. It is vital to the functioning of the immune system and crucial to the interaction of T cells, because MHC products are markers of "self" for T cells. The MHC contains two sets of genes coding for cell surface antigens, which are divided into Class I and Class II. Class I antigens are expressed on the surface of all nucleated cells. T cells only respond to antigens that are non-covalently bound to MHC gene products. CD8 T cells will only respond to antigen when they are complexed with Class I antigens. Class II antigens have a more limited cell distribution: B cells, macrophages, and dendritic cells. CD4 T cells can only react to antigens complexed with Class II molecules. Clinically, the MHC is important in transplantation, platelet transfusions, and associations with disease.

There are a variety of diseases—mostly autoimmune—associated with the MHC. The strongest association is with a Class I HLA–B antigen, HLA–B27, which is associated with ankylosing spondylitis (AS). HLA–B27 is also increased in patients with Reiter's syndrome; however, the association is not as strong. While more than 90% of Caucasian patients with AS have HLA–B27, only a small percentage of individuals with HLA–B27 actually have AS. The remainder of disease associations are with Class II antigens, primarily with the HLA–D/DR antigens. Associations with various rheumatic diseases are listed in Table 1. The significance of an HLA disease association is generally expressed as a relative risk, which is the risk of an individual with the particular HLA type of developing the disease as compared to an individual without the antigen. For example, an individual with HLA–B27 is 90 times more likely to develop AS than someone who is HLA–B27 negative. The relative risks listed in Table 1 are reported as a range of figures, representing data from numerous studies.

When examining the association of HLA and disease, there are several caveats. First, the association with a particular HLA antigen may not be with the gene itself, but the actual disease-associated gene could be a non-HLA locus that is closely linked to the MHC. There are many reports of weak associations with HLA antigens, with relative risks ranging from 1.5 to 2. The significance of these associations is unclear. In SLE, for example, the association with the HLA is not strong; however, there are clearly genetic factors that are important in susceptibility to the disease. Other genes also play a role. Lastly, it must be emphasized that possession of a particular HLA allele is not diagnostic of a particular disease, it simply means that an individual has an increased risk for developing that disease. Many of the HLA associations are epidemiologic data from large groups of individuals, and they may not significantly impact individual patients. As our ability to examine genes on the molecular level expands, we can further elucidate the role of genes in rheumatic diseases.

AUTOIMMUNITY

Autoimmunity is defined as pathologic changes that occur due to the immune reaction against autologous antigens (1–3), representing a loss of self-tolerance. *Tolerance*, or the unresponsiveness of the immune response to antigens, occurs both peripherally and centrally. Central tolerance occurs in immature lymphocytes in the thymus and bone marrow. Immature lymphocytes, which can recognize self, "see" these antigens in the thymus and bone marrow and are deleted or inactivated. Peripheral tolerance occurs in mature lymphocytes that "see" self-antigen in peripheral tissues. It provides for maintenance of self-tolerance for clones that escape destruction in the thymus or bone marrow, which is important for tolerance to tissue-specific self-antigens not found in the generative organs.

If tolerance is present, then how does autoimmunity occur? There are many theories to explain autoimmune disease. One explanation relates to changes in lymphocytes. Individuals may have autoreactive B cells, but without self-reactive CD4 T cells to provide help to these B cells, no immune response can occur. Because most of the potentially self-reactive T cells have been deleted or rendered inactive, these cells must be "tricked" into providing help to the self-responsive B cells. This can occur via stimulation with microbial antigens that cross-react with self-antigens. Another mechanism of autoimmunity involves the widespread activation of previously unresponsive self-reactive lymphocytes by substances that stimulate many clones of lymphocytes—so-called polyclonal activators. Substances such as lipopolysaccharides from gram-negative bacteria are polyclonal activators. In addition, tissue injury and inflammation can lead to autoimmunity by causing the release of normally sequestered self-antigens, which are seen as foreign upon release. There can be alterations of self antigens by either a microbial agent or by injury or inflammation, so that they are recognized as foreign. As discussed in the section on the HLA system, there are a variety of genetic factors that have a role in the autoimmune system. In summary, there is no one theory that explains all autoimmune diseases. In most situations, it is likely a complex interplay between environmental factors, including exposure to microbial antigens in a genetically susceptible host, that determines the development of autoimmune disease.

Autoimmune diseases may be classified as organ specific or non-organ specific, depending on whether the response is primarily against antigen localized to one or a limited number of organs, or whether the autoimmune reaction is directed against many tissues of the body. Common targets of organ specific autoimmune responses include thyroid, adrenals, stomach, and pancreas. The non-organ specific reactions include rheumatic diseases that involve primarily the skin, joints, kidney, and muscle. However, this classification is not absolute; within each group there is considerable overlap.

Many rheumatic diseases are characterized by detectable circulating levels of autoantibodies (15). These are useful in diagnosis, following disease activity, and in prognosis. For example, the presence of antibody against double stranded DNA (anti-DNA) in SLE is used both for initial diagnosis, and for following disease activity. Anti-DNA immune complexes may be deposited along the glomerular basement membrane in the kidney and along the dermal–epidermal junction in the skin. They are believed to be an important factor in the pathology of SLE (16). Another common autoantibody is rheumatoid factor (RF), which is an IgM antibody directed against the IgG molecule. It is present in approximately 75% of patients with RA, but its presence does not establish the diagnosis of RA. Nearly 25% of patients who fulfill the criteria for RA do not have RF, while RF can be present in patients with no joint disease. The exact role of RF in the pathogenesis of RA has not been clearly established (17). While RF can be detected in the synovial fluid from RA joints, and cells producing RF can be found in synovial tissue, the majority of cells in the synovial tissue are not plasma cells but CD4 helper T cells. More studies are needed to define the role of RF in the pathogenesis of RA.

Caution should be used when evaluating the role of autoantibodies in disease states. The presence of autoantibodies does not mean that autoimmune disease is present. Low levels of autoantibodies are found in many normal individuals. Even when high levels of autoantibodies are found to be associated with disease, they may not necessarily have a pathogenic role. We know that age, sex, and genetics have an effect on autoantibodies. Many studies show that autoantibodies increase as we age. In addition, autoimmune disease is more common in females. Furthermore, our genetic background has an important effect on autoantibody production. For example, clinically normal relatives of patients with SLE have a greater number of positive autoantibodies than the general population. This should not dampen enthusiasm for evaluating autoantibodies, but they must be evaluated in the proper light.

REFERENCES

1. Abbas AK, Lichtman AH, Pober JS: Cellular and Molecular Immunology. Second edition. Philadelphia, WB Saunders, 1994
2. Stites DP, Terr AI, Parslow TG: Basic and Clinical Immunology. Eighth edition. Norwalk CT, Appleton and Lange, 1994
3. Roitt I, Brostoff J, Male D: Immunology. Third edition. St. Louis, Mosby, 1993
4. Ikuta K, Uchida N, Freidman J, Weissman IL: Lymphocyte development from stem cells. Annu Rev Immunol 10:759–783, 1992
5. Johnson RB: Monocytes and macrophages. N Engl J Med 381:747–752, 1988
6. Lehrer RI, et al: Neutrophils and host defense. Ann Intern Med 109:124–142, 1988
7. Trinchieri G: Biology of natural killer cells. Adv Immunol 47:187–376, 1989

8. Herberman RB, Reynolds CW, Ortaldo J: Mechanisms of cytoxicity by natural killer (NK) cells. Annu Rev Immunol 4:651–680, 1986

9. Arai K, Lee F, Miyajima A, Miyatake S, Arai N, Yokota T: Cytokines: coordinators of immune and inflammatory responses. Annu Rev Biochem 59:783–836, 1990

10. Elliott MJ, Maini RN, Feldmann M, et al: Treatment of rheumatoid arthritis with chimeric monoclonal antibodies to tumor necrosis factor α. Arthritis Rheum 36:1681–1690, 1993

11. Ruddy S: Complement. In, Textbook of Rheumatology. Third edition. Edited by WN Kelley, ED Harris, S Ruddy, CB Sledge. Philadelphia. 241–252, 1989

12. Cotran RS, Kumar V, Robbins SL: Pathologic Basis of Disease. Fifth edition. Philadelphia, WB Saunders, 52–92, 199

13. Campbell RD, Trowsdale J: Map of the human MHC. Immunol Today 14:349–352, 1993

14. Salazar M, Yunis EJ: MHC: Gene structure and function. In, Samter's Immunologic Diseases. Fifth edition. Edited by MM Frank, KF Austen, HN Claman, ER Unanue. New York, 101–116, 1995

15. Naparstek Y, Poltz PH: The role of autoantibodies in autoimmune diseases. Annu Rev Immunol 11:79–104, 1993

16. Kotzin BL, O'Dell JR: Systemic lupus erythematosus. In, Samter's Immunologic Diseases. Fifth edition. Edited by MM Frank, KF Austen, HN Claman, ER Unanue. New York, 667–697, 1995

17. Winchester R: Rheumatoid arthritis. In Samter's Immunologic Diseases, Fifth edition. Edited by MM Frank, KF Austen, HN Claman, ER Unanue. New York, 699–757, 1995

Psychosocial Aspects

KATHLEEN M. SCHIAFFINO, PhD; and TERESA J. BRADY, PhD

For many people the word *arthritis* conjures up an image of grandparents with the minor aches and pains inevitably associated with aging. While osteoarthritis, the most common form of arthritis, does tend to occur in old age, the reality is that rheumatic disease can be found at every stage of life. Although sometimes mild, arthritis can also severely limit individuals' activities and affect their ability to perform the life tasks before them. This chapter will attempt to provide a theoretical perspective concerning the potential psychosocial impact of rheumatic disease at each stage in the life cycle.

THEORETICAL APPROACHES TO NORMAL DEVELOPMENT

Erikson's theory of psychosocial development through the life cycle (1) emphasizes the development of adaptive strengths through the ongoing balancing of competing predispositions. The opposing forces that create this dynamic balance are both essential to adaptation and growth; the over-development of one aspect at the expense of the other contributes to adjustment difficulties. Erikson identifies eight key conflicts that commonly influence development at specific stages of life and play a role throughout the lifespan. At each new stage, and with each substantial change in circumstance, earlier conflicts must be re-integrated to accommodate the new circumstances. Thus, these conflicts do not represent eight independent processes as much as themes that are perpetually intertwined.

According to Erikson, infancy is the time for balancing the opposing predispositions of *trust versus mistrust*. Their eventual equilibrium creates the adaptive strength of hope. A basic sense of trust emerges from confidence in the predictability of one's world. Infants who do not develop a sense of the world as safe and dependable learn to approach the world with fear and suspicion.

The move from infant to toddler introduces the individual to the next two life stage tasks: *autonomy versus shame/doubt* and *initiative versus guilt*. The balance between autonomy and shame/doubt results in the capacity to exercise free choice as well as self-restraint, and emerges out of early exploration of the child's environment which is encouraged by the parent and which contributes to feelings of independence and confidence. Overprotectiveness and denied autonomy, on the other hand, can contribute to doubt and later difficulties in assuming responsibility and control. Initiative develops in response to pleasurable accomplishment in socially approved activities—from play activities arise a set of idealized goals and a sense of purpose. Experiences that curtail the development of initiative and its resulting sense of freedom can induce feelings of guilt for wanting to do things that are not allowed. The lessons learned at this stage are reflected in adulthood as one continues to temper self-interest and expansiveness with cooperation and concern for others.

The school-age child is confronted with the task of balancing *industriousness versus inferiority*. Successful resolution of this conflict, resulting from the learning of facts and mastery of skills, will contribute to an adaptive sense of competence. With adolescence and young adulthood comes the need to balance *identity versus identity confusion*. Young adults struggle with the question of "Who am I?" and attempt to develop a coherent sense of self. The resulting self will incorporate social and professional identities and will facilitate the capacity to develop enduring and faithful relationships.

Critical to the development of adult relationships is the resolution of the conflict between *intimacy versus isolation*. Only after establishing a sense of identity is the young adult ready for intimacy that involves the capacity for commitment to lasting friendships and companionship, in general, and to partnership and sexuality, in particular. Resolution of this conflict results in a capacity for love and selective intimacy and prepares the adult for the next developmental task of *generativity versus stagnation and self-absorption*. Generativity refers to procreation, productivity, and creativity, and successful resolution of this stage is associated with the adaptive capacity for care in relation to family and society. Typically, resolution of this stage means becoming involved in something outside of oneself, such as work, family, or volunteer activities, while maintaining good self-care practices.

The final task confronted by individuals at the end of the life cycle concerns the balance of *integrity versus despair*, the ability to take stock of one's life; recognize successes, failures, and missed opportunities; and to make sense of this all without succumbing to feelings of failure and despair.

During the movement through life, Erikson suggests that individuals are confronted with challenges to resolve and opportunities for growth. More recent theoretical approaches have reflected a lifespan developmental perspective (2), which suggests that development takes place at multiple levels and assumes that these levels influence each other on a continuing basis. The levels considered in lifespan models include the biological, individual, dyadic, family, community, and cultural (see Chapter 8, Social and Cultural Assessment). According to lifespan developmental theory, the multiple levels at which development takes place are known as *embeddedness,* and the ability of each of these levels to influence the other levels is called *dynamic interactionism* (3).

Lifespan developmental theories underscore the fact that development involves the following: 1) normative age-related processes (things that occur at specific ages, such as puberty); 2) normative history-related processes (things that influence normal development for almost everyone at a given time, such as computers in schools and dual-career families); and, 3) non-normative life events, such as accidents, illness, or divorce (4). Included within this last set of experiences would be events that are perceived by the individual, and possibly by the larger social system, as non-normative events in that they "should not be happening to me now." Because of lay representations of arthritis, a diagnosis of rheumatic disease is commonly seen as non-normative for all but the older patient. This sense of arthritis as normal for the older person and not normal in middle adulthood or childhood can contribute to problems in adjustment.

IMPACT OF RHEUMATIC DISEASE AT EACH LIFE STAGE

Rheumatic disease has a differing impact on individuals at different life stages. Some of the factors that might affect persons with rheumatic disease at each of the recognized life stages are outlined below.

Infancy and Pre-school

Infants and toddlers confront and master many tasks in a short period of time. Infants learn to sit, stand, walk, and talk; they learn to smile, laugh, and calm themselves. As they grow, they learn to navigate an ever-widening social environment, progressing from family to neighborhood and from solitary to parallel to interactive play. They also learn to follow rules and take direction. Children emerge from this period, hopefully, with a sense of trust, autonomy, and initiative that will serve them throughout their lives.

More than 160,000 children in this country have been diagnosed with juvenile rheumatoid arthritis (5). The potential impact of this diagnosis on a young person and his/her family is clear. At a time when an infant is ideally surrounded by a supportive, predictable, and nurturing environment, the infant with juvenile arthritis may be presented with inexplicable pain; unpredictable failures when attempting to learn the most basic skills such as rolling over, sitting up, standing, and walking; and parents and family members who are overprotective. Even more difficult are situations in which the toddler—either unaware of or oblivious to pain and limitations—makes forays into the world of independence and initiative and is greeted by a negative reaction from loved ones that might easily engender shame, doubt, and guilt.

Research on the experience of pain in children has long been controversial. It was traditionally thought that children either do not experience pain or somehow perceive pain as less distressing than their adult counterparts (6). More recently, it has been acknowledged that children do experience pain and that the pain perception is modulated by a variety of psychological and socioenvironmental factors (7). It is now generally conceded that family resources predict adjustment in the child with arthritis, and that many families adjust quite well after an initial period of adaptation (8). The coping efforts of parent and child do not occur in a vacuum, however. These families are embedded in a larger social context including medical professionals, child care professionals, and community. The parents' own understanding of how to help their child is a function of other messages, which are often mixed. The challenge facing the rheumatology professional working with infants and toddlers is to help the family help their child master the developmental tasks identified above.

Primary School and Pre-adolescence

The task of the school age pre-adolescent child is to develop a realistic sense of competence based on activities both in and out of school. At this stage, the role of larger social structures can have a strong impact on a young person's sense of mastery. Moreover, earlier issues of trust, autonomy, and initiative can re-emerge in the face of a less than sympathetic social context. School systems unresponsive to limitations that the youngster is confronting, or resentful of demands on their own limited resources, can contribute to a sense of hopelessness, helplessness, and futility in the student precisely when he or she needs to develop a sense of mastery.

Children with juvenile arthritis may experience a variety of school-related problems such as impaired mobility, late arrival, difficulties moving from class to class on time, poor stamina, difficulties with fine and gross motor skills, difficulties with medication, and need for physical therapy, among others (9). These children miss 25% more days of school than do children with other chronic illnesses, and 300% more than children with acute illnesses (9). Because the pain and fatigue experienced by the youngster often are not visible to others, and because symptoms can be highly variable even within a given day, the child with juvenile arthritis may encounter skepticism from both classmates and teachers. The health professional working with grade school patients may find that the educational system plays a key role in successful treatment.

Adolescence and Young Adulthood

With adolescence come efforts to define identity; these efforts are commonly associated with a need to rebel against the rules of parents, teachers, and other authority figures (10). The adolescent with juvenile arthritis may be willing to sacrifice control of the illness for control of his/her life. Adolescent rebellion may be pursued on the playing field of arthritis management, and the young person may become unexpectedly recalcitrant. It has been reported that restrictions associated with juvenile arthritis are least during pre-school age and increase through adolescence, when the forced dependency on parents can significantly affect adjustment (11).

A crucial task for the young adult with arthritis is determining how to incorporate this illness within an overall sense of identity. At a time when being different from one's peers is hardly a preferred state of affairs, the adolescent may take any risk just to "fit in." A particular difficulty for the adolescent with arthritis is that medications to control the disease can contribute to a delayed onset of puberty and related growth difficulties. This assault on sexual development may seriously challenge the adolescent's efforts to define a sense of self (12). The rheumatology professional must help the young patient balance personal independence with treatment adherence. A crucial part of this challenge often involves helping parents let go of treatment management and helping the young adult comfortably take charge.

Mid-life

Although there are over 100 different types of rheumatic disease, the most common are osteoarthritis (OA), rheumatoid arthritis (RA), systemic lupus erythematosus, ankylosing spondylitis, and most recently fibromyalgia. It is ironic that, with the exception of OA, these rheumatic diseases often begin between the ages of 25 and 40. For most adults confronting the middle of their life, the specter of chronic illness is hardly considered normative. Nevertheless, these and other chronic illnesses tend to strike at precisely the time when people are beginning jobs, relationships, and families. The identity and sense of competence formed at earlier stages may be seriously threatened; both the individual and his or her social system may be more or less able to make the accommodations demanded by the illness.

Research examining the impact of RA has shown that pain is associated with higher levels of stress and depression among patients, and that these problems can have negative consequences for patients' families and for other members of their social network (13). The impact on family functioning includes increased frequency of arguments with marital partners and increased sexual problems. According to some research in patients with RA (14), 28% to 36% of spouses report frustration with the physical limitations of their partners, and 21% expressed concern over the future of the marriage as a result of health problems.

Rheumatic disease can affect the new mother's ability to parent as well as her ability to perform in valued professional roles. The struggle with disease limitations is accompanied by a struggle to incorporate this new patient identity into one's overall identity in a meaningful and acceptable way. Lupus patients who were unable to resolve this conflict, and who clung instead to their cherished "me before lupus" identity experienced greater amounts of depression (15).

Women with rheumatic disease, like their healthier counterparts, report high levels of psychological demands both at paid work and family work; autonomy was important in reducing family demands, and social support reduced the effects of work demands (16). It is important to define disability not only in terms of paid work, but also in terms of family responsibilities and unpaid activities (17).

Some studies have examined factors that appear to mediate the relationship between disease severity and psychological functioning and have found that cognitive variables such as a perception of control or self-efficacy, as well as a sense of mastery or competence, contribute to better psychological status (13,18). Feelings of helplessness and hopelessness contribute to poorer adjustment (13). These cognitive components are consistent with life tasks identified by Erikson and demonstrate the need to revisit these issues throughout the lifespan.

The health professional should help the adult patient prioritize more important roles and goals and communicate which parts of the self are most worth protecting and preserving. At the same time, the professional should look for indications that this patient is a "high self-efficacy" patient, one who is confident in the ability to manage the illness. In the absence of this ability, the process of sharing responsibility for treatment decisions will need to proceed more slowly.

Retirement and Older Adulthood

Because arthritis is thought of by many as "normal" in older adults, its impact on development would seem to be less. However, this stereotype of old age has negative consequences,

causing some individuals to restrict their activities in ways that may not be necessary. Patient and practitioner may jointly conclude that slowing down is normal and necessary at this stage of life. Retirement among individuals with arthritis is often premature: 10 years after disease onset, over 50% of people with RA and 30% of people with OA were found to be no longer working (19). Although changes in activity level at this stage of development may be quite normal, decisions that are made by the patients, drawing from their own wisdom and understanding of themselves, will contribute most effectively to coherence and integrity in the later stages of life.

Research has shown that as individuals age, a wide variety of limitations and personal failings are attributed to old age. The older a patient is, the more likely that they and others will attribute even mild short-term symptoms to aging; this attribution is associated with the utilization of passive rather than active coping strategies (20, 21). This kind of explanation carries with it the message that there is nothing that can be done about the older person's failings.

Because age cannot be changed, an explanation that says "I can't go out with my friends because I'm old and have arthritis" suggests that there is nothing one can do but accept the situation. On the other hand, an explanation that says "I can't go out with my friends because I get tired easily" allows for the possibility of alternative plans and suggests that things are not hopeless. Health professionals may fall prey to these kinds of ageist conclusions as well. Younger patients tend to be evaluated more positively in the clinic setting and older patients are seen less positively, exacerbating the likelihood of the older patient to revert to a passive role (22). Just when rheumatic disease might finally feel normal, the need to confront and challenge these assumptions is most compelling.

GUIDELINES FOR THE HEALTH CARE PROVIDER

The theoretical models on which this chapter is based suggest some factors to be considered in the individual with rheumatic disease.

Age-related Processes. Age is merely a marker for developmental changes that typically occur in a certain order; great individual variability exists with respect to when and if specific events will occur. Motor skills develop at different rates in children, adolescents pursue their efforts to separate from their parents at their own pace, not all adults marry and/or have children, and older adults vary greatly in their desire to remain active and involved in the world. Recognizing the variability in patients' lives will help prevent the professional from communicating to them a lack of "normalcy" if their course is somewhat different from the typical. It may also protect the professional from too quickly concluding that variations from the norm are a result of the disease.

History-related Processes. For each generation, at each stage of life, the world offers different experiences. Many young women currently struggle to balance marriage, family and profession in a way that was less common for the wives and mothers who preceded them. Similarly, a patient's mental image of a severely disabled grandparent and his/her own likelihood of becoming similarly disabled does not take into consideration advances in medical care. It may sometimes be necessary to uncover and then dispel preconceived notions that are no longer relevant but may block progress in treatment.

Table 1. Questions to aid the health care provider in understanding the patient's current needs.

1. Where is the patient on the continuum of life tasks? A child preparing for school? A young adult setting off on a career or relationship? A mature adult facing midlife challenges? An elder facing retirement?
2. How is the person spending their limited time, energy, and attention? Has arthritis become the sole focus of life?
3. What is the individual's current psychosocial development task? What opposing forces is he or she seeking to balance?
4. How does rheumatic disease complicate the person's current life stage and psychosocial developmental tasks? For example, how does arthritis make it more difficult to fulfill their particular career or family objectives?
5. What adaptive strengths has the patient developed, and how will the resolution of previous life tasks impact circumstances changed by rheumatic disease? For example, the adaptive strengths of competence and purpose will assist in adapting to arthritis, but will also need to be revisited due to this new challenge.

Developing a Treatment Plan

The ability of individuals to manage their disease will be, to an extent, a function of the social context in which they are embedded. The demands of family, school, and work must be considered in the development of a treatment plan. The efforts of the professional to implement a successful treatment plan should include recognition that the patient's understanding of his or her disease comes from the social context, and that treatment will, in turn, influence that context. Successful treatment efforts will ascertain the individual's current illness representations (23), providing clarification and facts as necessary but also acknowledging and respecting deeply held beliefs. Of particular importance are cultural beliefs (see Chapter 8, Social and Cultural Assessment), which may be more or less at odds with traditional Western medicine. Both professional and patient must work together to resolve the disparity. Ignoring these cultural beliefs will likely doom the traditional treatment plan to failure.

In addition, the successful treatment plan will ascertain the individual's current life goals. Each individual brings strengths and weaknesses to the experience of rheumatic disease, and an identity made up of a variety of valued roles and abilities. A treatment plan that specifies no tennis may be fine for the marginally athletic patient but would be a serious blow to the professional tennis coach. To design a plan that respects the needs of the individual and maximizes the likelihood of success, it is essential to determine patient expectations regarding the management of this illness and its place in his or her life. Finally, the plan should develop treatment goals, in conjunction with the patient, that are based on the realities of the disease and the realities of the patient's life. The five questions outlined in Table 1 can help the health care professional assess the patient's needs.

The Chinese symbol for crisis is a combination of the symbols for danger and opportunity. Development of a rheumatic disease can precipitate a life crisis and present the danger of losses of identity, competence, or productivity; it can also provide an opportunity to reintegrate psychosocial strengths and reprioritize family, work, and leisure activities. This can lead to new equilibrium which is even more satisfying as individuals continue "composing" their lives.

REFERENCES

1. Erikson EH, Erikson JM, Kivnick HQ: Vital Involvement in Old Age: The Experience of Old Age in Our Time. New York, WW Norton & Company, 1986
2. Bornstein MH, Lamb ME: Developmental Psychology: An Advanced Textbook. Hillsdale, NJ, Lawrence Erlbaum, 1992
3. Lerner RM: Developmental contextualism and the life-span view of person-context interaction. In, Interaction in Human Development. Edited by M Bornstein, JS Bruner. Hillsdale, NJ, Lawrence Erlbaum, 1989
4. Baltes PB, Reese HW, Lipsitt LP: Life-span developmental psychology. Annu Rev Psychol 31:65–110, 1980
5. Cassidy JT, Petty RE: Textbook of Pediatric Rheumatology. Second edition. New York, Churchill Livingstone, 1990
6. Varni JW, Bernstein BH: Evaluation and management of pain in children with rheumatic diseases. Rheum Dis Clin North Am 17:985–1000, 1991
7. Hagglund KJ, Schopp LM, Alberts KR, Cassidy JT, Frank RG: Predicting pain among children with juvenile rheumatoid arthritis. Arthritis Care Res 8:36–42, 1995
8. Varni JW, Wilcox KT, Hanson V: Mediating effects of family social support on child psychological adjustment in juvenile rheumatoid arthritis. Health Psychol 7:421–431, 1988
9. Bartholomew LK, Koenning G, Dahlquist L, Barron K: An educational needs assessment of children with juvenile rheumatoid arthritis. Arthritis Care Res 7:136–143, 1994
10. Manaster GJ: Individual Psychology: Theory and Practice. Itasca, IL, FE Peacock Publishers, Inc., 1982
11. Ungerer J, Horgan G, Chartow J, Champion GB: Psychosocial functioning in children and young adults with juvenile arthritis. J Pediatr 81:195–202, 1989
12. Eiser C, Berenberg JL: Assessing the impact of chronic disease on the relationship between parents and their adolescents. J Psychosom Res 39:109–114, 1995
13. Bradley LA: Psychological dimensions of rheumatoid arthritis. In, Rheumatoid Arthritis: Pathogenesis, Assessments, Outcomes, and Treatment. Edited by F Wolfe, T Pincus. New York, Marcel Dekker, 1994, pp. 273–295
14. Revenson TA, Majerovitz SD: The effects of chronic illness on the spouse: social resources as stress buffers. Arthritis Care Res 4:63–72, 1991
15. Kobasa SCO, Bochnak E, McKinley PS: Patient identity in women with SLE. Arthritis Care Res 4:S22, 1991
16. Reisine S, Fifield J: Family work demands, employment demands and depressive symptoms in women with rheumatoid arthritis. Women Health 22:25–45, 1995
17. Reisine S, Fifield J: Expanding the definition of disability: implications for planning, policy, and research. Milbank Q 70:491–508, 1992
18. Smith CA, Dobbins CJ, Wallston KA: The mediational role of perceived competence in psychological adjustment to arthritis. J Appl Soc Psychol 15:1218–1247, 1991
19. Boutaugh M, Brady T, Callahan L, Gibofsky A, Haralson K, Lappin D, Lautzenheiser R, Leong A, McAsey P, Rutkowski R: Quality of Life Action Plan. Atlanta, Arthritis Foundation, 1993
20. Leventhal E, Prohaska TR: Age, symptom interpretation, and health behavior. J Am Geriatr Soc 34:185–191, 1986
21. Erber JT, Szuchman LT, Rothberg ST: Age, gender, and individual differences in memory failure appraisal. Psychol Aging 5:600–603, 1990
22. Greene MG, Adelman R, Charon R, Hoffman S: Ageism in the medical encounter: an exploratory study of the doctor-elderly patient relationship. Lang Commun 6:113–124, 1986
23. Schiaffino KM, Cea CD: Assessing chronic illness representations: the Implicit Models of Illness Questionnaire. J Behav Med 18:531–548, 1995

SECTION B: ASSESSMENT AND EVALUATION OF THE PATIENT

<table>
<tr><td>CHAPTER
4</td><td># History and Physical Examination</td></tr>
</table>

LISA A. NICHOLS, MSN, RN, FNP-C

Over the past few decades, our understanding of rheumatic diseases has increased greatly from technologic advances in joint imaging and clinical immunology. However, an extensive history and complete physical examination remain the basis of a sound evaluation of the patient with musculoskeletal complaints. It is estimated that one of every six visits to a primary care provider is motivated by a musculoskeletal problem. Complaints exhibited by individuals can range from straightforward sprains and strains to complicated systemic diseases, such as systemic lupus erythematosus (SLE) or rheumatoid arthritis (RA). The examiner must have a working knowledge of the rheumatic diseases in order to recognize the appropriate path to follow when first questioning and examining the patient (1–5).

THE RHEUMATIC HISTORY

The history should be obtained from the patient in a private setting, before the physical examination is conducted. When possible, the interviewer should face the patient with no barriers between. If the patient is in pain or has difficulty sitting without support, he or she can sit in a chair with arms and a back, or perhaps recline rather than sit on the examining table. Attending to the patient's comfort at the outset will help establish a positive patient–provider relationship. Providing a non-threatening environment can aid in gaining the patient's trust and help allay fears. The interview should begin with a general open-ended question such as "What is it that brings you in to see me today?" This will help elicit the chief complaint. It is important to listen to the exact words the patient uses to describe the symptoms, as well as note any nonverbal clues. The clinician should resist the temptation to hurry the patient along by offering language to describe the problem. If the patient is reluctant to give information spontaneously, or has difficulty describing symptoms, more direct questioning by the interviewer may be needed. When assessing the pediatric patient, both the child and the child's parent or guardian should be questioned about current complaints and past examination findings (6).

Assessing the Chief Complaint

A systematic approach should be used when attempting to elicit information about the patient's chief complaint. Assess-

ment of seven particular symptom details can provide clues of diagnostic importance: location, character, quantity, course, aggravating and alleviating factors, setting, and associated manifestations (6). The pain associated with rheumatic conditions most frequently causes patients to seek out a health care provider. The precise *location* of the pain is essential to determine whether the pain is articular or nonarticular. Pain described as "deep" or difficult to pinpoint with one finger is likely to be articular, whereas pain described as "superficial" and/or easily pinpointed along tendons or to adjacent joint structures is likely to be extra-articular. The *character* or quality of the pain may best be described by the patient in comparison to another type of pain, such as "like a toothache" or "similar to labor pains." The origin of the pain can often be inferred from the patient's description. Muscular pain or myalgia is usually described as "crampy" or "throbbing", whereas neurologic pain is described as "pins and needles" or "electric shocks."

The *quantity* or intensity of pain is sometimes difficult to assess, as patients have different pain thresholds. Some patients, because of a need to convince the provider of the severity of the pain, may actually inflate the pain intensity. Children may best express their perception of pain by use of a cartoon pain assessment scale with several faces ranging from smiling to crying. The child chooses the face that best represents how he/she feels (7). The *course* of the pain, including date and type of onset (e.g., insidious or sudden), duration and progression may be of diagnostic importance. For example, pain may be acute (less than 6 weeks duration) with conditions such as gout or infectious arthritis, or it may be chronic (greater than 6 weeks duration) in osteoarthritis (OA) or RA. Joint pain may be intermittent (as in gout), additive (RA or OA), or migratory. Migratory articular pain implies a rapidly changing pattern of joint involvement and should suggest either rheumatic fever or viral or gonococcal arthritis. Nocturnal pain in a child may suggest growing pains, osteoid osteoma, or an inflammatory condition.

Aggravating and alleviating factors, such as rest or activity, heat or cold, should be assessed. The setting in which pain occurs may provide clues to causality, such as pain related to the performance of repetitive physical movements on the job in a patient with wrist pain. Musculoskeletal pain in a child that occurs only during the school week may suggest a school-related stressor. Associated manifestations, whether local (bony enlargements), constitutional (weight loss), or emotional (depression), can help determine the nature of the underlying process.

Joint swelling is an important component to many rheumatic diseases. Swelling may be subjective (i.e., perceived by the patient) or objective. As with pain, patients should be questioned about the location, pattern of onset, and aggravating or alleviating factors related to the swelling. Location is important in determining whether the swelling is localized to a discrete structure, as in a bursa, or to a broader area, such as a dependent limb. The pattern of onset may give clues to the acuteness of the problem, such as a traumatic injury. Aggravating and alleviating factors may include activity, rest, and response to medications.

Limitation of motion is commonly described by the patient in terms of interruption in their activities of daily living. Questions about the patient's ability to bathe, toilet, feed, dress, ambulate at home, and perform normal work or play activities should be addressed. Length of time the limitation has persisted, as well as how the patient has adapted are important. Assessment of the use of adaptive aids, such as canes or crutches, and assistive devices such as jar openers and dressing aids is necessary. The pattern of onset may have diagnostic importance. Sudden limitation of motion may be related to a tendon rupture, whereas a gradual limitation, as in contracture formation, may be caused by a chronic inflammatory condition.

Stiffness is the feeling of discomfort and/or restriction of movement after a period of inactivity. Morning stiffness of greater than 1 hour is a hallmark symptom of inflammatory arthritis such as RA and is usually systemic. Stiffness that occurs after brief periods of inactivity and lasts less than 60 minutes may occur in noninflammatory conditions such as OA. This sensation is most often perceived close to the affected joints. Patients may have difficulty quantifying the amount of stiffness they experience. Many are unclear as to what the interviewer means by stiffness. Some patients liken stiffness to pain, soreness, weakness, or fatigue. A generally accepted method of questioning patients about the duration of morning stiffness is to ask if they feel stiff upon awakening in the morning and the time stiffness is first noted. This is followed by inquiries to determine when the patient is most limber. The duration of stiffness is the time elapsed. The patient may feel more stiff on some days and less on others. It is best to have the patient give an average of morning stiffness for the past week, rather than just on the day of the interview.

Weakness is defined as a decrease in, or loss of, muscle strength. It may coexist with other constitutional symptoms, such as stiffness and fatigue; therefore, it is sometimes difficult for patients to separate weakness from other symptoms. Actual muscle weakness is noted only when muscles are being used, and it is frequently noted by an inability to carry out activities of daily living. Questions should focus on the patient's ability to perform the following functions: ambulating, gripping, chewing, swallowing, and toileting. The weakness manifested in inflammatory myopathies is usually present in proximal muscles, whereas neuropathies cause distal muscle weakness. Patients with true myopathies have little trouble distinguishing between muscle weakness and generalized fatigue.

Fatigue is one of the most common constitutional complaints associated with rheumatic disease (see Chapter 20, Fatigue). It is defined as a feeling of "weariness, exhaustion, or lassitude . . . frequently associated with a decreased capacity for work" (8). Fatigue is assessed by determining the time of onset, frequency, degree of severity, and impact on activities of daily living. Accompanying psychosocial stressors, diet, sleep patterns, and activity level should be determined. Fatigue is often prominent in inflammatory and noninflammatory conditions (e.g., RA and fibromyalgia, respectively).

Other Pertinent History

A history of any previous therapy for the current problem should be sought. If similar symptoms have occurred before, it is likely that other providers have been consulted. Use of previous prescription or nonprescription medications, physical therapies, natural or home remedies, and other nontraditional treatments should be elicited. Questions might encompass length of previous therapy, adherence, presence of side effects, acceptability of cost, and the patient's perception of success or failure of these modalities. In addition, all of the patient's current medications for seemingly unrelated illnesses should be reviewed to rule out potential drug interactions or the possibility of drug-induced rheumatic symptoms such as drug-induced lupus.

Exploring the patient's past medical and sexual history can help determine previous serious illnesses and surgeries, as well as identify conditions pertinent to the current illness. For example, urethritis that predates the onset of heel pain may be a significant clue to a diagnosis of Reiter's syndrome. The family history may also reveal information of diagnostic importance. Some rheumatic diseases have a genetic basis. For example, the HLA–B27 associated spondylarthropathies (ankylosing spondylitis, Reiter's syndrome, psoriatic arthritis, and enteropathic arthritis) can occur in several family members, even children. A family history of lupus in a child with SLE is not unusual, although chronic rheumatic diseases of childhood are seldom familial. A negative family history should also be noted. Potential environmental triggers, occupational exposure, travel, or recent viral or bacterial infection should not be overlooked. Finally, a careful developmental history should be obtained.

Review of Systems

The final part of the history is the review of systems. Because many rheumatic diseases are systemic in nature, a complete review of all body systems is another opportunity to identify important diagnostic symptoms or comorbid conditions. Examples of positive findings in the review of systems relevant to rheumatic diseases are included in Table 1.

THE PHYSICAL EXAMINATION

As with the history, the physical examination should take place in a private setting. Often patients with rheumatic complaints are unable to seat themselves on the examination table without assistance. Conventional tables may have too high a step for the patient with muscle weakness or lower extremity disease to master. If necessary, the majority of the physical examination can be performed with the patient seated in a chair. A motorized examination table that can be lowered to a height of approximately 24–36 inches is preferable. Physical examination of the child is similar to an adult, with two notable

Table 1. Positive findings in the review of systems relevant to rheumatic diseases.

System	Symptoms/Complaints	Diagnosis to Consider
Integument	Nail pitting	Psoriatic arthritis
	Nodules	Rheumatoid arthritis
	Tophi	Gout
	Photosensitivity	Systemic lupus erythematosus
	Rashes	Vasculitis, dermatomyositis, Lyme disease, psoriatic arthritis
Head and Neck	Alopecia	Systemic lupus erythematosus, scleroderma
	Dysphagia	Scleroderma, polymyositis
	Dry eyes/mouth	Sjögren's syndrome
	Jaw claudication	Temporal arteritis
	Nasal ulceration	Wegener's granulomatosis, systemic lupus erythematosus
Chest	Cough	Interstitial pulmonary fibrosis
	Chest pain	Pericarditis, pleuritis, costochondritis
Abdomen	Abdominal pain	Mesenteric vasculitis, peptic ulcer
Genitourinary	Penile ulceration	Behcet's disease, Reiter's syndrome
	Penile/vaginal discharge	Reiter's syndrome
	Microscopic hematuria	Lupus nephritis
Neurologic	Paresthesias	Carpal tunnel syndrome
	Seizures	Lupus cerebritis
	Headache	Temporal arteritis
Other	Fever	Systemic juvenile arthritis, septic arthritis, vasculitis
	Fatigue	Fibromyalgia, rheumatoid arthritis, systemic lupus erythematosus
	Weakness	Polymyositis

exceptions. First, a developmental assessment of the child should be made to determine whether the child is maturing at an age-appropriate pace. Second, it is wise to modify the order of the examination, saving potentially painful or distressing aspects of the examination until last. Most of the examination can be conducted with the child sitting on the parent or guardian's lap.

The General Physical Examination

Examination of the patient with rheumatic complaints should not be limited to the musculoskeletal system. As with the history, particular attention should be paid to other organ systems that may be involved. Concomitant illnesses, such as peptic ulcer disease, may also affect treatment selections.

The examination should begin with vital signs, including temperature, respirations, pulse, blood pressure, and weight. Unintentional weight loss may be a feature of neoplasia, chronic infection, or inflammatory disorders. Weight loss may be insidious early in the disease course, and is often only noted through serial evaluation. The adult patient should change into a gown and remove the shoes and socks to allow for complete inspection and evaluation of skin, nails, and extremities. It may not be necessary to thoroughly undress the child. Exposing small areas as they are assessed helps keep the child warm and feeling more in control.

The skin, hair, scalp, and nails are usually examined first. Special attention is paid to the presence of any nodules, tophi, rashes, ulcerations, telangiectasias, alopecia, or Raynaud's phenomena. A thorough pulmonary and cardiac examination are required and are of particular importance when progressive systemic sclerosis, SLE, or vasculitis are suspected. Careful neurologic examination is necessary when assessing for SLE, vasculitis, or nerve entrapment syndromes.

The Musculoskeletal Examination

Examination of the musculoskeletal system is best undertaken in a systematic manner. Many examiners begin at the head and move downward, while others begin with the upper extremities, move towards the trunk and then downward to the feet. The latter approach is less threatening to the patient, as the examination begins in a socially neutral location, the hands. Throughout the examination, the patient should be as comfortable as possible. Support should be provided above or below an inflamed joint when moving it through range of motion, rather than holding on to the joint itself. Movements should be slow and fluid, not sudden or forceful. A relaxed patient is better able to tolerate a thorough examination and will allow for more accurate assessment.

The basic maneuvers of a musculoskeletal examination include inspection, palpation, range of motion, and assessment of function. Inspection and palpation are usually performed simultaneously. Similarly, range of motion and function can often be assessed together. For example, while a patient is demonstrating active range of motion of the shoulder, the examiner can ask if the patient is able to style her hair.

Joint Findings

The most common joint abnormalities are swelling, tenderness, warmth, crepitus, limitation of motion, and sometimes deformity. Swelling can result from several causes such as bony overgrowth, joint effusion, or synovial proliferation, and it may be assessed by inspection and direct palpation of the joint. Tenderness is assessed by direct gentle, yet firm, palpation over the joint. Using both hands, the examiner should palpate the joint in all planes, anterior to posterior and medial to lateral. Enough pressure is exerted when the nail beds of the examiner's fingers or thumbs blanch. The amount of pain elicited should be weighed against the emotional state of the patient. Observing the patient's facial expressions, as well as listening to verbal cues, is often useful. Warmth of the joint is best confirmed by comparison with the opposite joint. Skin color changes may also be present.

Crepitus is the palpable or audible grating sensation produced by roughened articular or extra-articular surfaces rubbing against each other. Some crepitus is appreciated in normal joints, but severe cracking or grating is usually indicative of chronic degenerative processes. When assessing for limitation of motion, it is helpful to understand the normal ranges of joint motion. Range of motion should be assessed actively as well as passively. The only exception is the cervical spine, which should never be passively moved. Limitation of motion can occur either actively or passively; however, because patients are limited by their own pain, passive range of motion is usually greater, and therefore is a more accurate measure. Deformity denotes malalignment of the joint and may be the result of various causes, such as bony enlargement, joint subluxation, contracture, or destruction of ligamentous support.

Examination of Specific Joints

The Small Joints. The temporomandibular (TM), acromioclavicular (AC), sternoclavicular (SC) and sternomanubrial (SM) joints deserve inclusion in the examination. Despite their size, these joints can exhibit pain, swelling, and crepitus. The TM joint is located at the junction of the articular tubercle of the temporal bone and the condyle of the mandible. It is assessed for warmth, pain, and swelling by direct palpation over the joint directly anterior to the tragus. Crepitus can be discerned by inserting the index fingers just inside the external ear canal and gently pulling forward while the patient opens and closes the mouth. Range of motion is adequate if the patient is able to insert the width of two fingers inside the mouth. The AC joint is located by tracing the clavicle laterally to the acromion process. The SC joint is medial, where the clavicle meets the sternum. These two joints are assessed for tenderness, swelling, and crepitus. Motion of the AC is assessed by firmly pulling down on the forearm. The SC joint has minimal motion, but can be assessed by having the patient shrug the shoulders. The SM joint is located where the manubrium articulates with the body of the sternum. This joint has no motion, but it may be tender or swollen.

Shoulder. The shoulder is a ball and socket joint formed by the head of the humerus and the glenoid fossa of the scapula. Knowledge of shoulder anatomy is essential to assess the origin of symptoms. Pathology can occur in the glenohumeral joint, the rotator cuff, the subacromial bursae, the bicipital tendon, or the axillae. The shoulder is best examined from the front, so that both shoulders can be compared. The shoulder is inspected and palpated for warmth, swelling, tenderness, muscle spasm, or atrophy. Range of motion is assessed by having the patient perform the following procedures: raise arms forward in a wide arc and touch palms together above the head; with elbows flexed and hands on head, move arms posteriorly; raise arms extended in sideways arc and touch palms together above head; and rotate the arm internally behind the back and touch between the scapulae. Normal ranges of motion are forward flexion 90°; backward extension 45°; abduction 180°;

adduction 45°; internal rotation 55°, and external rotation 40° to 45°(3).

Elbow. The elbow is a hinge joint formed by three bony articulations: the humero-ulnar, radiohumeral, and the proximal radio-ulnar. The elbow is surrounded by one large (the olecranon) and several small bursae. This joint should be inspected for subcutaneous nodules, tophi, and the presence of olecranon bursitis. Palpation is conducted with the elbow flexed to approximately 70°. Synovitis is best appreciated in the medial paraolecranon groove. Normal elbow extension is 0° to 5°, while flexion is 135° or greater. Synovitis can cause loss of full extension, and if chronic, may result in flexion contracture (inability to fully extend to 0°).

Wrist and Hand. The wrist contains eight carpal bones arranged in two rows; the proximal row articulates with the radius. The wrist normally has 60° to 70° of extension and 80° to 90° flexion. Ulnar to radius deviation at the wrist is 30° and 20°, respectively. The wrist is inspected and palpated for synovitis, warmth, thickened tendons, cystic swelling, and deformity. Mild synovitis may manifest as pain on movement. Dorsal/ventral instability with or without bogginess of the ulnar styloid is known as the *piano key sign*. Compression of the median nerve in the carpal tunnel is tested by placing the wrist in severe flexion (60°) for at least 1 minute. When numbness or paresthesias are noted along the distribution of the median nerve (first three digits and medial half of the fourth), it is known as a positive *Phalen's sign*. This maneuver may be difficult for the patient with acute synovitis. An alternative maneuver is to percuss repeatedly along the volar aspect of the wrist. A tingling or feeling of electric shock in the same median nerve distribution is known as *Tinel's sign*.

Another clinical sequelae of prolonged median nerve compression in the carpal tunnel is thenar muscle atrophy, noted on the palm at the base of the thumb. *Dupuytren's contracture* may be noted as thickening and contracture of the palmar aponeurosis causing severe flexion of the fourth and fifth fingers. *De Quervain's tenosynovitis* is a common cause of wrist pain due to inflammation and stenosing of the tendon sheaths at the base of the thumb near the radial styloid. It is assessed by having the patient flex the thumb into the palm, then grip the fingers over the thumb and move the hand downward (ulnar deviated). If tenosynovitis is present, this maneuver may produce exquisite tenderness on the radial side of the wrist.

The metacarpophalangeal (MCP), proximal interphalangeal (PIP), and distal interphalangeal (DIP) joints comprise the small joints of the hands. They are hinge joints held in place by tendons and ligaments. Range of motion of these joints is most easily assessed by having the patient slowly flex the fingers to form a fist. Loss of extension in any single digit is best expressed as the number of degrees lacking full extension. Hands should be inspected for swelling, deformity, and skin and nail changes. Rheumatoid arthritis predominately affects the MCP and PIP joints. Common deformities include *swan neck deformity*, involving hyperextension of the PIP joint and flexion of the DIP joint, and *boutonnière deformity*, or flexion contracture of the PIP joint with hyperextension of the DIP joint. Osteoarthritis predominately affects the first carpometacarpal joint and the DIP joints. Osteophytic nodules that form on the PIP and DIP joints are known as *Bouchard's nodes* and *Heberden's nodes*, respectively. Scleroderma can cause the skin over the fingers to have a tight, shiny, atrophic appearance *(sclerodactyly)*. Pitting of the nails and dystrophic changes *(onycholysis)* may be seen in psoriatic arthritis.

Hip. The hip is a major weight-bearing ball and socket joint, formed by the head of the femur and the pelvic acetabulum. It is surrounded by strong ligaments and bursae. Inspection of the hip begins with gait assessment. Before palpating the hip, instruct the patient to indicate where pain is located. Often patients will point to the lateral side and describe the pain as being in the "hip joint", when in reality they are pointing over the trochanteric bursa. True hip pain is manifested anteriorly in the groin fold. The hip has a wide range of motions. Extension (normal 30°) can be measured several ways, including having the patient drop the leg off the table; or from a standing position moving one leg backward; or lifting the leg off the table while lying supine. Flexion (normal 120°) is done with the patient supine and drawing one knee up to the chest without bending the back. While in this position, the opposite hip can be checked for a flexion contracture. Abduction (normal 45°) is moving the leg away from the midline. Adduction (normal 20° to 30°) is moving the leg across the midline. Internal and external rotation are performed with the knee and hip flexed to 90°. Rotating the heel medially causes external rotation (normal 45°) and outwardly causes internal rotation (normal 35°). Hip movement can be quickly measured by placing the heel medially to the opposite knee and slowly lowering the flexed knee toward the table.

Knee. The knee is a large diarthrodial joint supported by a series of ligaments and surrounded by several bursae. Normal knee extension is 0°; normal flexion is 135°. The knee is inspected for swelling, deformity such as *genu varum* (bow legs) or *genu valgum* (knock knees), flexion contracture, locking or buckling, Baker's or popliteal cysts, and skin changes. The knee is palpated with the patient supine and in full extension. The patella should move easily medially and laterally, and may ballot if a large effusion is present. Minor knee effusions are best palpated after milking the fluid away from the medial side and then tapping the lateral aspect of the knee with the other hand. If an effusion is present, a small wave or bulge of fluid will reappear on the medial aspect *(bulge sign)*.

Stability of the collateral ligaments is tested by placing the patient supine with the knee at full extension. One hand stabilizes the femur on either side of the knee and acts as a fulcrum, while the other hand grasps the ankle and moves the lower extremity in the direction of the braced hand to assess the contralateral collateral ligament. Excess movement may indicate collateral ligament laxity or damage. The cruciate ligaments are tested by having the patient flex the hip to 45° and the knee to 90°. The examiner fixes the foot position. The fingers are then placed posteriorly in the popliteal space behind the knee, with the thumbs anteriorly over the joint line. The lower extremity is pulled forward or pushed backward to assess the cruciate ligaments. Increased forward motion denotes pathology with the anterior cruciate ligament. Increased posterior motion may indicate posterior cruciate damage. A positive finding is known as a *drawer sign*. Other findings related to knee pathology are quadriceps atrophy, crepitation on movement secondary to cartilage degeneration, and tenderness over the anserine bursa, on the anteromedial tibial plateau below the knee.

Ankle and Foot. The ankle is a hinge joint formed by the distal ends of the tibia and fibula and the proximal talus. This joint is limited in motion to plantar flexion (50°) and dorsiflexion (20°). The subtalar joint (articulation of the talus and the calcaneus) is responsible for inversion and eversion (5° each direction). The foot includes the intertarsal joints (midfoot), and the metatarsophalangeal (MTP) and interphalangeal (IP) joints of the toes. The metatarsal heads and the calcaneus are the weightbearing portions of the foot. Midfoot range of motion is assessed by stabilizing the calcaneus and inverting and everting the forefoot (MTP and IP joints). Forefoot range of motion can be checked by having the patient flex and extend the toes.

The foot and ankle should be inspected in weight-bearing and nonweight-bearing positions, both with and without footwear. Assessment should include swelling, deformity, nodules, tophi, nail changes, and calluses. Swelling of the ankle joint is sometimes difficult to differentiate from generalized edema. True ankle joint effusions are noted as a non-pitting fullness anteriorly and/or posteriorly around the malleoli. Ankle synovitis causes tenderness on movement. The feet and toes are commonly affected in RA, OA, and gout; deformities may include lateral deviation of the great toe *(hallux valgus)*, hyperextension of the MTP joint *(hammer toe)*, and dorsal subluxation of the MTP joint *(cockup deformity)*. Calluses and abnormal patterns of shoe wear can be important clues in assessing foot problems.

Spine. The spine supports the upright posture of the body and provides protection for the spinal column. Spinal range of motion provides flexibility for the trunk. The vertebral column as a whole produces 90° of flexion. The trunk (minus the cervical spine) extends to 30° posteriorly, and 50° laterally in either direction. The cervical spine provides 45° of flexion, 50° to 60° of extension, 60° to 80° of rotation, and 40° of lateral bending. In the RA patient, cervical range of motion is always done actively, as there is a possibility for subluxation of C1 and C2. The spine should be inspected first as a whole and then by section. A thorough examination requires the patient to be standing, with the entire back, shoulders, hips, legs, and feet visible. The spine is inspected for symmetry, abnormal curvature (scoliosis, kyphosis, lordosis), and paravertebral spasm. Palpation is performed systematically from the top down and from side to side. Ankylosing spondylitis commonly affects the thoracic and lumbar spine, causing forward protrusion of the head, decreased chest expansion, thoracic kyphosis, and loss of lumbar lordosis. The *Wright-Schöber test* measures forward flexion of the lumbar spine. A line is drawn at the level of the posterior superior iliac crests, with a second line 10 cm above the first. The distance between the two marks increases 5 cm or more in the case of normal lumbar mobility and less than 4 cm in the case of decreased lumbar mobility.

The sacrum is a triangular bone formed by the union of five sacral vertebrae. The lateral aspect of the sacrum has a large auricular surface for articulating with the ileum of the hip. These sacroiliac joints are assessed with the patient lying on his/her side. The examiner exerts steady downward pressure over the upper iliac crest. Localization of pain to the sacroiliac area is a positive sign of sacroiliitis, a common feature of ankylosing spondylitis. The *straight-leg raising test* is a screening tool for neurologic or muscular low back pain. This is done with the patient supine and one knee in full extension. The leg is gradually raised until symptoms occur, usually within 30° to 80° of flexion. Pain is aggravated by forced dorsiflexion of the foot, and relieved with flexion of the knee.

SUMMARY

A thorough history and physical examination of the musculoskeletal and selected other systems are the most important components of the evaluation of rheumatic complaints. Too much reliance on or inappropriate interpretation of laboratory testing and radiologic procedures may cloud the diagnostic picture, rather than guide the evaluation and plan of care. Early assessment and intervention can positively impact the morbidity and mortality of patients with rheumatic diseases. A careful history and physical examination can also yield the economic benefits of better utilization of clinician time and resources and decreased costs to patients.

REFERENCES

1. Cush JJ, Lipsky PE: Approach to articular and musculoskeletal disorders. In, Harrison's Principles of Internal Medicine. Thirteenth edition. Edited by KJ Isselbacher, E Braunwald, JD Wilson, JB Martin, AS Fauci, DL Kasper. New York, McGraw Hill, 1994, pp. 1688–1692
2. Polly HF, Hunder GG: Rheumatologic Interviewing and Physical Examination of the Joints. Second edition. Philadelphia, WB Saunders, 1978
3. Hoppenfeld S: Physical Examination of the Spine and Extremities. New York, Appleton-Century-Crofts, 1976
4. Fries JF: Assessment of the patient with rheumatic disease. In, Textbook of Rheumatology. Third edition. Edited by WN Kelly, ED Harris, S Ruddy, CB Sledge. Philadelphia, WB Saunders, 1989, pp. 417–441
5. American College of Rheumatology Ad Hoc Committee on Clinical Guidelines: Guidelines for the initial evaluation of the adult patient with acute musculoskeletal symptoms. Arthritis Rheum 39:1–8, 1996
6. Bates B: A Guide to Physical Examination and History Taking. Sixth edition. Philadelphia, JB Lippincott, 1995
7. Cassidy J, Petty R: Textbook of Pediatric Rheumatology. Third edition. Philadelphia, WB Saunders, 1995
8. American Rheumatism Association Glossary Committee: Dictionary of the Rheumatic Diseases. Volume I: Signs and Symptoms. New York, Contact Associates International Ltd, 1982

Audiovisual Resources

Title: The Joint Exam and You
Copyright: University of Texas Southwestern Medical Center, 1991
Write to: University of Texas Southwestern Medical Center
            Division of Rheumatic Diseases
            Dallas, Texas 75235
            214-648-3466

Title: Physical Examination of the Musculoskeletal System
            (Third edition)
Copyright: JB Lippincott Company, 1995
Write to: 227 East Washington Square
            Philadelphia, PA 19106-3780
            800-523-2945
            ISBN: 0397-55225-4

Health Status Assessment

DONNA J. HAWLEY, EdD, RN

Health status characterizes both the long- and short-term outcomes of chronic disease. It summarizes outcomes that go beyond the physiologic damage caused by a disease to encompass the consequences of the disease from the perspective of the individual's daily functioning. During the last 30 years, reliable, valid, and sensitive instruments and methods (Table 1) have been developed to evaluate health status. Initially such assessments were used only in research studies and clinical trials; however, evaluation of health status as a disease outcome has become an important component of routine clinical care. Third party payers, health policy makers, clinicians, and patients want information about how interventions affect the outcome of disease over time. Measurement of health status is a major method of providing such information.

DEFINITIONS

Health status includes functional status and health-related quality of life (HRQL). The three terms have similar meanings, but differ in the scope of disease outcomes described. *Functional status* is the ability to carry out the usual daily self-care activities including both basic activities of daily living (ADL) and instrumental activities of daily living (IADL). The ADL include daily personal self-care activities of eating, dressing, grooming, and toileting. In contrast, IADL include more complex daily activities such as running errands, shopping, walking outside, and preparing meals. Limitations in either ADL or IADL can result from disease pathology; however, functional status is determined by factors other than physical damage. Psychosocial factors such as coping skills, motivation, family support, formal education, and family income play a role. Environmental influences such as geographic location, transportation, and assistive devices are also important (1). Motivation, family support and various assistive devices may actually improve functioning and mediate the physical damage. For example, walkers and canes may assist someone walking without altering the disease course. Zipper pulls, Velcro openings, and special eating utensils maintain independent functioning when physical signs indicate that assistance from others would be necessary. Individual motivation and determination sometimes compensate for physical limitations. Thus, environmental and psychosocial factors must be considered when evaluating the ability to manage the activities of daily living.

Health status is broader than functional status and encompasses the total physical, mental, and social well-being (1). In addition to functional status, health status includes important aspects of health such as emotions and mood, symptoms (such as pain, sleep disturbance, fatigue), cognitive abilities, and social activities and roles (2). Numerous self-report questionnaires such as those described in this chapter are available to measure health status.

Quality of life is more comprehensive and abstract than either functional or health status. Quality of life is influenced by numerous factors unrelated to an individual's health or disease, such as safe water, adequate housing, crime, and educational opportunities. Further, the perception of one's quality of life has meanings, preferences, and priorities unique to the individual (3). The totality of quality of life is very difficult to define and measure. For these reasons, evaluation of the effect of disease on a person's quality of life has become more narrowly focused on health-related quality of life (HRQL) (3,4). Although HRQL is more comprehensive than health status, the terms are frequently used interchangeably. Both refer to the aggregate effects of disease on the individual's total life (1). In this chapter, "health status" will be used to refer to both HRQL and health status. "Functional status" will refer to the ability to perform activities of daily living.

ASSESSMENT OF FUNCTIONAL STATUS AND HEALTH STATUS

Assessment of functional and health status supplements the information obtained through more traditional assessments of health history, physical examination, laboratory tests, and radiography. Traditional assessments provide data about disease status. Data such as the number of tender joints, the current degree of inflammation, and the number of erosions are documented by physical examination, laboratory tests and x-rays, respectively. Health status assessments provide additional information about how the patient is managing the disease and the consequences of the disease on the individual's everyday life. They provide information from the patient's viewpoint. The ability to eat, dress, and walk outside independently may be more important to the patient than a decrease in the erythrocyte sedimentation rate or even an increase in the number of joint erosions. Direct observation, physician estimation of functioning, and self-report questionnaires have been used to assess both functional status and health status.

Direct Observation

There are several standardized observational methods that may be used to evaluate one or more aspects of functional status. Hand function (button test), hand and arm strength (grip strength), lower extremity movement (walk time and timed-stands test) and range of motion (Keitel index) are described in Table 2. With the exception of the time to walk 50-feet test (5,6), these measures have been shown to be valid and sensitive to change in clinical studies. Each relies on the motivation and cooperation of the patient. The amount of time needed to complete the Keitel index (10 minutes using a health professional's time) limits its use in routine clinical practice. The specially designed equipment needed for the button test and the

Table 1. Terms used in evaluating assessment methods and instruments.

Term	Definition	Example
Reliability	Extent of agreement when there are repeated measurements of the same sample (consistency) or degree of agreement among different evaluators or instruments (equivalence)	An elastic ruler is not a reliable tool for measuring distance.
Validity	Degree to which an instrument or method measures what it is intended to measure.	Grip strength may be a valid measure of hand, wrist and forearm strength, but not lower extremity strength.
Sensitivity	Degree to which an instrument records changes or responds to variation in the concept being measured.	Scores on functional status instruments increase or decrease in response to changes in a person's functional ability.

timed-stands test requires an initial expenditure. Grip strength can be assessed quickly within a busy clinic setting at minimal cost. It is a standard outcome measure for many clinical trials and is sensitive to improvement in inflammation as well as function for a person with rheumatoid arthritis (RA) (6).

Clinician Estimation

Two common methods for assessing function are physician global estimate of disease activity and the American College of Rheumatology (ACR) Revised Criteria for Classification of Functional Status in Rheumatoid Arthritis. Physician global assessment is based on the subjective interpretation of the patient's symptoms, apparent functioning, and laboratory tests. Assignment of scores from 0 (no disease activity) to 4 (very severe activity) is recommended by some authors (5). While this measure has been shown to be sensitive to short-term change during clinical trials (6), similar findings have not been reported for practice situations (7). Physicians tend to overestimate physical limitations compared to patients' perceptions, especially at higher levels of impairment in persons with RA (7). If health care professionals plan to use professional judgment to evaluate functioning, validating one's judgment through discussion with the patient would be appropriate and wise.

Functional status may be classified using the ACR Revised Criteria for Classification of Functional Status in Rheumatoid Arthritis. These criteria, as listed in Table 3, may be used for the "rapid, global assessment of functional status by health professionals" (8). They are helpful in classifying groups of RA patients at one specific point in time; however, using these criteria to monitor change over time for individual patients is not recommended (8,9). More detailed assessments are needed to determine important clinical change over time.

Self-Report Questionnaires

During the last three decades, numerous instruments and questionnaires have been developed to measure health status. These instruments vary in complexity from those measuring a single domain (such as ability to do ADL or self-report pain levels) to more comprehensive instruments having several subscales that measure different aspects of health status. In addition to functional status, the multidimensional instruments contain measures of pain, mood, and emotional well-being; symptoms such as sleep disturbance, fatigue (energy level), gastrointestinal distress, and morning stiffness; social activities and role; cognitive ability; and work and work disability. Patients' global perceptions of health and disease and their satisfaction with their overall health are included in several instruments. Less commonly evaluated are perceived priority areas for health, attribution of health problems, indirect and direct costs of a disease, and drug side effects.

Instruments are classified as generic or disease specific. Generic instruments may be used to evaluate a variety of chronic conditions and to compare across diseases. Comparisons with the general population or with "healthy" groups is also possible (10). Disease-specific instruments are more sen-

Table 2. Standardized direct observation measures for evaluating physical functioning in chronic rheumatic diseases.

Measure	Purpose	Measurement Method	Comments
Grip Strength (5)	Measurement of hand, wrist, and forearm strength	A sphygmomanometer with a mercury column is used. The patient squeezes the cuff inflated to 30 mm/HG as hard as possible. The highest level on the mercury column of three attempts is recorded. Record arm tested.	Motivation, handedness, pain threshold and muscle weakness will affect score as well as involvement of any joint from the elbow to the hand. Grip strength has been shown to be sensitive to change in clinical trials (6).
Time to Walk 50 Feet (5)	Measurement of lower extremity function	Individual walks 50 ft on a flat surface using any aids or assistive devices. Time is recorded in the nearest 0.1 second.	Patient motivation is influential. Low reliability and insensitive to changes in disease (6).
Button Test (47)	Measurement of hand function	Standard board with 5 buttons. Patients are timed while they unbutton and button both right and left hand separately. Mean of 2 scores recorded.	Motivation is an important factor. Useful in disorders with direct effect on hand function (e.g., rheumatoid arthritis).
Timed-Stands Test (48)	Measurement of lower extremity function	Number of seconds used in standing up and down 10 times from a chair using only the lower extremities.	Motivation, age, and non-musculoskeletal co-morbid conditions may affect scores. Sensitivity to change has not been determined.
Keitel Index (49)	Upper and lower extremity function with emphasis on range of motion	Measures 24 standard tasks of peripheral and axial joint motion performed by patients. Evaluation is by trained observer. Time: 10–15 minutes.	Motivation may be a factor. Time and personnel to observe and score tasks are a factor in its use. Scale is sensitive to short-term change.

Table 3. American College of Rheumatology revised criteria for classification of functional status in rheumatoid arthritis (8; used with permission).

Class	Description*
Class I	Completely able to perform usual activities of daily living (self-care, vocational, and avocational)
Class II	Able to perform usual self-care and vocational activities, but limited in avocational activities
Class III	Able to perform usual self-care activities, but limited in vocational and avocational activities
Class IV	Limited ability to perform usual self-care, vocational, and avocational activities

* Usual self-care activities include dressing, feeding, bathing, grooming, and toileting. Avocational (recreational and/or leisure) and vocational (work, school, homemaking) activities are patient-desired and age and sex-specific.

sitive to particular problems or symptoms (11). For example, pain is more important to evaluate in the rheumatic diseases than it is for patients with hypertension. Lower extremity function is especially important following hip or knee replacement for osteoarthritis (OA); however, limitations in activities related to hand functioning may be especially significant in early RA. The severity of a particular disease may be evaluated

best by disease-specific instruments (11). Table 4 lists the common health status instruments used in rheumatology research and clinical practice and the domains included within each instrument.

Disease-Specific Instruments

Health status instruments have been developed and validated for use across the rheumatic disorders and more specific instruments for use in a particular rheumatic disease. The Health Assessment Questionnaire (HAQ) and its modifications, the Arthritis Impact Measurement Scales (AIMS) and its revision (AIMS2), and the Functional Status Index (FSI) are the more general of the disease-specific instruments. The Western Ontario and MacMaster University Osteoarthritis Index (WOMAC) and the Fibromyalgia Impact Questionnaire (FIQ) are examples of instruments for use with OA and fibromyalgia patients, respectively. Each of these instruments is briefly described below; the domains included in each instrument are listed in Table 4.

Health Assessment Questionnaire. The full HAQ is an extensive questionnaire that evaluates economic costs, medi-

Table 4. Domains of health status questionnaires (adapted from 19, used with permission).*

Domain	F-HAQ	HAQ	CLINHAQ	MHAQ	FSI	AIMS	AIMS2	WOMAC	SF-36	SIP	NHP	FIQ
Functional Disability	X	X	X	X	X	X	X	X	X	X	X	X
Eating										X		
Body Care					X		0			X		
Mobility					X	0	0			X		
Dexterity						0	0					
ADL/Self-care						0	0					
Arm Function					X		0					
Physical Function						0	0					
Pain	X	X	X	X	O	X	X	X	X		X	X
Social Activities & Roles					X	X	X		X	X	X	
Social Roles/Function						0	0		0			
Home Management					X					X		
Social Activities						0	0		0			
Recreation/Pastime										X		
Social Interaction/Isolation										X	0	
Social Support							0					
Communication										X		
Work/Work Disability	X		X				X		X	X		X
Symptoms Sleep/Rest			X							X	X	X
Stiffness				X				X				X
Fatigue/Energy			X	X					X		X	X
GI Problems			X	X								
Alertness/Cognition										X		
Adverse Drug Reactions	X		X									
Global Measures												
Global Disease Severity	X	X	X	X								
Global health/well-being			X	X					X			X
Satisfaction			X	X			X					
Emotions/Mood			X	X	X		X		X	X	X	X
Depression			0			0	0					0
Anxiety			0			0	0					0
Helplessness/Attitude				0								
Financial Aspects	X											
Indirect Costs	0											
Direct Costs	0											
Other Areas												
Attribution of problems							X					
Priority areas: Self-stated							X					

* F-HAQ = Full HAQ; HAQ = Health Assessment Questionnaire; CLINHAQ = clinical HAQ; MHAQ = Modified HAQ; AIMS = Arthritis Impact Measurement Scales, Original Version; AIMS2 = Arthritis Impact Measurement Scales, Version 2 clinical; WOMAC = Western Ontario and MacMaster University Osteoarthritis Index; SF-36 = Medical Outcome Study 36-Item Short Form health Survey; SIP = Sickness Impact Profile; NHP = Nottingham Health Profile; FIQ = Fibromyalgia Impact Questionnaire; X = A Major Section or scale of the instrument; 0 = Subsection or subscale of the instrument.

cations and their side effects, use of health care services, co-morbidity as well as functional disability, pain, and global disease severity. Although the long version of the HAQ (20 pages) has been used in long-term outcome studies, it has never been published. In fact, the instrument periodically changes to reflect changes in both treatments and health care delivery practices. The full HAQ is not suitable for use in clinical practice due to its length.

The HAQ, as described extensively in the literature and used in clinical practice, refers to the short functional disability scale (24 questions) of the full HAQ. This instrument evaluates eight activities of daily living including dressing, arising, eating, walking, hygiene, reach, grip, and general activities such as running errands and getting in and out of a car (12). Scores range from 0 (able to perform all activities without difficulty) to 3 (unable to do activities even with help). Visual analogue scales measuring severity of pain during the last week and global disease severity are also included frequently as part of the HAQ. In contrast to the full questionnaire, this instrument may be completed and scored in less than 5 minutes and is suitable for use in both research and clinical practice. The HAQ functional disability scale has been translated into several languages (13). The instrument is sensitive to change in clinical trials and in long-term outcome studies, and it has been shown to predict mortality and future disabilities. Modifications have been made for use with children (14), and for patients with ankylosing spondylitis (15), systemic sclerosis (16), and psoriatic arthritis (17).

Modified Health Assessment Questionnaire (MHAQ). The MHAQ includes a shortened version of the HAQ functional disability scale (8 items) plus items related to patient satisfaction with function and patient interpretation of his/her change in ability to perform routine activities over the previous 6 months. By reducing the number of items related directly to functional status, the authors developed an instrument that measures satisfaction and attitude as well as daily functioning, but is short enough to be incorporated into routine clinical practice (18). The MHAQ has been used extensively in clinical trials and long-term observational studies. Additional revisions have resulted in a total assessment instrument that includes a functional status scale plus items related to activity levels (walking, running, climbing stairs), sleep disturbance, stress, depression, anxiety, stiffness; visual analogues scales for pain, gastrointestinal distress, fatigue; the learned helplessness scale; and items related to co-morbidity, medication side effects, and demographics (19).

CLINHAQ. The CLINHAQ, developed for use in both clinical practice and observational studies, evaluates multiple domains important in the care of persons with chronic rheumatic disease (20). It contains the HAQ functional disability scale, five visual analogue scales (pain, global disease severity, sleep disturbance, gastrointestinal distress, and fatigue), a pain diagram, and the anxiety and depression subscales from the original AIMS instrument.

Functional Status Index. This index assesses both ADL and IADL with 18 items in five categories including gross mobility (walking inside, climbing stairs, and chair transfer), personal care (hygiene and dressing), hand activities (opening jars and writing), home chores (laundry, reaching, yardwork, and vacuuming), and social/role activities (driving and performing one's job). The patient rates the degree of assistance, the degree of difficulty, and the pain involved in each activity

(21). The FSI has been used in clinical trials, as a program evaluation instrument, and within routine clinical practice.

Arthritis Impact Measurement Scales. The AIMS, a comprehensive rheumatic disease health status instrument, has been published in two versions. The original AIMS examined the "impact" of arthritis in terms of both physical function (scales for mobility, physical activity, dexterity, and activities of daily living) and psychosocial aspects of chronic arthritis (subscales for social role, social activities, pain, depression, and anxiety) (22). The instrument has been extensively validated. It has been translated into several languages, employed in both clinical trials and observational studies, and used with adults who have had a variety of rheumatic diseases (23). Its length (20 minutes to complete) and complexity of scoring have limited its use in clinical practice.

AIMS2, published in early 1992, added new components that addressed issues of patient satisfaction, patient preference or priority areas for health status improvement, and attribution of symptoms/problems to arthritis (23). Three new subscales were added, and revisions were made in other subscales. AIMS2 contains renamed and new domains of mobility level, walking and bending, hand and finger function, self-care, household tasks, social activities, support from family and friends, arthritis pain, work, level of tension, and mood (23). The instrument is the most comprehensive of all disease-specific health status instruments and was designed primarily for use in clinical research.

Western Ontario MacMaster Universities Osteoarthritis Index. The WOMAC is a self-administered instrument designed to measure dimensions particularly relevant in OA. It specifically measures pain, stiffness, and physical function activities associated with OA of the hip or knee (24). The instrument has been used in trials of nonsteroidal anti-inflammatory drugs (25) and following hip and knee arthroplasty (26). Its brevity (<10 minutes to administer), availability in both questionnaire or visual analogue formats, and sensitivity to change make it appropriate for use in specialized clinical practice settings.

The Fibromyalgia Impact Questionnaire. The FIQ is a brief, 19-item questionnaire designed specifically for the assessment of fibromyalgia. Items included are physical function, work status, pain, fatigue, morning tiredness, stiffness, anxiety, depression, and general well-being (27). The instrument has been used in studies of fibromyalgia; however, its narrow focus limits its clinical use in other populations.

Generic Health Status Measures

Generic health status measures are not disease specific; they are designed to assess and compare functioning and associated well-being across chronic conditions. These instruments are usually multidimensional, and they provide comparisons between "healthy" or "non-diseased" controls and facilitate descriptions of chronic disease outcomes controlling for co-morbidity (10). International use of some of these instruments permits comparisons of chronic disease outcomes across cultures. Table 4 includes common generic health status instruments.

Nottingham Health Profile (NHP). The NHP was developed in England and has been translated and tested in several languages. It includes 38 true–false questions evaluating physical abilities, pain, sleep, social isolation, emotional reactions, and energy level (28). Completion time is about 10 minutes. Results are similar to the AIMS and HAQ on most similar scales, but it is less sensitive to change (29). The instrument is best used to measure major disabling conditions rather than minor disorders or small degrees of physical limitation (30).

Sickness Impact Profile (SIP). The SIP has been widely used across numerous chronic diseases including the rheumatic disorders and in several European countries (30). It contains 312 items within the dimensions of physical and psychosocial functioning. Specific sections include sleep and rest, eating, work, home management, recreation and pastimes, ambulating, mobility, body care and movement, social interaction, alertness behavior, emotional behavior, and communication (31). The SIP can be self-administered or administered by an interviewer and takes 20 to 30 minutes to complete. While the SIP is one of the most comprehensive generic multidimensional health status questionnaires, it does not include a pain scale.

The Medical Outcome Study Short Form 36 (SF-36). The Medical Outcome Study SF-36 was developed in the United States as part of the Medical Outcomes Study (32), a comprehensive study of "physicians' practice styles and patients' outcomes in competing systems of care" (10). The instrument evaluates eight areas of health status including physical functioning, role limitations due to physical and emotional problems, pain, general health perceptions, vitality (energy and fatigue), social functioning, emotional well-being, and change in health (30). The instrument can be completed in 5 to 10 minutes, scored quickly, and may be used in clinical practice, research, health policy studies, and population surveys. The SF-36 has been tested in large populations, and normative information is available (33). Questions concerning sensitivity of the pain scale and functioning scales in severely ill or impaired populations have been raised. The SF-36 is an important instrument due to its use as an outcome measure for U.S. health services research, as well as major ongoing efforts to translate and validate the instrument in 15 other languages (30).

HEALTH STATUS ASSESSMENT IN CHILDREN

While there are numerous reliable and well-validated instruments for the assessment of health status in adults, such instruments are not available for children with chronic rheumatic diseases. Functional classifications systems, including the ACR Functional Class and the Chronic Activity Limitations Scale (CALS), have been used to describe functional limitations in children with rheumatic diseases; however, they do not describe adequately the physical limitations of these children. With both instruments, over 85% of the disabilities of children with juvenile rheumatoid arthritis (JRA) have been categorized in classes indicating no or only minor disruptions in functional status (34). Several pediatric rheumatology tertiary care centers are working on assessment instruments that are age-appropriate and provide comprehensive information about the functional abilities of children with chronic rheumatic diseases (35). Published instruments assess functional status and pain only.

The Juvenile Arthritis Functional Assessment Scale (JAFAS) includes 10 activities of daily living (such as buttoning a shirt or blouse, cutting food, walking, and bending) that are observed and evaluated by a health professional. The

instrument has been tested in children aged 7 and older. It has been shown to discriminate between healthy children and children with JRA and between different ability levels of chronically ill children (36). The Juvenile Arthritis Functional Assessment Report (JAFASR), an adaptation of the JAFAS, includes 23 items and is designed as a self-report instrument with separate versions to be completed by parents and children. The child form is administered by a health professional. Because these two instruments may be self-administered, they could be used in clinical practice. Sensitivity of these instruments to change has not been established. At what age the child is capable of completing the questionnaire independently, when administration by a health professional is required, and when the parent best serves as the child's proxy has yet to be determined (37).

The Child HAQ (C-HAQ), adapted from the functional status scale of the HAQ, assesses functional status, pain, and global severity. Items related to each of the functional areas on the original HAQ (e.g., dressing, eating, arising) were added so that there is at least one item for each functional area that could be completed by children of all ages. For example, able to remove socks was added to the dressing and grooming area, because a healthy 1-year-old child can perform this activity but could not accomplish the other listed activities. The instrument may be completed by either the child or parent as appropriate (14). Sensitivity to change has not been determined.

USE OF HEALTH STATUS MEASURES IN PRACTICE

Many health status instruments have been developed and validated in clinical studies. They have been used as outcome measures in clinical trials of medications (38,39), educational interventions (40), and joint replacement surgery (41). These measures predict health care costs, length of stay in rehabilitation facilities, and even mortality (42,43). They are now being integrated into routine practice (44–46).

In selecting an instrument for use in clinical care, the length of the instrument and appropriateness to the practice setting are the major concerns. For routine monitoring of outpatients in a rheumatology practice, the HAQ functional status scale, the MHAQ, and the CLINHAQ are the instruments of choice. The MHAQ and CLINHAQ measure the important aspects of health status, such as functional status, pain, psychological distress, fatigue, and satisfaction; however, responding to all items takes less than 5 minutes. Patients may complete the questionnaires while sitting in a waiting room. Administration does not disrupt clinic routine and requires a minimum of staff and patient time. Scoring can be accomplished quickly so that important information (depression level, pain severity, functional status) is available immediately for use during the clinic visit (46).

In rehabilitation settings and evaluations following orthopedic surgery, other instruments may be used to assess the outcome of treatment. Perhaps the more comprehensive AIMS or AIMS2 would be helpful, especially if repeated administrations are not required. Time for completion is longer than for the HAQ, MHAQ, FSI, or the CLINHAQ; however, more comprehensive information is obtained. If one is studying outcome in OA following orthopedic surgery, the WOMAC might provide the most useful and meaningful information.

The trade-off between costs of administration and comprehensive information remains the issue.

In primary care clinics, where a variety of chronic health problems are seen in addition to rheumatic diseases, the SF-36 may be the best choice. Domains included in the SF-36 are similar to the AIMS1 and AIMS2 and to aspects of the FSI, HAQ, CLINHAQ, and MHAQ. The availability of normative data and the extensive use of the SF-36 in health policy research in the U.S. make adoption of this instrument for a primary practice clinic appealing. Like the disease-specific HAQ, the CLINHAQ and the MHAQ, patients can complete the SF-36 in a few minutes without assistance. Rapid scoring is feasible and provides the health professional with ready access to important information. Sensitivity to serious physical limitations remains a concern, however.

REFERENCES

1. Liang MH: The historical and conceptual framework for functional assessment in rheumatic disease. J Rheumatol 14 (Suppl 15):2–5, 1987
2. Froberg DG, Kane RL: Methodology for measuring health-state preferences—I: measurement strategies. J Clin Epidemiol 42:345–354, 1989
3. Gill TM, Feinstein AR: A critical appraisal of the quality of quality-of-life measurements. JAMA 272:619–626, 1994
4. Testa MA, Nackley JF: Methods for quality-of-life studies. Annu Rev Public Health 15:535–559, 1994
5. Decker JL, McShane DJ, Esdaile JM, Hathaway DE, Levinson JE, Liang MH, Medsger TA, Jr, Meenan RF, Mills JA, Roth SH, Wolfe F: Dictionary of the Rheumatic Diseases: Volume I: Signs and Symptoms. New York, Contact Associates International, Ltd., 1982
6. Anderson JJ, Felson DT, Meenan RF, Williams HJ: Which traditional measures should be used in rheumatoid arthritis clinical trials? Arthritis Rheum 32:1093–1099, 1989
7. Kwoh CK, O'Connor GT, Regan-Smith MG, et al: Concordance between clinician and patient assessment of physical and mental health status. J Rheumatol 19:1031–1037, 1992
8. Hochberg MC, Chang RW, Dwosh I, Lindsey S, Pincus T, Wolfe F: The American College of Rheumatology 1991 revised criteria for the classification of global functional status in rheumatoid arthritis. Arthritis Rheum 35:498–502, 1992
9. Stucki G, Stoll T, Bruhlmann P, Michel BA: Construct validation of the ACR 1991 revised criteria for global functional status in rheumatoid arthritis. Clin Exp Rheumatol 13:349–352, 1995
10. Stewart AL, Greenfield S, Hays RD, et al: Functional status and well-being of patients with chronic conditions: results from the Medical Outcomes Study. JAMA 262:907–913, 1989
11. Fowler FJ, Cleary PD, Magaziner J, Patrick DL, Benjamin KL: Methodological issues in measuring patient-reported outcomes: the agenda of the work group on outcomes assessment. Med Care 32:JS65-JS76, 1994
12. Fries JF, Spitz P, Kraines RG, Holman HR: Measurement of patient outcome in arthritis. Arthritis Rheum 23:137–145, 1980
13. Ramey DR, Raynauld J-P, Fries JF: The Health Assessment Questionnaire 1992: status and review. Arthritis Care Res 5:119–129, 1992
14. Singh G, Athreya BH, Fries JF, Goldsmith DP: Measurement of health status in children with juvenile rheumatoid arthritis. Arthritis Rheum 37:1761–1769, 1994
15. Daltroy LH, Larson MG, Roberts WN, Liang MH: A modification of the Health Assessment Questionnaire for the spondyloarthropathies. J Rheumatol 17:946–950, 1990
16. Poole JL, Steen VD: The use of the Health Assessment Questionnaire (HAQ) to determine physical disability in systemic sclerosis. Arthritis Care Res 4:27–31, 1991
17. Husted JA, Gladman DD, Long JA, Farewell VT: A modified version of the health assessment questionnaire (HAQ) for psoriatic arthritis. Clin Exp Rheumatol 13:439–443, 1995
18. Pincus T, Summey JA, Soraci SA, Jr, Wallston KA, Hummon NP: Assessment of patient satisfaction in activities of daily living using a modified Stanford Health Assessment Questionnaire. Arthritis Rheum 26:1346–1353, 1983
19. Wolfe F: Health Status Questionnaires. Rheum Dis Clin North Am 21:445–464, 1995
20. Wolfe F: Data collection and utilization: a methodology for clinical practice and clinical research. In, Rheumatoid Arthritis: Pathogenesis, Assessment, Outcome, and Treatment. Edited by F Wolfe, T Pincus. New York, Marcel Dekker, 1994, pp. 463–514
21. Jette AM: The functional status index: reliability and validity of a self-report functional disability measure. J Rheumatol 14 (Suppl 15):15–19, 1987
22. Meenan RF, Gertman PM, Mason JH: Measuring health status in arthritis: the Arthritis Impact Measurement Scales. Arthritis Rheum 23:146–152, 1980
23. Meenan RF, Mason JH, Anderson JJ, Guccione AA, Kazis LE: AIMS2: the content and properties of a revised and expanded Arthritis Impact Measurement Scales Health Status Questionnaire. Arthritis Rheum 35:1–10, 1992
24. Bellamy N, Buchanan WW, Goldsmith CH, Campbell J, Stitt LW: Validation study of WOMAC: a health status instrument for measuring clinically important patient relevant outcomes to antirheumatic drug therapy in patients with osteoarthritis of the hip or knee. J Rheumatol 15:1833–1840, 1988
25. Bellamy N, Kean WF, Buchanan WW, Gerecz-Simon E, Campbell J: Double blind randomized controlled trial of sodium meclofenamate (Meclomen) and diclofenac sodium (Voltaren): post validation reapplication of the WOMAC Osteoarthritis Index. J Rheumatol 19:153–159, 1992
26. Bellamy N, Buchanan WW, Goldsmith CH, Campbell J, Stitt L: Validation study of the WOMAC: a health status instrument for measuring clinically-important patient relevant outcomes following total hip or knee arthroplasty in osteoarthritis. J Orthop Rheumatol 1:95–108, 1988
27. Burckhardt CS, Clark SR, Bennett RM: The Fibromyalgia Impact Questionnaire: development and validation. J Rheumatol 18:728–733, 1991
28. Hunt SM, McKenna SP, McEwen J, Backett EM, Williams J, Papp E: The Nottingham Health Profile: subjective health status and medical consultations. Soc Sci Med 15A:221–229, 1981
29. Fitzpatrick R, Ziebland S, Jenkinson C, Mowat A: A generic health status instrument in the assessment of rheumatoid arthritis. Br J Rheumatol 31:87–90, 1992
30. Anderson RT, Aaronson NK, Wilkin D: Critical review of the international assessments of health-related quality of life. Qual Life Res 2:369–395, 1993
31. Bergner M, Bobbitt RA, Carter WB, Gilson BS: The Sickness Impact Profile: development and final revision of a health status measure. Med Care 19:787–805, 1981
32. Ware JE, Sherbourne CD: The MOS 36-item short-form health survey (SF-36) (abstract). Med Care 30:473–483, 1992
33. Mchorney CA, Ware JE, Lu JFR, Sherbourne CD: The MOS 36-Item Short-Form Health Survey (SF-36): 3 tests of data quality, scaling assumptions, and reliability across diverse patient groups. Med Care 32:40–66, 1994
34. Lovell DJ: Newer functional outcome measurements in juvenile rheumatoid arthritis: a progress report. J Rheumatol 19 (Suppl 33):28–31, 1992
35. Tucker LB, DeNardo BA, Abetz LN, Landgraf JM, Schaller JG: The Childhood Arthritis Health Profile (CHAP): validity and reliability of the condition-specific scales (abstract). Arthritis Rheum 38 (suppl 9):S183, 1995
36. Lovell DJ, Howe S, Shear E, et al: Development of a disability measurement tool for juvenile rheumatoid arthritis: the Juvenile Arthritis Functional Assessment Scale. Arthritis Rheum 32:1390–1395, 1989
37. Howe S, Levinson J, Shear E, et al: Development of a disability measurement tool for juvenile rheumatoid arthritis: the Juvenile Arthritis Functional Assessment Report for Children and their Parents. Arthritis Rheum 34:873–880, 1991
38. Bombardier C, Ware J, Russell IJ, Larson M, Chalmers A, Read JL: Auranofin therapy and quality of life in patients with rheumatoid arthritis: results of a multicenter trial. Am J Med 81:565–578, 1986
39. Meenan RF, Anderson JJ, Kazis LE, et al: Outcome assessment in clinical trials: evidence for the sensitivity of a health status measure. Arthritis Rheum 27:1344–1352, 1984
40. Lorig KR, Mazonson PD, Holman HR: Evidence suggesting that health education for self-management in patients with chronic arthritis has sustained health benefits while reducing health care costs. Arthritis Rheum 36:439–446, 1993
41. Liang MH, Fossel AH, Larson MG: Comparisons of five health status instruments for orthopedic evaluation. Med Care 28:632–642, 1990
42. Pincus T, Brooks RH, Callahan LF: Prediction of long-term mortality in patients with rheumatoid arthritis according to simple questionnaire and joint count measures. Ann Intern Med 120:26–34, 1994
43. Wolfe F, Mitchell DM, Sibley JT, et al: The mortality of rheumatoid arthritis. Arthritis Rheum 37:481–494, 1994

44. Greenfield S, Nelson EC: Recent developments and future issues in the use of health status assessment measures in clinical settings (abstract). Med Care 30:MS23-MS41, 1992
45. Deyo RA, Carter WB: Strategies for improving and expanding the application of health status measures in clinical settings—a researcher developer viewpoint. Med Care 30:MS176-MS186, 1992
46. Wolfe F, Pincus T: Data collection in the clinic. Rheum Dis Clin North Am 21:445–464, 1995
47. Pincus T, Callahan LF: Rheumatology function tests—grip strength, walking time, button test and questionnaires document and predict long-term morbidity and mortality in rheumatoid arthritis. J Rheumatol 19: 1051–1057, 1992
48. Newcomer KL, Krug HE, Mahowald ML: Validity and reliability of the timed-stands test for patients with rheumatoid arthritis and other chronic diseases. J Rheumatol 20:21–27, 1993
49. Kalla AA, Smith PR, Brown GMM, Meyers OL, Chalton D: Responsiveness of Keitel functional index compared with laboratory measures of disease activity in rheumaoid arthritis. Br J Rheumatol 34:141–149, 1995

Diagnostic Tests

THOMAS D. BEARDMORE, MD, FACP, FACR

Diagnostic tests in rheumatic diseases have great importance. They are an integral part of the American College of Rheumatology (ACR) classification criteria for many of the common rheumatic diseases, including rheumatoid arthritis (RA), systemic lupus erythematosus (SLE), and degenerative joint disease (DJD). Sometimes negative results of tests are useful, as in the diagnosis of fibromyalgia and exclusion of inflammatory joint disease. In spite of the usefulness of diagnostic tests, it is important to remember that no rheumatic disease is established by tests alone. The careful integration of history, physical examination, and laboratory tests is necessary to establish diagnosis.

Health care providers and patients benefit when testing is utilized and understood. The optimal diagnostic test should be *sensitive* (able to identify a disease when present) and *specific* (able to identify that the disease is not present). An evaluative or monitoring test should be sensitive to change in the disease state over time. Additionally, tests should be inexpensive, easily performed, and readily available. Diagnostic testing is of great importance in establishing treatment modalities, whether these are medicines, exercises, or lifestyle adjustments. Testing is closely associated with prognosis, including the development of disability.

GENERAL LABORATORY TESTING

Rheumatic disorders and treatments can affect major body systems. General laboratory testing reveals multi-system organ involvement and specific organ function. It is important to test the patient at baseline and periodically during the course of treatment to detect disease improvement, progression, and medication toxicity. A flow sheet for laboratory data is a valuable tool for the health care provider to assess the overall disease state and toxicity.

Hematology

A complete blood count including hemoglobin, hematocrit, white blood cell count with differential, and platelet count is one of the most common baseline tests in systemic rheumatic diseases. It is used not only for rheumatic disease diagnosis and monitoring, but also for detection of anemia. Understanding the etiology of anemia is important both for the disease and for treatment. Hemolysis resulting in anemia occurs on an immune basis in SLE. Many rheumatic diseases such as RA, SLE, and systemic sclerosis, may be associated with an anemia termed *anemia of chronic disease*. In this anemia, the red cells have normal shape and hemoglobin content (normocytic and normochromic). This is in contrast to the anemia that develops as a consequence of gastrointestinal bleeding from nonsteroidal anti-inflammatory drugs, in which the cells are small and the hemoglobin content low, a microcytic anemia resulting from iron deficiency. Therapy with drugs such as methotrexate may result in an anemia where red cells are large, that is, a macrocytic anemia. Modest anemia (hemoglobin levels of 10 g/dl) is commonly seen in rheumatic diseases and is ascribed to anemia of chronic disease when normocytic and normochromic. More severe anemia should always be investigated to determine whether or not it is related to drug toxicity or serious complications of the underlying rheumatic diseases.

Knowledge of hematologic abnormalities is important in designing exercise programs, education, activities of daily living, and medical treatment. For example, the provider needs to be aware when prescribing medications that bleeding may occur when platelet counts are low, or infections may occur when white cell counts are low. When the patient has an anemia, he or she may experience general loss of energy and endurance.

Urinalysis

Urinalysis is one of the most informative, easy to perform, and cost-effective laboratory tests. Analysis for protein and microscopic presence of cells is important as a diagnostic aid in SLE, which has a high incidence of nephritis. Proteinuria is one of the ACR classification criteria for SLE. Nephritis can be reflected as increased urinary protein, white or red cells, and the presence of casts on microscopic analysis. When present, proteinuria should be quantitated by a timed collection (typically 24 hours).

Urinalysis is used to monitor for toxicities related to gold or penicillamine treatment of RA because of the associated renal toxicity manifested by proteinuria (both drugs) and hematuria (gold). Trace and modest proteinuria frequently can be managed by reducing the dosage of medications. Large amounts of proteinuria may require cessation of drugs and renal biopsy to understand the renal histopathology that is resulting in the protein loss.

Chemical Analysis of Blood

Routine blood chemistries are commonly measured as a panel of tests. Included are serum electrolytes, liver function, renal function, and mineral metabolism. Most medications are metabolized by the liver and excreted by the kidneys, and the effects of early toxicity may be seen in chemistry panels. Toxicity may be reflected as a decrease in albumen, a rise in liver function tests such as alanine aminotransferase (ALT) and aspartate aminotransferase (AST), or an increase in blood urea nitrogen or creatinine (renal function). For example, the doubling of ALT and AST in a patient taking methotrexate for RA is an indication of potentially significant liver toxicity, which may require reduction or cessation of the drug.

Elevated serum uric acid is useful in the diagnosis of gout, which primarily affects men. There is a direct relationship between the level of serum uric acid, the development of gout, and the development of renal uric acid stones. Patients with serum uric acid markedly above the normal (2.5 to 8 mg/dl) have a greater chance of developing gout. They should have periodic testing of uric acid and evaluation for gouty arthropathy. However, it is important to remember that transient hyperuricemia is common, a minority of patients with hyperuricemia develop gout, and a normal uric acid may be seen in patients with gout.

Serum measures of muscle function, including creatine phosphokinase (CPK) and aldolase, are used to diagnose and monitor patients with polymyositis and dermatomyositis. The highest and most persistent levels of CPK and aldolase are seen in the inflammatory myopathies and can be used as a therapeutic indicator, because they will decrease with disease improvement. These measures can be elevated in conditions involving muscle breakdown or necrosis, such as intramuscular injections, extreme exercise, or myocardial infarction. Lactate dehydrogenase and AST may be elevated in muscle disease and mistaken for abnormalities of liver function.

COMMON SEROLOGIC TESTS

Autoantibodies

An autoantibody is an immunoglobulin that is directed against a normally occurring protein or cellular component (see Chapter 2, Overview of Immunology and Inflammation). They may react with soluble serum proteins, such as antibodies directed against immune globulin (rheumatoid factor), or they may be against cell components such as cytoplasmic or nuclear antigens (antinuclear antibody). Autoantibodies are common in RA, SLE, and diffuse connective tissue diseases. Tests for autoantibodies are commonly performed in patients with musculoskeletal complaints.

Rheumatoid Factor

The first autoantibody discovered, rheumatoid factor, is an antibody directed against an immunoglobulin. The commonly observed rheumatoid factor in RA is an IgM antibody that is directed against the constant portion of IgG. It is detected by an agglutination test utilizing latex particles. In this test, latex particles are coated with IgG and reacted with the patient's serum. If IgM rheumatoid factor is present, it will agglutinate the latex particles, which are then interpreted as the value equal to the dilution at which agglutination no longer occurs. Rheumatoid factor is also measured by nephelometry, which provides better quantification and may be automated.

Rheumatoid factor is not diagnostic of RA; in early RA, many patients will test negative for rheumatoid factor. However, 80% of patients with RA will become rheumatoid factor positive (1). The test cannot be used alone to diagnose RA, but it is one of the ACR classification criteria. A positive rheumatoid factor is associated with increased disease severity, the development of erosions, extra-articular manifestations, and greater disability (2). Rheumatoid factor does not change with

treatment unless a remission occurs, hence, there is no reason to repeat this test on a frequent basis.

The incidence and titer of rheumatoid factor increase with age until patients reach the age of 70 or 80, after which it tends to decrease (3). Many other rheumatic diseases, as well as bacterial endocarditis, tuberculosis, osteomyelitis, viral and parasitic infections, and chronic liver disease have a high frequency of rheumatoid factor.

Antinuclear Antibodies

Antinuclear antibodies (ANA) are commonly seen in rheumatic diseases. A positive ANA test is not diagnostic of any connective tissue disease, but ANA are seen with a high frequency in SLE, systemic sclerosis, Sjögren's syndrome, polymyositis, and RA. Ninety-nine percent of patients with SLE will be ANA positive (4).

The ANA test is usually performed as an indirect immunofluorescent test using the patient's serum overlaid onto a substrate. The human cell line HEp-2 (an immortalized laryngeal epithelial cancer) is commonly used as a screening test and has a high degree of sensitivity but low specificity. It is associated with a greater number of false positives than other fixed cell preparations such as liver or polymorphonuclear white cells. The health care provider should understand the laboratory and cell preparation used in order to interpret the importance of the test.

In general, ANA titers of less than 1/80 have less significance than those which are of greater titer. However, positive tests must also be coupled with the appropriate history and physical examination to establish diagnosis, because patients with SLE may have low titers. The ANA patterns have some importance, but are not diagnostically specific. Rim or peripheral patterns are most commonly associated with SLE; nucleolar or centromere patterns are most commonly associated with systemic sclerosis. The diffuse and speckled patterns have less diagnostic significance. When present in low titer, these ANA are the pattern most commonly seen in patients without any underlying disorder.

If ANA are present, more specific testing for the related protein antigen is indicated (5) (Table 1). The anti-double stranded DNA antibody is most closely associated with the rim pattern and has high specificity but low sensitivity for SLE. The anti-Sm antibody has similar sensitivity and specificity for SLE (Sm or Smith is an RNP antigen). Anti-DNP is most commonly associated with the homogeneous pattern ANA. However, this test, though common in SLE, has low specificity and may be seen in other rheumatic diseases. The specific antibody test SCl-70 (anti-topoisomerase I) and anticentromere antibodies are seen in diffuse scleroderma and the CREST variant of scleroderma respectively. Anti-U_1RNP may be seen as a speckled pattern ANA; the highest titers are seen in mixed connective tissue disease. Although ANA tend to decrease in titer with treatment, they cannot be used as a guide for prognosis and should not be repeated as therapeutic indicators.

COMPLEMENT

The complement system is a series of proteins that constitute 2% to 3% of serum protein. It is important in the handling of infections through lysis of bacteria, promotion of phagocytosis,

Table 1. Useful autoantibody tests in rheumatic disease (5).*

Autoantibody	Disorder	Frequency	Other
RF	Rheumatoid arthritis	70–80%	IgM antiglobulin
Anti-dsDNA	SLE	40–70%	High specificity, Native DNA antigen
Anti-ssDNA	Drug-induced SLE	80%	Denatured DNA antigen, 70% of SLE
Anti-Sm	SLE	20–30%	High specificity
Scl-70	Diffuse scleroderma	70%	Topoisomerase antigen (DNA uncoupling enzyme)
SS-A, SS-B	Primary Sjogren's syndrome	70–90%	35–40% of SLE
Anti-U_1RNP	MCTD	>95%	Very high titers are common

* RF = rheumatoid factor, IgM = immunoglobulin M, dsDNA = double stranded DNA, SLE = systemic lupus erythematosus, ssDNA = single stranded DNA, MCTD = mixed connective tissue disease.

and enhancement of inflammation (6). This system is of importance in disorders which involve immune complexes such as SLE or vasculitis, because it indicates immune complex clearance from the system. When immune complexes are formed and cleared from the body, the complement level is decreased.

There are three common measurements for serum complement. These include the protein components C3 and C4, which measure the direct and indirect pathways, and CH_{50} (total hemolytic complement), which is a biologic measure of the entire complement pathway. In the rheumatic diseases, low levels of CH_{50}, C3, and C4 are usually related to consumption of complement by immune complex activation of the classical pathway (6). Rarely, reductions are related to an absence of one of the complement proteins. Complement measurement is particularly useful in SLE, an immune complex disease, due to its association with active disease. A decrease in complement level may precede the development of disease flares, particularly renal disease.

HLA ANTIGENS

Currently only one human leukocyte antigen, HLA–B27, is commonly measured in the rheumatic diseases. This antigen is found in 8% to 10% of the U.S. population, but it is present in 95% of patients with ankylosing spondylitis, 80% of patients with Reiter's syndrome, and a high percentage of patients with other spondylarthropathies and acute anterior uveitis (7). This test is not diagnostic for ankylosing spondylitis, but because of its high specificity, it has utility in early disease when x-ray changes have not yet occurred. It should not be used as a screening test, because it is also seen in patients without disease. In the future, other HLA antigens such as HLA–DR4 may have some usefulness. Current investigation seems to indicate that it is more common in RA and is associated with severe disease (7,8).

SYNOVIAL FLUID ANALYSIS

Aspiration and examination of synovial fluid is an integral part of diagnosis of joint pain. It is a time-honored method of establishing correct diagnosis and treatment. Synovial fluid is usually clear, acellular, viscous, and low in volume. Alterations in the appearance, volume, and cellular content of synovial fluid are useful in diagnosis.

Based on a visual inspection of clarity and color, the synovial fluid is classified into one of four groups (9). Group I is non-inflammatory, Group II inflammatory, Group III pyogenic, and Group IV hemorrhagic (Table 2). This grouping is a continuum. Depending on the severity of the disorder and the timing of the aspiration, a patient may have fluids in different groups. This is particularly true for the inflammatory disorders. A good example occurs in gout: during a quiescent period, synovial fluid could be in Group I, in Group II in early disease, and with severe gout attacks, could be opaque with cell counts as high as 100,000/mm³ (Group III).

The microscopic examination and culture of synovial fluid is extremely important. All synovial fluids in Groups II, III, and IV should be cultured when the diagnosis is unknown if infection is suspected. The culturing of organisms from synovial fluid establishes a diagnosis of infectious arthritis and allows treatment (specific antibiotics), which can result in cure.

In addition to cell counts and differentials, synovial fluid should be examined for crystals. Gout and calcium pyrophosphate deposition disease, two naturally occurring crystalline arthropathies, are easily diagnosed by the demonstration of birefringent crystals using polarized light microscopy. In each of these conditions the crystals may be ingested by a polymorphonuclear leukocyte (PMN), an indicator of its role in inflammation. The calcium pyrophosphate dihydrate (CPPD) crystal will have a rhomboid or rectangular shape and be weakly birefringent. If a first order red compensator is used, CPPD will show positive birefringence demonstrating blue color. Gouty crystals (monosodium urate) are needle-shaped and show

Table 2. Synovial fluid analysis in rheumatic disease.*

	GROUP			
	I	II	III	IV
Clarity	Clear	Translucent	Opaque	Bloody
Type	Non-inflammatory	Inflammatory	Infectious	Traumatic
Cell count/type	<2000/mono	2K–20K/mono, PMN	20K–200K/PMN	RBC
Disorder	DJD, ONB	RA, SLE, Crystalline arthritis	Infectious, Crystalline arthritis	Trauma, Bleeding disorders

* PMN = polymorphonuclear, mono = mononuclear, ONB = osteonecrosis of bone, SLE = systemic lupus erythematosus, RA = rheumatoid arthritis, DJD = degenerative joint disease.

strong negative birefringence, having a bright yellow appearance with the red compensator. Hydroxyapatite crystals will occasionally be seen in synovial fluid, but they must be stained because they are not birefringent. Talc from the provider's glove will appear as birefringent Maltese crosses, and crystalline corticosteroid may have positive and/or negative birefringence.

Blood within the synovial fluid is seen in trauma, bleeding disorders such as hemophilia or iatrogenic overcoagulation, tumors, and neuro-arthropathy.

ACUTE PHASE REACTANTS

One of the body's internal responses to inflammation, infection, or other major insult is to synthesize proteins that are involved in the body's response. These proteins are called acute phase reactants (10,11). Many acute phase reactants are synthesized by the liver, including fibrinogen, prothrombin, haptoglobin, C-reactive protein (CRP), serum amyloid A protein, and others. Some of the acute phase proteins (e.g., fibrinogen) are normal serum components and may increase modestly. Others may be newly synthesized (e.g., CRP) and may increase dramatically in concentration. Acute phase reactants are a common component of acute inflammation, but they also accompany chronic inflammation seen in the rheumatic diseases. Measurements of these reactants are done directly, through measurement of CRP, and indirectly, through measurement of the erythrocyte sedimentation rate (ESR).

The ESR is the most common measurement of acute phase proteins in the rheumatic diseases. This simple test can be performed in the office with minimal equipment and requires only 1 hour for the red cells to sediment in a measured tube. The Westergren ESR uses a 100-mm tube to measure the sedimentation rate of cells over a 1-hour period. Sedimentation of the red cells is directly related to the quantity of acute phase proteins that are synthesized by the liver, particularly those with an asymmetrical shape such as fibrinogen. However, this test is nonspecific, and positive findings may be seen in people who have no illness or who have illnesses such as anemia, which are not related to development of acute phase proteins.

The measurement of acute phase reactants is important in rheumatic diseases, because it corresponds with chronic inflammation and, when elevated, may be used to monitor the disease course to some degree. It may be very helpful in RA, polymyalgia rheumatica, and giant cell arteritis, but less important in SLE and ankylosing spondylitis. The ESR is one of the diagnostic criteria for polymyalgia rheumatica, when coupled with the appropriate history, and for giant cell arteritis when there is a positive biopsy of an affected artery. In these two conditions the sedimentation rate may be exceedingly high.

Another measure of the acute phase response directly related to this phenomenon is the measurement of CRP. The changes in CRP occur more quickly and return to normal more quickly than the ESR. However, CRP testing takes 1 day to perform and requires an enzyme-linked immunoadsorbent assay (ELISA) or radioimmunodiffusion equipment. The CRP can also be used to monitor disease course because it reflects inflammation. Very high CRP values are seen when infection is present, and they may occur before ESR elevations are noted.

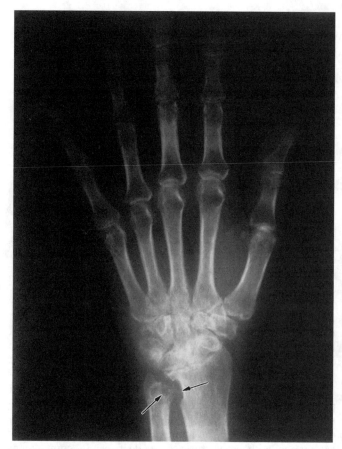

Figure 1. Radiographic features of rheumatoid arthritis. Diffuse and periarticular osteopenia, symmetric joint space loss, and multiple erosions are present in this advanced case. Large erosions are seen at the distal radial-ulnar articulation (arrows).

IMAGING TECHNIQUES

Radiography

The routinely performed radiograph, or x-ray, is the basic imaging technique for diagnosis and staging of all rheumatic diseases. Radiographs form the basis for monitoring disease progression. Plain x-rays are a component of the ACR classification criteria for RA and DJD, and are integral components of the diagnosis of ankylosing spondylitis, diffuse idiopathic skeletal hyperostosis, all the spondylarthropathies, and osteoporosis. Radiographs have the advantage of ready availability, low cost, and the absence of a need for specialized equipment or diagnosticians.

Radiographic changes in the rheumatic diseases are best exemplified by inflammatory arthritis and DJD. The classic example of inflammatory arthritis is RA, in which there is symmetric joint disease with soft tissue swelling, the development of periarticular osteopenia, marginal erosions, and loss of articular cartilage (Figure 1). Coupled with this are the development of joint malalignment and characteristic deformities.

Degenerative joint disease (Figure 2) also has articular loss; unlike RA however, it is in an asymmetric pattern. There is increased subchondral bone density or sclerosis and the development of marginal osteophytes. Involvement of weight-bearing joints is a common finding. However, some forms of DJD may occur in non-weight bearing joints, as exemplified by

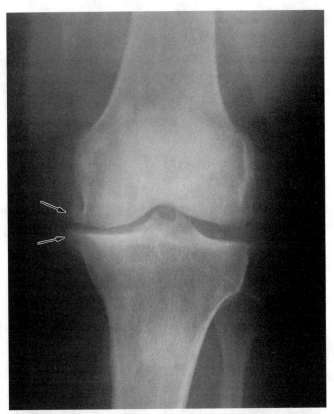

Figure 2. Radiographic features of degenerative joint disease. Osteophytes (arrows) and asymmetric medial cartilage loss are present in this knee x-ray.

the degenerative changes in the proximal interphalangeal and distal interphalangeal joints of the hands.

Plain x-ray technique may be enhanced by the use of arthrography, in which radiocontrast dye (usually an iodinated water soluble material) is injected into a joint. Arthrography is useful in diagnosing cysts and other herniations from joints (Figure 3A).

Ultrasonography and Radionuclide Imaging

The use of ultrasound in the diagnosis of musculoskeletal disorders has the advantage of being inexpensive and readily available. It is most valuable in assessment of soft tissues and in superficial parts of the body. A common use of ultrasound is in the diagnosis of cysts at the knee (Figure 3B) or in cardiac examination in SLE or RA where pericardial effusions may be seen.

Radionuclide imaging or scintigraphy is used in the rheumatic diseases, primarily with two radionuclides, Technetium[99] and Gallium[67]. Technetium is primarily used for bone scans; however, in the early test phase it is an indicator of blood flow and transudation of fluid from vascular areas. Later in the test it is deposited in bone. Early phase studies are of value in the assessment of inflammation, because increased radionuclide uptake occurs in areas of inflammation related to the rheumatic diseases.

If infection is present, radionuclide scanning allows visualization of structures that are not readily accessible to physical examination or arthrocentesis, such as the spine and sacroiliac joints. In these cases, Gallium is concentrated in infectious sites and scanning would show increased uptake in these areas.

The disadvantages of radionuclide scans are high cost, prolonged examination time, and the need for special facilities. Its value compared to magnetic resonance imaging (MRI) when diagnosing deep infections is yet to be determined.

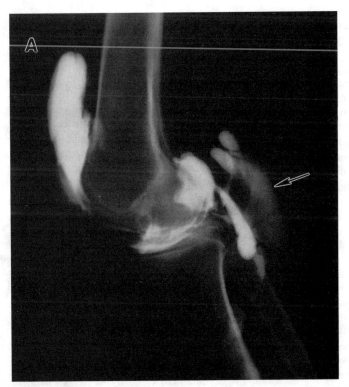

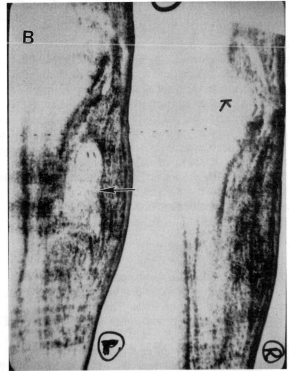

Figure 3. Popliteal cysts. A) Arthrography clearly demonstrates the small popliteal (Baker's) cyst (arrow) on this lateral knee x-ray. B) Ultrasonography in a dissecting Baker's cyst shows an echogenic free mass in the mid calf (arrow), L = left leg, R = right, K = knee.

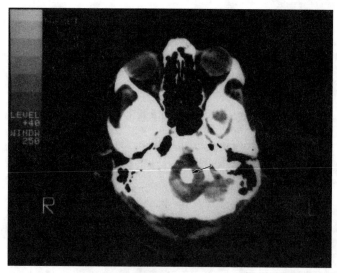

Figure 4. Computed tomography of the base of the skull showing migration of the dens of C2 (arrow) into the foramen magnum in a patient with rheumatoid arthritis.

Computed Tomography and Magnetic Resonance Imaging

The development of computed tomography (CT) and MRI has greatly enhanced the diagnostic potential of imaging techniques in the rheumatic diseases. They better visualize soft tissues and deep structures within the body such as the spine and pelvis.

In CT, computer reconstruction in the axial plane permits greater resolution between bone and soft tissue. Structures that previously were only seen in the frontal, two-dimensional plane now can be seen in an axial plane. Thus, more precise anatomical diagnosis can be made (Figure 4). Spinal inflammatory and degenerative disease, osteonecrosis of bone, and cysts within deep joints such as the hip, which are not easily seen on plain x-rays, are easily diagnosed with CT.

Magnetic resonance imaging has the advantages of showing greater soft tissue contrast and being free of radiation. Because of its greater soft tissue resolution, it is of particular value for osteonecrosis of bone and soft tissue lesions, such as inflammatory synovitis in deep structures of the body like the spine and pelvis. It is also of great value in soft tissue pathology such as rotator cuff tears, spinal disk disease (Figure 5), and other ligamentous and tendon pathology. Because of the high soft tissue contrast, MRI is supplanting arthrography and myelography in the rheumatic diseases. However, its high cost and need for special facilities are disadvantages.

Dual X-ray Absoptiometry

Osteoporosis is an extremely common problem in the rheumatology practice, and may be idiopathic, related to rheumatic disease, or iatrogenic from drugs. This is especially true in patients with RA in the perimenopausal age who may be taking corticosteroids, all of which result in increased bone loss. A measurement of the bone mineral content or bone density is imperative to monitor treatment of these patients, because studies show that fracture rate is directly related to bone mineral density.

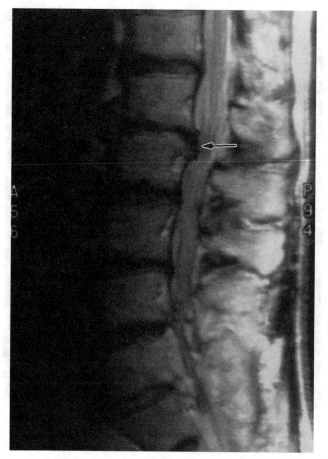

Figure 5. Magnetic resonance imaging of the lumbar spine. This sagittal view shows severe degenerative disk disease with a large herniated disc at L1–2 (arrow) and canal stenosis. Disc herniation is also seen at L2–3 and L3–4.

There are many ways to measure bone density including dual x-ray absorptiometry (DXA), single and dual photon absorptiometry, and quantitative computed tomography. Dual x-ray absorptiometry was introduced in 1987 and is becoming the preferred test for clinical practice (12). These scans are most commonly used to measure trabecular bone of the lumbar vertebrae and the hip, but they can be used for the forearm, calcaneus, and total body. The hip and lumbar spine are the most important measurements due to the increased morbidity associated with fractures in these areas. The DXA scan can also be used in the lateral projection of the lumbar spine, avoiding artifactual elevations from osteophytes, stress fractures, and calcifications of the aorta.

Bone mineral density should be measured in all patients who are at risk for osteoporosis and fracture. It will have the greatest utility in patients with RA, menopausal women, and patients taking corticosteroids. Testing at baseline and yearly thereafter permits assessment of disease progression and response to treatment.

REFERENCES

1. Arnett FC, Edworthy SM, Bloch DA, McShane DJ, et al: The American Rheumatism Association 1987 revised criteria for the classification of rheumatoid arthritis. Arthritis Rheum 31:315–324, 1988
2. Harris E: Clinical features of rheumatoid arthritis. In, Textbook of Rheu-

matology. Edited by WN Kelley, ED Harris, S Ruddy, CB Sledge. Philadelphia, WB Saunders Co, 1993, pp. 874–911

3. Carson D: Rheumatoid factor. In, Textbook of Rheumatology. Edited by WN Kelley, ED Harris, S Ruddy, CB Sledge. Philadelphia, WB Saunders Co., 1993, pp. 155–163

4. Tan EM, Cohen AS, Fries JF, Masi AT, et al: The 1982 revised criteria for the classification of systemic lupus erythematosus. Arthritis Rheum 25: 1271–1277, 1982

5. Von Muhlen CA, Tan EM: Autoantibodies in the diagnosis of systemic rheumatic diseases. Semin Arthritis Rheum 24:323–358, 1995

6. Moxley G, Ruddy S: Immune complexes and complement. In, Textbook of Rheumatology. Edited by WN Kelley, ED Harris, S Ruddy, CB Sledge. Philadelphia, WB Saunders Co., 1993, pp. 188–200

7. Arnett FC: Histocompatibility typing in the rheumatic diseases. Rheum Dis Clin North Am 20:371–390, 1994

8. Van Zeben D, Hazes JMW, Zwinderman AH, et al: Association of HLA-DR4 with a more progressive disease course in patients with rheumatoid arthritis: results of a followup study. Arthritis Rheum 34:822–830, 1991

9. McCarty D: Synovial fluid. In, Arthritis and Allied Conditions. Edited by D McCarty, W Koopman. Twelfth edition. Lea and Febiger, Philadelphia, 1993, pp. 63–84

10. Kushner I, Rzewnicki DL: The acute phase response: general aspects. Baillieres Clin Rheumatol 8:513–530, 1994

11. Volanakis J: Acute phase proteins in rheumatic disease. In, Arthritis and Allied Conditions. Edited by D McCarty, W Koopman. Twelfth edition. Lea and Febiger, Philadelphia, 1993, pp. 479–494

12. Lane N, Genant H: Osteoporosis and bone mineral assessment. In, Arthritis and Allied Conditions. Edited by D McCarty, W Koopman. Twelfth edition. Lea and Febiger, Philadelphia, 1993, pp. 133–149

Psychological Assessment

JERRY C. PARKER, PhD; and GAIL E. WRIGHT, PhD

Characterizing the psychological aspects of the rheumatic diseases is difficult due to the diversity of diagnostic categories. Arthritis almost always results in pain and restricted movement, but some acute conditions such as gout and septic arthritis respond quickly to treatment and have minimal long-term psychological impact. However, in chronic conditions such rheumatoid arthritis (RA) and systemic lupus erythematosus (SLE), years of pain, functional losses, and deteriorated health are a major challenge to the coping process. Many persons with chronic, debilitating arthritis manage to cope successfully. In some cases, however, either the disease-related stressors are too severe or the environmental resources are not sufficient to sustain a successful coping effort. Consequently, some persons with arthritis display psychological symptoms secondary to disease. In other cases, persons with arthritis present with pre-existing psychological problems.

The prevalence of psychological distress is difficult to estimate across a diversity of arthritic conditions and socioeconomic settings. Useful data, though, can be obtained from the primary care literature, where the prevalence of psychological problems has been shown to be relatively high. One national survey found that 25% of all patients seen by primary care physicians had disabling psychiatric disorders (1). In a rural Wisconsin primary care clinic, 35% of patients screened positive for a mental disorder (2). Another study found that 15% to 40% of primary care patients met the criteria for a diagnosable mental disorder (3). There is little doubt that primary care settings are confronted with a high prevalence of mental, emotional, and behavioral problems.

In most rheumatology settings, psychological problems appear to be similarly prevalent. Estimates suggest that approximately 20% of persons with RA present with major depression (4). Approximately 40% of persons with either RA or SLE have elevated MMPI (Minnesota Multiphasic Personality Inventory) profiles (5), and approximately one-half of persons with either RA or osteoarthritis (OA) may experience losses in social relationships (6), which is a risk factor for depression (4). Although such psychological problems are far from universal, the literature convincingly shows that a substantial number of persons with arthritis encounter psychological distress at some point in their lives. Those providing care to arthritis patients should be both vigilant regarding psychological problems and familiar with the process of psychological assessment.

IMPORTANCE OF PSYCHOLOGICAL PERSPECTIVE

Beyond recognizing the relatively high prevalence of psychological problems in medical settings, arthritis health professionals also need a keen appreciation of psychological concepts in order to optimally care for patients. Three broad psycholog-

ical perspectives are important in the management of rheumatic disease: 1) the biopsychosocial model of illness; 2) the Institute of Medicine model of disability; and 3) the empirical foundations for psychological interventions.

Biopsychosocial Model

For the past 400 years, the conceptualization of physical illness has been dominated by a biomedical framework. Illness has been viewed as a physicochemical abnormality requiring biologic management. The biomedical model is highly valid under many circumstances, and it has led to impressive therapeutic breakthroughs in acute illnesses such as infectious disease. Increasingly, though, the inadequacy of the biomedical model has been recognized, especially in chronic diseases such as arthritis. In these conditions, there is an intermingling of biological, psychological, and sociological determinants with regard to the onset, course, and outcomes of illness. Engel (7) coined the term, biopsychosocial model, to convey the multiple determinants of physical illness. For optimal health care, the psychological and social aspects of rheumatic disease must be thoroughly assessed and treated.

Institute of Medicine Model of Disability

Another psychological concept derives from the Institute of Medicine (National Academy of Sciences) model of disability (8). Traditionally, tissue abnormalities and/or physiologic imbalances have been viewed as the primary determinants of disability. However, many persons with abnormalities at the cellular level never develop a failure of an entire organ system. Even persons who experience organ system failure do not necessarily develop functional limitations, due to personal resilience (e.g., effective coping) and/or prosthetic devices. Finally, even persons who encounter functional limitations are not necessarily disabled, unless the society in which they live is unable to accommodate alternative methods of functioning, such as wheelchairs. Disability is not a purely biologic phenomenon; it is also determined to an extent by the psychosocial processes of coping and adaptation. Consequently, from the disability perspective, the psychological symptoms of persons with arthritis should be carefully assessed.

Psychological Interventions

The effectiveness of psychological interventions should also be considered by health care providers. In general, psychological treatments work reasonably well. A meta-analysis of the effectiveness of cognitive therapy for depression found that the average therapy patient did better than 98% of the control subjects (overall effect size = .99) (9,10). In comparison, the average effect size for drug treatment in arthritis ranges from only .45 to .77 (11). Even in severe psychiatric disorders such as major depression, behavioral treatments are effective in approximately 55% of cases (12).

Regarding arthritis, a recent literature review on cognitive-behavioral treatments for RA found nine studies with positive outcomes in areas such as pain and functional status (13). In addition, a stress management program for persons with RA has been shown to decrease helplessness, improve confidence in coping ability, and reduce pain, with benefits lasting up to 15 months (14). Evidence for the effectiveness of psychological interventions for persons with arthritis is impressive. Thus, psychological assessment can be viewed as an important prelude to beneficial psychological treatment.

APPROACHES TO PSYCHOLOGICAL ASSESSMENT

Psychological assessment is not a uniform procedure; it is a variety of approaches to the characterization of psychological/behavioral processes. There are three general approaches to psychological assessment: 1) diagnostic criteria; 2) unstructured clinical interviews; and 3) psychometric assessment. These approaches are not mutually exclusive. In fact, they can often be used in combination.

Diagnostic Criteria

A common approach to the assessment of psychological/psychiatric difficulties is the use of specific diagnostic criteria. In this approach, the symptoms characteristic of a given syndrome are systematically elaborated. The most common example is the Diagnostic and Statistical Manual-IV of the American Psychiatric Association (15), in which a classification of psychological/psychiatric states has been developed. The person conducting an assessment can search for the constellation of symptoms that characterize a particular diagnosis.

Diagnostic criteria have several advantages. The assessment process takes place in the context of a broad diagnostic classification system. Structured interviews guide the data gathering process and minimize errors of omission. Also, when a psychological/psychiatric diagnosis is formulated, the associated clinical characteristics of the syndrome, such as natural history and prognosis, can usually be inferred. However, there are disadvantages to this approach. Many psychological manifestations do not conveniently fit into a structured diagnostic framework. Especially in the case of subclinical conditions, standard diagnostic frameworks simply may not apply. Diagnostic criteria are most useful in the case of moderate to severe psychological/psychiatric conditions.

Clinical Interviews

Psychological assessment also can be approached through the use of unstructured clinical interviews. The examiner seeks to create a comfortable environment in which the examinee will feel free to discuss any psychological problems. The client-centered concepts of Carl Rodgers provide the theoretical foundation for this approach (16). The interviewer asks open-ended questions and then listens in an accepting, nonjudgmental way. Subsequently, most examinees will articulate their individualistic, psychological concerns. The interviewer is thus able to gain an in-depth understanding of the patient's unique circumstances.

One advantage of the unstructured interview is the opportunity to access highly personal information that might otherwise be overlooked in a structured search for signs and symptoms. Another advantage is the rapport-building which usually occurs during a client-centered assessment; an excellent foundation may be established for future provider–patient interactions. The primary disadvantage of the client-centered approach is the lack of standardization of the data-gathering process. Judging the severity of a patient's psychological problems in comparison to other people may be difficult. Additionally, some patients are unable to articulate their personal problems, because they do not fully recognize and/or understand them. Therefore, unstructured clinical interviews are most valuable when augmented by other structured approaches.

Psychometric Assessment

Psychometric assessment refers to the examination of psychological characteristics and/or related behaviors through the use of psychological tests. A psychological test is defined as an "objective and standardized measure of a sample of behavior" (17). The behavioral characteristic to be examined must be objective and must be observable by others. The collection of test data must be standardized so that the stimuli and demands of the test can be reproduced. A psychological test is typically restricted to a sample of behavior, because the full-range of an examinee's responses is not accessible. In short, psychological testing is simply a rigorous way of observing behavior.

There are several advantages to this approach. The quantification inherent in psychological testing permits an assessment of how much of a specific psychological or behavioral characteristic exists. Thus, the establishment of norm groups is possible. A second advantage is that the error inherent in psychological tests can be estimated, which permits a confidence interval to be established for a test score. Third, the psychometric approach is rigorous in terms of statistical and quantitative methodology. However, only a narrow range of behaviors are sampled; a psychological test may not adequately focus on a person's primary psychological concerns. The effectiveness of psychological tests may vary across populations due to ceiling or floor effects (i.e., scores primarily at the top or bottom of the scale). In general, such tests are most useful when complemented by other types of clinical data.

PREREQUISITES FOR PSYCHOMETRIC ASSESSMENT

In general, diagnostic criteria and clinical interviews can be used by anyone who learns the specific procedures. Psychometric assessment, however, requires more specialized training and is usually performed by psychologists or others with knowledge of psychometric theory. There are several prerequisites for accurate psychological assessment. First, there is the issue of *reliability*, or the assurance that a test yields similar results on successive administrations. Second, psychological tests must be *valid* in the sense of measuring what they, in fact, purport to measure. Third, psychological tests should have a *small standard error*. Multiple administrations of the test should cluster tightly around the "true" score. Next, psychological tests must be interpreted in the context of *appropriate norm groups*. Fifth, psychological tests must be *standardized*, with procedures, stimuli, and task demands that are consistently reproducible. Finally, psychological tests must be used *ethically* with careful attention to confidentiality and respondents' rights to privacy. When these prerequisites are met, examiners who are skilled in psychometric theory can obtain valuable clinical data.

Types of Psychometric Assessment

There are literally hundreds of well-validated psychological tests that could be used in a rheumatology setting. However, the psychological domains most applicable for persons with arthritis include helplessness, depression, self-efficacy, coping/adaptation, social support, marital/family functioning, life stress, vocational preference, personality, and cognitive functioning. Each of these assessment domains warrants brief discussion. References for specific tests are found in Parker and Wright (18).

Helplessness. The concept of helplessness is particularly relevant to the care of persons with arthritis and is related to health outcomes (19). For many forms of arthritis, symptoms wax and wane; flares are generally unpredictable. Similarly, treatments for many forms of arthritis are only palliative. Therefore, persons with arthritis may perceive themselves as helpless and as having minimal control over their disease. Helplessness can be measured with the Arthritis Helplessness Index.

Depression. Although not universal, depression is a significant clinical problem for some persons with arthritis. Persons with chronic diseases have a higher probability of developing depression than do persons who are healthy (20). Social isolation and economic distress have been identified as factors that can contribute to depression (21). Several measures have been developed to assess depression, including the Center for Epidemiologic Studies-Depression Scale, the Beck Depression Inventory, and the Hamilton Rating Scale for Depression.

Self-efficacy. Self-efficacy refers to a person's belief in his or her ability to accomplish a task or cope with a stressor (22). Self-efficacy for function, for pain, and for other symptoms have all been found to be related to important clinical outcomes such as functional capacity and health status. In addition, it is an important factor in the success of patient education interventions (23). Self-efficacy can be measured with the Arthritis Self-efficacy Scale.

Life Stress. *Stress* is a common but potentially confusing term. Sometimes it can refer to environmental stimuli that are judged to be taxing by the individual. At other times, stress may refer to a person's biologic response to taxing stimuli. Lastly, it can refer to a person–environment interaction that is dependent on a person's perception of his or her situation, rather than on the situation itself. Despite this diversity of definitions, stress can be considered a common problem for many persons with arthritis. Disease-related problems such as chronic pain, functional losses, employment difficulties, and economic worries contribute to life stress. Paper-and-pencil measures of stress include the Social Readjustment Rating Scale, the Life Experiences Survey, the Hassles Scale, and the Daily Stress Inventory.

Coping and Adaptation. In the face of numerous stressors, persons with arthritis must adapt to rapidly changing circumstances. The coping process usually involves a primary appraisal or judgment as to whether a stressor poses a risk of threat or harm. If a threat or harm is perceived, a secondary appraisal typically occurs, involving a judgment as to whether sufficient resources exist to cope with the stressor. If persons perceive that they do not possess sufficient coping resources, then the stressfulness of the situation dramatically intensifies. Thus, assessment of the coping/adaptation process is important in the care of persons with arthritis. Measures of the coping process include the Ways of Coping Scale, the Coping Strategies Questionnaire, and the Vanderbilt Pain Management Inventory.

Social Support. Social support refers to interpersonal relationships that are beneficial to a person's well-being. At best, social relationships offer support and understanding. At worst, they may offer criticism and blame. High levels of social support are generally associated with better adherence to medical regimens and more effective coping (24), although such findings are not universal (25). Social support can be measured with the Social Support Questionnaire and the Social Relationship Questionnaire.

Marital and Family Functioning. In chronic illness, marital and family functioning is often severely challenged. When health status changes for one family member, adaptation is often required by other family members as well. In arthritis, changes in work capacity or the ability to perform social roles can contribute to marital/family distress. Therefore, assessment of marriage and family functioning is important and can be accomplished with measures such as the Locke-Wallace Marital Adjustment Test and the Spanier Dyadic Adjustment Scale.

Vocational Assessments. One of the greatest challenges in the care of persons with arthritis is the maintenance of gainful employment. Work-related difficulties and economic losses are common occurrences in the context of rheumatic diseases such as RA (26). Vocational rehabilitation can lead to dramatically improved quality of life. Vocational measures such as the Strong-Campbell Interest Inventory and the Holland Self-Directed Search can be useful. In addition, vocational assessments can elucidate aptitudes and functional work capacities.

Personality Testing. Personality testing refers to the examination of enduring psychological or behavioral traits of an individual. In rheumatology settings, personality testing is typically reserved for situations in which serious psychological problems appear to be developing or when mental health difficulties pre-date rheumatic disease. The most common measure of personality is the MMPI-II. This lengthy questionnaire yields ten clinical scales and three validity scales that are used to assess overall psychological status. For persons with arthritis, the MMPI-II has distinct disadvantages, because some items overlap with the signs and symptoms of rheumatic disease (27). For example, symptoms such as "tiring easily" or "having aches and pains" are associated with rheumatic disease, so they do not necessarily reflect mental health problems. Alternative measures of global psychological functioning include the Symptom Checklist-90-Revised and the Millon Clinical Multiaxial Inventory-II.

Cognitive Functioning. Rheumatic diseases do not typically involve cognitive dysfunction. The most notable exception is SLE, in which cognitive functioning and psychiatric symptomatology may become prominent. Cognitive dysfunction also may occur in patients taking high-dose corticosteroid or certain other medications. In addition, arthritis patients may present with comorbidities that affect cognitive status, such as strokes, head injuries, or dementias. In these situations, neuropsychological testing can be helpful. Global intellectual functioning can be assessed with the Wechsler Adult Intelligence Scale-Revised and the Kaufman Adult Intelligence Test-Revised. Memory can be assessed with the Wechsler Memory Scale-Revised and the Rey Auditory Memory Scale. Comprehensive neuropsychological examination can be accomplished with the Halstead–Reitan Neuropsychological Test Battery, which samples a wide range of cognitive, motor, and sensory capacities.

INDICATIONS FOR PSYCHOLOGICAL/MENTAL HEALTH CONSULTATION

Beyond an awareness of specific psychological tests, health care providers also need to know when and how to request psychological/mental health consultations. An initial step in the process is to carefully explain the rationale for psychological referral to the patient. Understandably, persons with arthritis view their health-related problems as primarily medical, so a psychological referral may seem dissonant if not carefully explained. Conversely, a majority of persons with arthritis recognize that their chronic disease constitutes a major challenge to their coping capacities. When psychological referral is presented as being secondary to their arthritis, most patients easily accept, or even welcome, the opportunity to receive help. There are five key questions for which psychological/mental health consultation may be helpful: 1) psychiatric diagnosis; 2) psychotropic medications; 3) chronic psychological distress; 4) acute adjustment reactions; and 5) psychoeducational treatments.

Psychiatric Diagnosis. In the management of rheumatic disease, a well-formulated psychiatric diagnosis is sometimes critical. For example, treatments for depression vary widely depending on the specific diagnosis. For major depression, pharmacologic treatment is usually indicated. Conversely, for adjustment reaction with depressed mood, supportive counseling is typically the treatment of choice. Similarly, cognitive dysfunction may be secondary to such diverse etiologies as adverse effects of medication, major depression, or dementia; treatment varies depending on the specific etiology. Therefore, psychological assessment should be obtained in situations where psychological/psychiatric diagnoses may effect treatment strategies.

Psychotropic Medications. A related situation in which mental health assessment/consultation is indicated involves psychotropic medication. The typical rheumatology health professional does not possess extensive familiarity with either mental illness or psychotropic medications. A referral for psychological assessment or mental health consultation can result in more effective psychopharmacologic intervention for arthritis patients with concomitant psychiatric problems.

Chronic Psychological Distress. Persons with arthritis can present with an extensive history of psychological distress, even though they do not show evidence of full-blown psychiatric disturbance. For some patients, the burden of living with a chronic disease eventually overpowers their coping capacities. Patients who show signs of chronic psychological distress should not be overlooked; referral for psychological assessment and subsequent intervention can lead to improved quality of life.

Acute Adjustment Reactions. Acute adjustment reactions sometimes occur in persons with rheumatic disease, just as they do in the physically healthy population. Acute marital conflicts or family disturbances may develop. Concerns regarding employment, finances, or social circumstances may arise. Although acute life stressors are unavoidable, they are often particularly severe in the context of a chronic disease. Careful psychological assessment can lead to effective interventions.

Psychoeducational Treatments. There are numerous reports regarding the effectiveness of psychoeducational interventions (reviewed in 23). For example, the Arthritis Self-management Program has been shown to be beneficial for persons with arthritis (28), and rheumatology teams are increasingly using the services of psychologists, counselors, and educators. Psychological assessment can be helpful prior to implementing a psychoeducational intervention. For some arthritis patients, group treatments that enhance opportunities for socialization are indicated. For others, an individual treatment approach may be more viable. When there is uncertainty about the best psychoeducational strategy, psychological assessment should be considered.

COLLABORATIVE CARE

There are two ways in which rheumatologists and mental health professionals can work together. First, psychologists and other mental health professionals can be treated as consultants; arthritis patients with concomitant psychological problems can simply be referred to mental health professionals working outside the arthritis team. The consultant model is easy to establish, but the mental health consultants may have little understanding of the unique needs of arthritis patients. In addition, some arthritis patients may not be comfortable receiving care in a mental health environment.

The second strategy for collaboration involves the direct participation of mental health professionals as members of the arthritis rehabilitation team. In this model, mental health professionals gain the opportunity to develop a deeper understanding of the needs of arthritis patients, and they can deliver their interventions within the overall context of the rheumatology setting.

REFERENCES

1. Orleans CT, George LK, Houpt JL, Brodie HKH: How primary care physicians treat psychiatric disorders: a national survey of family practitioners. Am J Psychiatry 142:52–57, 1985
2. Kessler LG, Cleary PD, Burke JD: Psychiatric disorders in primary care. Arch Gen Psychiatry 42:583–587, 1985
3. Jencks SF: Recognition of mental distress and diagnosis of mental disorders in primary care. JAMA 253:1903–1907, 1985
4. Creed F, Ash G: Depression in rheumatoid arthritis: aetiology and treatment. Int Rev Psychiatry 4:23–34, 1992
5. Liang MH, Rogers M, Larson M, et al: The psychosocial impact of systemic lupus erythematosus and rheumatoid arthritis. Arthritis Rheum 27:13–19, 1984
6. Yelin E, Lubeck D, Holman H, Epstein W: The impact of rheumatoid arthritis and osteoarthritis: the activities of patients with rheumatoid ar-

thritis and osteoarthritis compared to controls. J Rheumatol 14:710–717, 1987

7. Engel GL: The need for a new medical model: a challenge for biomedicine. Science 196:129–136, 1977

8. Pope AM, Tarlov AR: Disability in America: Toward a National Agenda for Prevention. Washington, DC, National Academy Press, 1991

9. Dobson KS: A meta-analysis of the efficacy of cognitive therapy for depression. J Consult Clin Psychol 57:414–419, 1989

10. Lipsey MW, Wilson DB: The efficacy of psychological, educational, and behavioral treatment: confirmation from meta-analysis. Am Psychol 48:1181–1209, 1993

11. Felson DT, Anderson JJ, Meenan RF: The comparative efficacy and toxicity of second-line drugs in rheumatoid arthritis: results of two meta-analyses. Arthritis Rheum 33:1449–1461, 1990

12. Depression Guideline Panel: Depression in Primary Care. Vol. 2: Treatment of Major Depression. Clinical Practice Guideline, No. 5. Rockville, MD, US Department of Health and Human Services, Public Health Service, 1993

13. Parker JC, Iverson GL, Smarr KL, Stucky-Ropp RC: Cognitive-behavioral approaches to pain management in rheumatoid arthritis. Arthritis Care Res 6:207–212, 1993

14. Parker JC, Smarr KL, Buckelew SP, et al: Effects of stress management on clinical outcomes in rheumatoid arthritis. Arthritis Rheum 38:1807–1818, 1995

15. Diagnostic and Statistical Manual of Mental Disorders. Fourth edition. Washington, DC, American Psychiatric Association, 1994

16. Raskin NJ, Rogers CR: Person-centered therapy. In, Current Psychotherapies. Edited by RJ Corsini, D Wedding. Itasca, NY, FE Peacock Publishers, 1989

17. Anastasi A: Psychological Testing. Sixth edition. New York, Macmillan Publishing Co, 1988

18. Parker JC, Wright G: Psychologic assessment in rheumatology. Rheum Dis Clin North Am 21:465–480, 1995

19. Nicassio PM, Wallston KA, Callahan LF, Herbert M, Pincus T: The measurement of helplessness in rheumatoid arthritis: the development of the Arthritis Helplessness Index. J Rheumatol 12:462–467, 1985

20. Rodin G, Craven J, Littlefield C: Depression in the Medically Ill: An Integrated Approach. New York, Brunner/Mazel, 1991

21. Newman SP, Fitzpatrick R, Lamb R, Shipley M: The origins of depressed mood in rheumatoid arthritis. J Rheumatol 16:740–744, 1989

22. Bandura A: Self-efficacy: toward a unifying theory of behavioral change. Psychol Rev 84:191–215, 1977

23. Lorig K, Konkol L, Gonzalez V: Arthritis patient education: a review of the literature. Patient Educ Counsel 10:207–252, 1987

24. Wallston BS, Alagna SW, DeVellis BM, DeVellis RF: Social support and physical health. Health Psychol 2:367–391, 1983

25. Schiaffino KM, Revenson TA: Relative contributions of spousal support and illness appraisals to depressed mood in arthritis patients. Arthritis Care Res 8:80–87, 1995

26. Meenan RF, Yelin EH, Nevitt M, Epstein WV: The impact of chronic disease: a sociomedical profile of rheumatoid arthritis. Arthritis Rheum 24:544–549, 1981

27. Pincus T, Callahan LF, Bradley LA, Vaughn WK, Wolfe F: Elevated MMPI scores for hypochondriasis, depression, and hysteria in patients with rheumatoid arthritis reflect disease rather than psychological status. Arthritis Rheum 29:1456–1466, 1986

28. Lorig K, Lubeck D, Kraines RG, Seleznick M, Holman HR: Outcomes of self-help education for patients with arthritis. Arthritis Rheum 28:680–685, 1985

Additional Recommended Reading

1. Blalock SJ, DeVellis RF, Brown GK, Wallston KA: Validity of the Center for Epidemiological Studies Depression Scale in arthritis populations. Arthritis Rheum 32:991–997, 1989

2. Parker JC, Bradley LA, DeVellis RM, et al: Biopsychosocial contributions to the management of arthritis disability: blueprints from an NIDRR-sponsored conference. Arthritis Rheum 36:885–889, 1993

3. Pincus T, Callahan LF: Depression scales in rheumatoid arthritis: criterion contamination in interpretation of patient responses. Patient Educ Counsel 20:133–143, 1993

CHAPTER 8   Social and Cultural Assessment

LAURA ROBBINS, DSW, MSW

For the person living with a chronic illness, there are many emotional and physical challenges to everyday life activities and interpersonal relationships. These changes require a re-evaluation of goals and long-term commitments. Moreover, chronic diseases, like rheumatoid arthritis (RA) and systemic lupus erythematosus (SLE) are often unpredictable, resulting in the need for emotional and social support from family members, friends, and ultimately the health care team. While social workers are trained to assess a patient's social and cultural background, it is not unusual for other health professionals to conduct similar assessments. The professional should possess the basic knowledge, skill, and training to evaluate a patient's coping patterns and level of social adjustment, to make referrals to the appropriate member of the health care team, and to ensure optimal health outcomes. Understanding the patient in the appropriate social and cultural context can lead to referrals to education and support programs that have been demonstrated to affect health outcomes (1).

THE ASSESSMENT METHOD

A comprehensive social and cultural assessment begins with evaluation of the patient's physical status, emotional state, and support system. This approach, grounded in the social work concept of "the person in the situation," focuses on the person, the situation, and the interaction between them (2). In the health care setting, the person is the patient, the situation may be medical crisis, and the interaction can be considered to be the process that evolves between the patient and their support system when attempting to cope with the medical condition. In chronic illness, the emphasis is on the *process* by which people learn to cope or function within their social network. The method also emphasizes communication skills and the patient's ability to articulate emotional, social, and physical needs to other people within their environment (3).

The patient becomes an integral member of the medical team throughout the duration of the chronic illness. The patient brings a unique history and understanding of the disease and contributes to the treatment process. Optimal health outcomes, particularly effective emotional and social functioning, are more likely to occur because the patient becomes a part of the evaluation and influences the treatment plan. The goal for the health care worker is to gain an understanding of the patient's emotional, social, and physical reaction to their medical situation in order to provide appropriate care. Through patient information and participation, the health professional and the patient should work together to assess the impact of the disease over the course of the illness.

The first step in this process is a complete social and cultural assessment. Depending on the individual's experiences, social supports, and level of physical activity, an assessment may take from one to several sessions. A written evaluation is completed at the end of the assessment, which then becomes a part of the patient's medical record. Just as medications and treatments are re-evaluated and adjusted periodically, the assessment should be reviewed and updated to reflect the ongoing disease. This continual review is particularly pertinent for patients with rheumatic diseases, because there may be episodes of increased disease activity. An assessment should be done during each hospitalization and updated during routine office visits.

THE SOCIAL ASSESSMENT

The Patient as Person

A social assessment begins with the person diagnosed with the rheumatic disease. The goal is to evaluate the person's life history and the impact of the diagnosis on the individual's current functioning. Unless fully unable to communicate, the patient is the best source of information about the impact of their illness. Scheduling the assessment interview with the patient alone is optimal. If this is not possible, asking family members for privacy is appropriate. It is not unusual, however, for an older person to have family members present during the assessment who will answer questions addressed to the patient. When this occurs, patients must be encouraged to answer the questions themselves in order to obtain pertinent information. Scheduling an assessment interview with the family members will also demonstrate that the family is vital as the patient learns to cope and adjust to the medical situation. It also allows the health care professional to assess the family's adjustment to the changing physical and emotional situations.

Most assessments begin with demographic details and information, including definitive or concrete questions related to age, marital status, parental status, level of education, sexual identity, work history, medical insurance, and religious affiliation. The assessment should also explore prior and current alcohol and drug use. Additional areas should address patient concerns related to housing arrangements, geographic location and proximity to health care services, and modes of transportation. As illustrated in Table 1, these questions should be phrased to elicit concrete responses. As questions begin to produce information, the responses can be used to evaluate the family constellation, support systems, and the impact of arthritis on the patient's life.

Perhaps the most difficult part of evaluation involves assessing the significance of physical and emotional changes for the patient during interactions with people in their environment. Rapid, unplanned episodes of disease such as flares, increased pain, or medication side effects present unique challenges. To capture this process, it is helpful to begin by asking simple, direct questions aimed at evaluating changes that have occurred since the onset of the

Table 1. Social assessment sample questions.

Social Impact Questions
Do you live close to the medical center?
Who lives in your household with you?
How do you get to and from the medical center?
Are you presently working?
What has changed about your current work schedule?
Do you go to school?
Who in your family is responsible for the cooking, shopping, child rearing, or the well-being of aging parents?

Emotional Impact Questions
How has the relationship with your children changed since you learned that you have arthritis?
How has your family reacted to the fact that you can no longer contribute to the household responsibilities?
How do your friends react to you since you told them about your arthritis?

Interpersonal Impact Questions
What did you and your partner enjoy that you can't enjoy now due to your arthritis?
What do you discuss with your husband about your osteoarthritis?
What are the kind of things that you and your husband routinely discuss?
How does your spouse feel about the changes in your relationship since you developed arthritis?
Have your sexual relationships changed since being diagnosed?

Non-verbal Assessment Questions
Does the patient ask questions during the interview?
Does the patient indicate that he or she is listening by a head nod as I am talking?
Does the patient appear distressed and perhaps too emotional to respond to questions?

Effective Communication

Good communication skills are fundamental in the patient and health professional relationship. Learning how to enhance discussions and increase the exchange of information will facilitate the ability to ask questions that are personal and confidential. This includes not only spoken verbal language but nonverbal interactions as well.

To enhance the patient–physician relationship, health professionals need specific tools for better communication. These include role modeling through demonstration of the following: the ability to ask for help, knowing how to verbalize questions and concerns, listening, and having the confidence to ask for clarification and additional information. Questions that begin with "how," "what," and "why" are effective because they tend to elicit answers that require explanations. Questions that lead to "yes" and "no" answers tend to hinder a free exchange of information.

Evaluation of communication skills can be through observation as well as direct questions. You can observe if someone is listening by asking yourself a series of questions (see Table 1). Awareness of how you as the health professional ask questions can greatly enhance the outcome of the assessment. Encourage patients to fully express their concerns about their medical situation. Urge them to ask all their questions regardless of how relevant they seem. Good communication allows a meaningful exchange of information to be elicited during the assessment interviews.

The Social Environment

For people living with chronic illness, personal relationships are further broadened to include doctors, nurses, hospital personnel, and health insurance companies. Through this expanding social network, the patient is confronted with many new and unique situations that can be perceived as opportunities as well as obstacles. The way in which people cope with chronic illness depends largely upon their experience with other threats to their lives and lifestyles. Availability of food, shelter, transportation, medical care, employment, education, and recreational activities are examples of some resources required for basic survival.

However, patients also have psychosocial realities that are challenged when dealing with crisis (4). These realities are more obscure and include concepts such as role identity, self esteem, and perceived self worth. These qualities are expressed through interpersonal relationships. When chronic illness mandates changes in roles from full-time career woman, wife, and mother to full-time patient, and part-time wife and mother, the patients' role status changes. This challenges the individual's identity and perceived self worth. Family structure and family members' perceptions of the patient's roles also change. Psychosocial challenges, although intangible, are as important as the concrete realities of food and shelter, and can dramatically alter the former coping mechanisms of the person transformed to patient. While the individual exercises some control by choosing friends for social support, most social relationships with parents, siblings, and extended family members are inherited. The quality of these relationships can have a potent effect and create pressures over which the individual has no control (5). With chronic illness, there is an increased need for intermittent dependency, which can make a patient feel out of

diagnosis. These change questions (Table 1), when directed to the patient, also address the person's interpersonal relationships with the significant people in their immediate social network. Similar questions should be asked about other relationships in the patient's extended environment and may include casual relationships with work colleagues, school peers, religious congregations, and recreational contacts. Generally, these questions begin with *"What is different about . . . "*, or *"How has your life changed since . . . "*. Alterations in daily routines due to physical limitations can also shift social relationships and result in emotional distress. For example, the patient who has had to stop working due to RA may not only lose daily contact with colleagues but also the supportive listening of available friends. Questions targeted towards change in the patient's life will provide you with information to assess disease impact.

Comparable questions about the nature of intimate personal relationships and recent changes since adjusting to a chronic illness also need to be explored. Questions about role shifts in family responsibilities between spouses and children are essential and should focus on the daily responsibilities for the patient within the family system. Personal relationships and questions about sexual relationships must also be explored. Information about change in sexual activity due to the pain and discomfort associated with some rheumatic diseases can be extremely informative about the disease impact on marital relationships. A direct approach to questions is most effective, particularly when the information required is personal and private. Knowledge about changes in sexual functioning as part of the assessment will assist in appropriate referral and in the treatment process.

control and cause increased stress and anxiety. These feelings interfere with communication and normal interpersonal relationships.

Patients with rheumatic diseases often experience changes in physical mobility, financial status, and emotional health. The goal of social assessment is to evaluate the extent to which changes have occurred in relationships between the patient and their social supports, and how these changes affect the patient's self worth and self esteem. The assessment should focus on changes the patient can control and those affected by the attitudes, behaviors, and reactions of other people within their social environment. Questions should assess how family members, friends, and colleagues reacted to the patient's chronic illness—questions best addressed during the evaluation of the patient's cultural system.

THE CULTURAL ASSESSMENT

Health Beliefs and Behaviors

A social assessment is not complete without an evaluation of the patient's cultural background. It would be artificial to separate the social experience from the cultural one, because a person's cultural group is made up of the family and social support network. Culture has a significant impact on the outcomes of treatment and health management. People acquire their own perceptions and beliefs about the origin of diseases and treatments, which are sanctioned by their cultural group, learned in childhood, and expressed through behaviors. Through these shared cultural beliefs we come to value what is worthwhile, desirable, and important for our physical and emotional well-being. However, our cultural identity may differ from those of people we encounter in our daily contacts. Health professionals, for example, may not be of the same cultural background, and often have a tendency to view their own cultural orientation as the standard against which other cultures are judged (6). Therefore, assessment of the person diagnosed with a chronic disease requires a culturally enlightened and culturally sensitive approach.

Culture is a filter through which we interpret experiences. Health beliefs, attitudes, and behaviors are defined within the cultural experience. In modern Western societies, explanations for illness are typically rooted in natural phenomena, such as infection with micro-organisms, and mechanical dysfunction. More recently stress has been identified as an explanation for illness. However, there are groups of people who attribute disease and illness to very different causes (7). How a person defines and copes with chronic disease and the health care experience can greatly modify the treatment plan and delivery of services.

There is no consensus on whether society should support cultural adaptation, cultural diversity, or a multicultural society especially since the melting pot theory no longer shapes our society (8). Most health professionals do not have training in cultural diversity. Cultural sensitivity training exists, but often it is not required in academic programs. Although professionals may strive to be open-minded about different cultural groups, even the most well-intentioned professionals bring ethnocentric biases to the assessment of a person with different cultural attitudes and beliefs. Moreover, individuals who are not personally prejudiced or discriminatory may still distance

Table 2. Cultural self-assessment sample questions.

Health Professional Self-assessment
What is my cultural heritage?
What was the culture of my parents and my grandparents?
With what cultural group do I identify?
What values, beliefs, opinions, and attitudes do I hold that are consistent with the dominant culture? Which are inconsistent? How did I learn these?
What unique abilities, aspirations, expectations, and limitations do I have that might influence my relations with culturally diverse individuals?
How do I communicate with my patients?
Do I change my communication styles to enhance discussion with my patients who come from different cultures than I do?

culturally different groups if they avoid communication or fail to recognize how others interpret their own behavior (9). There is a need for practitioners to recognize that their health beliefs and practices differ from those of other populations. In the Anglo-American culture, values of mastery over nature, individualism, competition, and directness vary significantly from values of harmony with nature, group welfare, cooperation, and indirectness characteristic of some ethnocultural groups (10). Recognizing and understanding the differences in these values will lead to understanding of culture-specific behaviors that influence health behaviors. Thus, the goal of the cultural assessment is to provide sensitive and effective health care to patients from differing cultures (11).

A cultural assessment should begin by self-assessment on the part of the health professional to evaluate his or her own cultural values and beliefs. This step is essential in order to assess personal biases. Recognizing one's own cultural identity and how it influences personal values, beliefs, and behaviors is a precursor to understanding and being able to assess a patient's cultural orientation. This self-assessment of cultural awareness is based on the premise that awareness of self is the first step to understanding others (12). As illustrated in Table 2, basic questions for self-assessment are designed to help health professionals recognize their own cultural identity through key questions focusing on one's own cultural orientation. In addition to creating self-awareness, such questions also assist the health professional in a general understanding of the influence of culture-specific beliefs and attitudes on health behaviors.

The cultural assessment must emphasize the patient's global beliefs, practices, and behaviors as well as health-specific ones. However, the goal is not only to understand beliefs, attitudes, and subsequent behaviors, but to identify how they are important to the development of the individual's concept of self, the core for emotional and social functioning. Self-concept develops through socialization within the family unit, social networks, and community groups. Individuals develop a perception of self through interactions that are sanctioned and defined within their cultural group. Self-concept is formed by several factors, including language, gender identity, and behaviors. It is rarely a conscious trait and is often expressed through verbalized attitudes, beliefs, and behaviors. Questions focused on the patient's attitudes and beliefs about health care reveal information about health behaviors practiced by the patient. Table 3 lists sample questions for obtaining cultural information about the patient that can be utilized in developing the treatment plan. These questions also help the health professional to understand how a person within a cultural group defines and treats diseases as well as the patient's perception of how they cope and function.

Table 3. Patient assessment sample questions.

<u>**Cultural Identity**</u>
  To what ethnic group do you belong?
  What language do you speak most often with your family?
    With your friends?
  What religious group do you belong to? Do you attend services regularly? In what ways do you practice your religion?

<u>**Health Beliefs**</u>
  What do you believe caused your arthritis?
  How would you describe your arthritis symptoms?
  What does having arthritis mean to you?
  How do you believe that your arthritis can be treated?

<u>**Health Behaviors**</u>
  Who in the family makes the major decisions?
  Who do you go to in your community for advice about medical problems or treatment?
  When do you go for advice or treatment?
  Do you go to a healer or any other person for advice about your health (Chinese herbalist, spiritualist, minister)?
  What advice do you follow?
  What foods do you eat that you believe makes your arthritis better?
  What foods do you eat that you believe makes your arthritis worse?
  What other things do you do to deal with your arthritis?

For example, the concept of "machismo", or males as the strong, dominant family figure is common within the Latino culture (13). For most traditionally raised Latinos, machismo is an unquestioned cultural value, an expected trait and behavior that becomes the internalized self-concept males learn during the childhood experience. When working with Latinos in the health care setting, this cultural expression has to be recognized and respected in order to facilitate positive health outcomes. If you are assessing a Latino woman diagnosed with SLE who needs to start kidney dialysis, it is imperative to assess her family status. It is vital to invite the dominant male figure to the assessment interview. Without appealing to the male's cultural identity as the dominant family figure, the patient will likely have difficulty adhering to the treatment plan and may be labeled "non-compliant" because the key person within the cultural group was not consulted.

The importance of culture in patient assessment is further exemplified within the Asian population. It is common for patients in this cultural group to smile when told by a physician that the medical situation is serious. Patients of Asian background often present a "good face" when in crisis due to a culturally intrinsic value of respect and reverence to authority figures. This may appear to be inappropriate behavior during the assessment, when in reality it is an expression sanctioned by the cultural group. However, it may be difficult to assess the patient's emotional reaction to their illness if one does not have an understanding of this culture. The patient may be labeled as "inappropriate" because the behavior may appear inconsistent with the crisis situation.

Behaviors that are defined in relationship to other key family members or that may not overtly represent the patient's emotional state should be assessed. In African-American culture, the female may be the dominant family figure. Often it is the grandmother who should be consulted in any decisions regarding the health of family members in this cultural group. Similarly, the grandmother or aunt are the primary caregivers. There are many other cultures in which it is expected that the husband, or dominant male figure, be consulted about important decisions particularly if decisions will affect the family unit (14).

Verbal and Non-verbal Language

Language is another element that must be considered in any cultural assessment. While culture provides a sense of belonging and identification to a group of people and ascribes meaning and utilization to behaviors, it also provides meaning and function to language. Language shapes our world, defines our roles within society, and is the way in which we express our self-concept and identity (15). There can be severe handicaps to understanding the impact of chronic illness when language differences hinder communication.

Any patient whose primary language differs from the health care provider's has this as an additional barrier during an assessment (16). Language complicates assessment of health status because it serves a vital role in social and survival functions. When doing a cultural assessment ask the patients what language they primarily speak, read, write, and think in when at home or with friends and family. Response to this question usually indicates which language the patient uses most often in familiar social situations. In the health care setting, patients who speak different languages often attempt understanding physician questions, due to cultural values of respect for authority figures. Their marginal understanding of English can be conveyed by a head nod or responding "yes" or "no" to questions. However, the patient usually does not fully understand the question or the instructions. When asking questions of someone who speaks English marginally, refrain from using questions that result in yes/no answers, and always ask the patient to repeat the information, as an indicator of patient comprehension.

When there is any indication that the patient does not comprehend your assessment questions, you should use an interpreter. There are many concerns related to the use of third-party information gathering. First, it is inappropriate to use family members to translate during an assessment. Due to time constraints in hospital and office settings, family members—particularly young children—and close friends are used for communication during interviews. This method of translation results in a breach of patient confidentiality, leads to inaccurate translation of questions and responses, and causes emotional distress for family members who themselves are coping with the patient's medical condition (17). When family members are not present, hospital and office staff may be asked to translate if they speak the same language. This practice is also inappropriate, because staff who have a knowledge of the patient's condition will often paraphrase the questions asked during the assessment. Additionally, they will provide their own interpretation of the patient's medical situation in an earnest attempt to assist the patient. Important information can be misinterpreted and stripped of its significance, contributing to poor treatment outcomes.

However, translators can be effective if utilized appropriately. Models for the use of translators that include bilingual, bicultural people have been the most effective (18). Community-based agencies can provide professionally trained translators, and a growing number of agencies train translators to be available via phone to assist in the communication process. Another effective model is the use of bilingual, bicultural patient advocates who are trained as translators for other patients from the same cultural group. While this model may appear to be labor intensive, the training and supervision of a cadre of patients is worth the initial investment to ensure the well-being of new patients. This model also allows for assessment of the patient's level of language and communication skills, as well as a determination of cultural health beliefs and practices.

In addition to language differences, specific cultures have clearly defined folklore health beliefs and practices that differ from those of Western medicine. It would be unrealistic to expect that health professionals be knowledgeable about the plethora of cultures they may encounter. Cultural sensitivity is a place to start. To ensure ongoing cultural understanding, it may be necessary to engage a community leader as a key informant about the patient's culture to assist you in obtaining information (19). Community leaders often are identified within cultural groups as the informant for group-specific norms, beliefs, and attitudes. They also sanction culturally determined behaviors. There are large community health agencies serving Asian, Latino, African-American, and Native American groups that specifically train their constituents to serve cultural groups in a variety of roles. Enlisting a cultural informant to assist in a social and cultural assessment greatly enhances the communication process between health provider and patient. Moreover, it ameliorates the mistrust, fear, and intimidation that some cultural groups feel towards Anglo-American institutions (20). A cultural informant does not replace the patient; rather, the informant collaboratively serves as a verbal translator and advocate for the patient. The patient's consent and permission should always be obtained prior to engaging a third party in the assessment process.

Acculturation

Culturally determined health beliefs and practices may vary within cultural groups due to the length of time the patient has lived in the United States. Socialization in the patient's native homeland or within a different culture also affects the health beliefs and practices of patients. Therefore, acculturation becomes a factor in assessment, because people learn new behaviors when they are exposed to new cultures. It should be standard practice during an assessment to ask a brief question that addresses level of acculturation. A simple question, *"How long have you lived in . . ."* will provide a response that clarifies the patient's exposure to different cultural groups. If a patient from Russia has lived in the United States for 15 years, the patient is probably more familiar with Anglo-American health beliefs and behaviors. The response to this question should then guide you when conducting the full cultural assessment.

THERAPEUTIC INTERVENTIONS

Once a social and cultural assessment is completed, it may be necessary to refer the patient for psychosocial treatment. There are many therapeutic interventions available; however, the type of referral depends on the assessment. Casework is one of the most common treatments, which focuses on helping the patient cope with their medical situation. In this model, the social worker uses counseling to assist the patient in making emotional adjustments to chronic illness. Social workers can also help the patient with concrete needs, such as financial evaluations and referrals for assistance. They also assist with problems relating to housing, medical insurance, disability, and transportation. Additionally, if it is determined that the patient

is clinically depressed or has an existing personality disorder, a social worker can refer to a psychiatrist or psychologist as appropriate.

When the patient and family members assessment indicates interpersonal difficulties, family therapy may be needed. Referrals should be made to family social workers who can provide counseling and emotional support to the entire family. If more dysfunctional family problems are apparent, a family therapist with a psychology background is required.

For patients who are experiencing the normal problems in coping, such as mild depression, anger, or sadness due to the common adjustments of living with a chronic illness, a referral to a self-help or mutual support group can be extremely beneficial. The Arthritis Foundation, through its local chapters, offers support programs such as the Arthritis Self-Management Program, the Systemic Lupus Erythematosus Self-Help Program, and the Fibromyalgia Self-Help Program (21). Over time, participants in the Self-Management Program report a decrease in depression, an increase in self confidence, and an increase in self-management skills (22). Programs like these are excellent vehicles for empowering patients by providing educational information and social support.

Finally, traditional therapeutic interventions may not be relevant to some cultural groups. For many people, support and empathy originates from systems within the cultural group. For African-Americans, religious affiliations transcend spiritual support and are a source of comfort during medical crises. In some Latino cultures, curanderos and spiritualists are sought for support during medical illness. In some Asian cultures, patients in emotional distress will keep their concerns within the family, rather than seek outside assistance. When working with culturally diverse patients, the goal is to understand the client's emotional and social supports.

Utilizing a social and cultural assessment as a key component of evaluating the patient with rheumatic disease is a comprehensive model that ultimately enhances the treatment plan. This assessment is an important piece to the overall medical diagnosis, management, and treatment of the person who is challenged by a chronic disease.

REFERENCES

1. Robbins L: Patient education. In, Primer on the Rheumatic Diseases. Eleventh edition. Edited by J Klippel, C Weyand, R Wortmann (in press)
2. Hollis F: Casework: A Psychosocial Therapy. Second edition. New York, Random House, 1972
3. Turner F, editor: Social Work Treatment: Interlocking Theoretical Approaches. New York, Free Press, 1979
4. Perlman H: Social Casework: A Problem Solving Process. Chicago, University of Chicago Press, 1957
5. Billingsley A: Black Families in White America. Englewood Cliffs, NJ, Prentice-Hall, 1968
6. Locke D: Increasing Multicultural Understanding: A Comprehensive Model. Newbury Park, CA, Sage Publications, 1992
7. Airhihenbuwa C: Health and Culture: Beyond the Western Paradigm. Newbury Park, CA, Sage Publications, 1995
8. Marin G, Marin B: Research with Hispanic Populations. Newbury Park, CA, Sage Publications, 1991
9. Kavanagh K, Kennedy P: Promoting Cultural Diversity: Strategies for Health Care Professionals. Newbury Park, CA, Sage Publications, 1992
10. Sigelman L, Welch S: Black Americans' Views of Racial Inequity: The Dream Deferred. New York, Cambridge University Press, 1991
11. David-Randall E: Strategies for Working With Culturally Diverse Communities and Clients. Washington DC, US Department of Health and Human Services, Association for the Care of Children's Health, 1989
12. National Coalition of Hispanic Health and Human Services Organization

(COSSMHO): Delivering Preventive Health Care to Hispanics. Washington, DC, Provider Education Project, 1988

13. Locke DC: Cross-cultural counseling issues. In, Foundations of Mental Health Counseling. Edited by AJ Pakmo, WJ Weikel. Springfield, IL, Charles C. Thomas, 1986
14. McGoldrick M, Pearce J, Giordano J, editors: Ethnicity and Family Therapy. New York, Guilford Press, 1982
15. Steward E: American Cultural Patterns. La Grange Park, IL, Intercultural Network, 1972
16. Sotomayor M: Language, culture and ethnicity in developing self-concept. Soc Casework 41:195–203, 1977
17. Molina C, Aguirre-Molina M, editors: Latino Health in the US: A Growing Challenge. Washington DC, American Public Health Association, 1994
18. Robbins L: A Pilot Study of a Translated, Culturally Sensitive Systemic Lupus Erythematosus Self-Help Course for Latino Lupus Patients. Doctoral Dissertation, City University of New York, 1994
19. Breckon D, Harvey J, Lancaster R: Community Health Education: Settings, Roles, and Skills for the 21st Century. Gaithersburg, MD, Aspen Publication, 1994
20. Robbins L, Allegrante JP, Paget SA: Adapting the Systemic Lupus Erythematosus Self-Help (SLESH) course for Latino SLE patients. Arthritis Care Res 6:97–103, 1993
21. Arthritis Foundation, 1330 W. Peachtree Street, Atlanta, GA, 30309
22. Lorig KR, Mazonson PD, Holman HR: Evidence suggesting that health education for self-management in patients with chronic arthritis has sustained health benefits while reducing health care costs. Arthritis Rheum 36:439–446, 1993

Additional Recommended Reading

1. Braithwaite R, Taylor S, editors: Health Issues in the Black Community. San Francisco, Jossey-Bass Publishers, 1992
2. Journal of Multicultural Social Work. New York, The Haworth Press, Inc.
3. Carlson V: Social Work and General Systems Theory. School of Social Welfare, University of California, Berkeley, 1957
4. Ponterotto J, Casas J, Suzuki L, Alexander C, editors: Handbook of Multicultural Counseling. Newbury Park, CA, Sage Publications, 1995
5. Locke DC: Increasing Multicultural Understanding: A Comprehensive Model. Newbury Park, CA, Sage Publications, 1992

SECTION C: CLINICAL INTERVENTIONS

CHAPTER

9

Patient Education

MICHELE L. BOUTAUGH, BSN, MPH; and KATE R. LORIG, DrPH

There is considerable research evidence that patient education in the rheumatic diseases can result in positive changes in knowledge, health behaviors, beliefs, and attitudes that affect health status, quality of life, and possibly health care utilization (1–10). More recently attention has been focused on *how* patient education interventions work, and the transfer of what has been learned to clinical and field settings.

The Arthritis and Musculoskeletal Patient Education standards (11) define patient education as "planned, organized learning experiences designed to facilitate voluntary adoption of behaviors or beliefs conducive to health." While the standards do not prescribe specific educational strategies, they state that high-quality programs are based on the needs of the target population and demonstrate their effectiveness in maintaining or improving health status and/or psychological outcomes. Table 1 describes the major types of interventions that have had positive outcomes. The most commonly reported are self-management education (12–17) and cognitive-behavioral therapy (6,7). Other successful interventions are group exercise and education classes (18–20), telephone counseling (21–24), and mediated instruction (25–30).

Additional strategies include the provision of general information using materials and/or didactic lectures and the use of psychotherapy or mutual support groups. While such interventions have been used alone, they are being used more frequently as part of multi-intervention programs or as control or comparison groups. There is a growing recognition that while knowledge is certainly *necessary*, it is not usually *sufficient* to bring about desirable behavioral changes and improvement in health status outcomes. Therefore, programs that focus solely on providing information are usually of limited value (5). Data on psychotherapy and mutual support groups is inconclusive (5,10). However, interventions that incorporate social support as an adjunct (e.g., by involving family members and friends) often have better outcomes (31).

Consistent with good program design (2,32), successful programs utilize more than one type of intervention. For example, the Arthritis Self-Management Program (ASMP) not only includes self-management education, but also incorporates some cognitive-behavioral techniques, educational materials, and strategies to encourage social support.

EDUCATION PRINCIPLES AND STRATEGIES

While it is important to provide information to improve understanding of one's condition and treatment options, appropriate self-management of a chronic illness also involves the mastery of a complex set of beliefs, behaviors, and skills. Such mastery cannot be obtained by simply providing information, but requires a planned, multi-faceted approach. The content and strategies used should be based on the client's needs and characteristics. Because time is usually limited and multiple providers may be involved, there should be a protocol of possible topics to teach and educational methods for teaching each topic. If the protocol is in a checklist format, it can serve as a documentation tool. Protocols should include not only what the professionals want to teach, but more importantly, what the clients need and want to know. In general, comprehensive patient education should include attention to three major tasks faced by most people with any chronic illness, including rheumatic disease: 1) tasks necessary to deal with the chronic condition, such as taking medicine, exercising, dealing with fatigue, and communicating with health care providers; 2) tasks necessary to carry on or adapt one's social, work, family, and recreational roles; and 3) tasks necessary to deal with the emotional responses to rheumatic disease, such as depression, anger, fear, uncertainty, and frustration (33).

Patient education is a continuous process. It is not appropriate to cover everything in a single education session. Patients often feel overwhelmed at the time of diagnosis. Education at this time should be aimed at mitigating fears, suggesting immediate support resources, and arranging for another contact in the near future to deal with questions and to begin more formal education. Prioritize which topics to cover based on the preferences of the client. Determining the appropriate content, methods, and sequencing requires two-way communication. Effective patient education is an active process; it is not something done *to* the client, but rather must be done *with* the client as an active participant (34). There are several common strategies which may be useful to practitioners.

Provide Problem-based Education

One of the first steps of effective education is to identify the client's major concerns so you can tailor educational messages and recommendations (35–37). For example, exercise is often taught as a means of increasing mobility. However, a major concern of most people with rheumatic disease is pain (8). When clients identify pain as their major problem, then exercise should be taught as a means of managing pain by reducing

53

Table 1. Types of psychoeducational interventions (10, adapted with permission).

Type of Intervention	Characteristics	Representative Studies
Self-management/self-help programs	Group class series with sessions usually lasting about 2–2½ hours for 5–7 weeks; taught by trained professionals and/or lay leaders; emphasis on interactive methods/experiential learning Content provides a combination of (1) disease-related information and (2) training and support in learning and adopting new behaviors/skills: exercise, relaxation, energy-saving techniques, problem-solving, communicating with professionals and family, changing to positive self-talk. Recent programs emphasize improving self-efficacy (via goal-setting, contracting, feedback, use of positive role models, reinterpretation of symptoms, persuasion). Can include support component (involvement of family/peers, buddy system, allotment of time for group sharing/support)	Arthritis Self-Management Program (ASMP) (Lorig & Gonzalez, 1992, Lorig & Holman, 1993) ASMP adapted for Dutch (Taal et al, 1993) Australian arthritis education program (Lindroth et al, 1995) SLE Self-Help Course (Braden et al, 1991) OA education low-literacy program (Bill-Harvey et al, 1989)
Cognitive behavior therapy (CBT)/ behavior treatments or programs	Typical format is group sessions of 1–2 hours for 5–10 weeks; generally led by psychologists or specially trained professionals Content emphasizes learning new techniques for controlling or managing pain: (1) educational (e.g., explanation of pain theories and inter-relationship of emotional, cognitive, physical and behavioral components of pain; (2) learning new cognitive (e.g., relaxation, diversion, cognitive restructuring) and behavioral (e.g., activity-pacing, goal setting) coping skills, and (3) maintenance/relapse prevention strategies	See reviews by Parker et al (1993) and Keefe and Van Horn (1993) and Chapter 10, Cognitive Behavioral Interventions
Exercise/education classes	Group class series which includes exercise demonstration and practice and educational discussions; taught by fitness professionals or therapists Content focuses on promoting the adoption of regular physical activity including range of motion, muscle strengthening and/or low-impact aerobic exercises. May include self-efficacy enhancing strategies, problem-solving discussions and other activities to promote long-term maintenance of exercise	Educize (Perlman et al, 1990) Aerobic walking and aquatics (Minor & Brown, 1993) Walking program (Allegrante et al, 1993)
Telephone	Contacts by trained laypersons or professional counselors. Content may include: monitoring of joint pain or other symptoms related to arthritis or other co-morbid conditions; individualized counseling and support to address problems related to symptoms, patient-physician communication, medication compliance and side effects, barriers to medical care/appointment-keeping, self-care activities, and stress.	Indiana program (Rene et al, 1992; Weinberger et al, 1993; Mazzuca et al, 1995) Alabama program (Maisiak et al, 1995)
Mediated instruction	Format may include personalized, self-paced instruction using self-instructional workbooks and audiovisual aids, computer-assisted instruction (CAI) and/or computer tailored materials. May be augmented by individualized instruction and support from health professionals or trained lay persons. Content may be focused on one issue such as stress management or total joint replacement, or may include a variety of self-management and/or cognitive behavioral topics and strategies.	CAI-RA program (Wetstone et al, 1985) CAI-total joint replacement (Reisine & Lewis, 1993) Bone Up on Arthritis (Goeppinger et al, 1989; 1995) SMART computer-tailored program (Gale et al, 1994) CAI-stress management (Parker et al, 1995)

stiffness and relaxing muscles. If a client is concerned about not being able to do a particular activity, focus on the exercises that will improve that function. The subject matter has not changed, but the framing of the teaching is based on the perceived problem(s) of the client. A quick way of determining problems is to ask open-ended questions such as: "What do you think of when you think of arthritis?" or "What are the most important problems or concerns you have in managing your arthritis?" Encourage clients to bring a list of their concerns or problems with them to visits.

Accommodate Existing Beliefs

Most people come to a health care setting for treatment of their rheumatic condition with pre-existing and sometimes conflicting beliefs and self-care practices (see Chapter 8, Social and Cultural Assessment). Patients will judge the appropriateness and efficacy of suggested treatments based on these perceptions and experiences (12, 37).

Ask clients to explain the cause and meaning of their disease and symptoms and their goals for treatment (e.g., "What caused your problem? What consequences have resulted? What have you already done to treat this problem? What would you like to change? What activity would you like to be able to resume? What are you afraid might happen if you follow this treatment?") Determining these perceptions allows the health care provider to correct false expectations or other problematic misunderstandings, help motivate clients to adopt new behaviors relevant to their goals, and help set priorities for treatment options (37).

Do not try to change clients' beliefs or practices unless they are causing harm. If education conflicts with beliefs, the education will generally be rejected. For this reason, it is important not to fight against copper bracelets or people who think that grapefruit will cause a flare of their arthritis. Simply try to suggest new beliefs and practices as appropriate. Clients always have choices. There are often many paths to the same solution, and little is gained by being dogmatic.

Help clients reinterpret the causes of their symptoms. When discussing a symptom like fatigue, explain the many different possible causes. If clients believe that fatigue is solely due to their disease, they may only be willing to try medication or rest to deal with the symptom. However, when patients understand that fatigue can also be due to multiple causes like deconditioning, poor nutrition, or depression, they may be motivated to consider other strategies such as exercise, sleep hygiene, or improved nutrition (12).

Positive "self-talk" can have a beneficial effect on patients' feelings, beliefs, and behaviors. Conversely, negative statements like "I can't do anything anymore" or "I have so far to walk" arouse feelings of helplessness and inhibit behavioral changes. Suggest that clients write down their self-defeating statements and then change the negative talk to positive talk (e.g., "There's still a lot I *can* do," or "I'm nearly halfway finished") (20,38).

Provide Specific Instructions

For each recommended treatment, use simple, lay language to explain the purpose or benefits, particularly as they relate to the client's identified problems and goals. When rheumatologists made a clear statement about the purpose of a medication, 79% of the patients adhered to the regimen 4 months later, versus an adherence rate of only 33% among those patients who were not given this information (37). To participate actively in their self-management, clients should also be informed about their diagnosis, including test results, dosage and duration of pharmacologic therapy, possible side effects or other drawbacks of recommended treatments, how to judge treatment efficacy, and when to return for follow-up care. Summarize conclusions and instructions at the end of the visit to help the patient retain information. Write down the diagnosis and treatment plan and supplement it with written information, such as Arthritis Foundation patient education publications.

Use Multiple Educational Methods

Because knowledge is necessary but not sufficient to achieve behavior or health status change, the simple provision of verbal instruction or materials should not occupy more than one-third of all education time. Vary the activities in each educational session to include brief lectures, group discussion, brainstorming, problem solving, demonstration and practice opportunities, and other methods that involve the active client participation. Monitor comprehension by asking clients to repeat how they will follow the agreed-upon regimen—what they will do, when, and how often. Have them demonstrate any needed skills.

Pictures and other audiovisuals can reinforce key messages. Install educational posters and charts in the waiting room and in the examination rooms. A bulletin board can be used to display sample educational materials and news about upcoming educational programs. Utilize a lending library with videotapes and books. Anatomical models may help illustrate particular disease information.

Use Behavioral Techniques

When suggesting a treatment, adherence is more likely if the treatment takes into consideration client preferences (35, 36). For example, someone may have a very bad hip but be more concerned about stiff fingers because she is a concert pianist. In this case, attention to the hip, if the hands are ignored, will probably not result in full participation in treatment. Consider suggesting the addition of new behaviors rather than eliminating established behaviors. If weight is a problem, suggest adding some exercise, rather than major dietary changes.

Use the power of credible messengers to deliver messages such as "I want you to start exercising," or "I want you to cut down your fat intake." Find out who your clients consider a credible source of health information. For many people, it is the physician; for others, it may be more appropriate to use a peer educator.

New behaviors can be linked to old behaviors. For example, suggest to an individual that he or she take their medication after brushing their teeth. A stationary bicycle can be used while watching a favorite television program. To motivate people who are unsure about making a recommended change, help decision-making by using a pro and con worksheet to weigh the positive and negative reasons to continue the same behavior versus starting the recommended behavior.

Provide adequate opportunities for practice and repetition of new skills and behaviors over several weeks. Traditional education programs are often given as a lecture series with a different topic each week. This does not give participants the opportunity to try new skills and behaviors, discuss problems, and build new habits. It is better to provide a brief time each week to discuss and practice key skills and behaviors like relaxation techniques or exercise, beginning with simpler tasks and then building in complexity as the program progresses.

Anticipate problems with adherence and maintaining behavioral changes, and plan ways to overcome these problems. Potential barriers can be identified by asking in a non-threatening way: "Many of my clients find it difficult to follow all of their exercise program—what problems do you expect might keep you from doing your exercises as scheduled?" or "Many people miss taking their medication at times—what are some things that might keep you from taking yours?" Adherence can be assessed during follow-up visits by again asking in a non-threatening way how the client did with the targeted behavior and what factors seemed to help or hinder them. The provider may ask questions such as, "Was there any dose you were likely to miss? What did you do when you missed? Did you have any reminders? Did your spouse help or hinder? What made it difficult? Was it harder to do when your symptoms went away? What problems did you have?"

Help Clients Solve Problems

When your clients experience problems, try to avoid giving advice but rather help them problem-solve (38). Teach problem-solving skills by asking: "What have you already tried to solve that problem? What other alternatives do you see? What are the pros and cons of those options? What option do you want to try?"

Build Self-efficacy

Arthritis Self-Management Program evaluations revealed that there was minimal correlation between increased exercise and relaxation behaviors and improved outcomes such as pain and depression. Further research led to the identification of a psychological variable that did correlate strongly with health outcomes. This attribute, *self-efficacy*, is defined as a person's confidence that he or she can perform specific behaviors that will affect disease consequences. Subsequent studies documented that adding strategies to enhance self-efficacy to the ASMP increased the course's effectiveness related to health outcomes (12). Breaking down skills and behaviors into easily mastered components and helping clients reinterpret their symptoms are two ways of enhancing self-efficacy. Other key strategies include short-term goal setting and contracting, feedback, and modeling.

Clients should set realistic, short-term goals to accomplish what they want to achieve. Ask them how much they are doing now and then suggest that they set a goal to just do a little more. Build commitment by having clients write down their goals in a contract. The more specific the contract is, the more likely it is to be followed. Then ask how confident they are that they can carry out their commitment on a scale of 0 (not at all sure) to 10 (totally sure). If clients do not feel confident, help them modify the goal so that it is achievable or problem-solve to address any perceived barriers. Continually monitor progress toward goals and provide praise and positive feedback. Encourage clients to use self-monitoring tools, such as an exercise diary, to keep track of their progress.

Seeing others succeed in similar circumstances is a strong form of educational motivation. This "modeling" can be done by having people with arthritis teach others, as utilized in the ASMP. It can also be achieved by putting people with similar conditions in touch with each other, and by using materials that contain images of people who resemble your clients' ages, sexes, weights, and ethnic groups. In written materials, the use of real-life vignettes is often helpful. Modeling should always be considered when choosing or recommending audiovisual materials such as exercise videotapes. Health professionals also need to ensure that they are being good role models by practicing what they preach regarding exercise, weight control, smoking, and encouraging client involvement.

Help Clients Give and Receive Support

Structure group education classes in such a way that participants actively help others with such things as problem solving, goal setting, and other support as appropriate. The role of the group leader should be a facilitator of group interaction (31). Natural support networks can be nurtured by encouraging involvement of family members and significant others in clinical visits and patient education activities. The telephone is often overlooked as a way to reinforce information and provide support (21–24). Support groups may be helpful, if they are structured to foster mutual support rather than as a lecture series. Another means of fostering support is to utilize "experienced" patients who are successfully managing their disease as mentors for newly diagnosed patients.

Provide a Comfortable Learning Environment

In addition to addressing emotional concerns of the client, it is important to provide as much consistency as possible. The same instructor(s) should be used throughout an educational program, and all instructors should attend all sessions. Without continuity of instructors, continuity of instruction is very difficult. Use ritual as a way of providing security. People feel more in control when they know what to expect and how they are expected to participate. Therefore, each session or contact should have more or less the same structure.

Referral

Time and personal limitations usually prevent any one person from meeting all of the educational needs of someone with arthritis. Referrals do not have to be to other professionals, nor do they have to be disease-specific. Familiarize yourself with the self-management courses, cognitive-behavioral therapy programs, exercise classes, and support groups in your community. While the Arthritis Foundation is an obvious referral choice, other possibilities are senior centers, community exercise classes, videotapes, books, information and referral services, churches, service clubs and internet bulletin boards and news groups. Before referring, make sure that the service is appropriate. Your clients are more likely to use the service if you provide a contact person's name and phone number.

IMPACT OF ARTHRITIS PATIENT EDUCATION

Knowledge

While increased knowledge alone is no longer usually considered an adequate endpoint for patient education programs, the patient's right to informed consent does constitute an important rationale for providing information. Numerous studies document that patients are often inadequately informed (37). Participation in formal arthritis patient education programs can increase knowledge. Two sequential reviews (1,8) described a total of 42 patient education interventions that assessed knowledge change; of these, 36 (86%) reported significant increases in knowledge. Many of the studies included in these reviews showed success in increasing knowledge in long-term patients, indicating the potential for considerable improvement in patient education within clinical practice (4).

Behaviors

In one review, 37 of 48 studies (77%) showed positive behavior changes (1). A review (8) of an additional 34 studies included 29 that reported positive changes. In 12 of these studies, positive changes were of statistical significance. The most successful intervention studies focused on exercise, adherence, self-care behavior, general behavior, pain behavior, relaxation, work simplification practices, or sleep behavior.

Psychosocial Status

Statistically significant positive changes have been reported in depression, helplessness, anxiety, general attitude, self-efficacy, or locus of control (8,10). A meta-analysis of arthritis psychoeducational interventions found that, on average, the experimental groups experienced a 22% improvement in depression over controls (2). In another review, 10 of 14 interventions demonstrated improvement in depression (10), although in most of these studies the effect sizes were small. The largest effect sizes were seen in a study that compared cognitive behavioral therapy and a self-management program.

Health Status

A recent review of arthritis patient education included studies assessing 52 measures of physical health status. Positive change was reported in 40 of these measures, and 27 demonstrated statistically significant changes (8). Variables that were positively impacted included pain, functional disability, work capacity/work and exercise time, count of painful joints, physical activity level, disease activity, general health score, grip strength, quality of life, and stiffness level. In another review, 16 of 20 interventions resulted in reduced pain (10). The studies with the largest effect sizes utilized cognitive behavioral therapy, self-management, and/or support interventions. Ten interventions (out of 15) had a positive, although usually slight, impact on functional ability.

Most of the successful studies utilized a self-management intervention. A meta-analysis showed an average improvement of 16% in pain and 8% in disability in treatment groups versus controls (2). Because the subjects in these studies were already receiving medical care, results suggest that patient education can achieve clinically significant health outcomes over and above traditional medical care. In fact, while clinical studies of rheumatologic care offer 20% to 50% improvement in reported symptoms, patient education studies suggest an additional improvement of up to 30% (8). These findings provide strong support for establishing patient education as an integral part of quality clinical care.

Health Care Utilization and Costs

Data on the impact of arthritis patient education on health care utilization and costs remains limited (4,9). A 4-year follow-up study of ASMP participants showed a 43% decrease in physician visits (13). After subtracting the costs of the course, the 4-year cost benefit was projected to be about $650 per participant with rheumatoid arthritis, and about $190 for each participant with osteoarthritis. The authors further extrapolated that if just 1% of the target population successfully participated in the program, a cumulative, 4-year savings to the economy of $33 million could be achieved.

The annual cost of a telephone intervention for patients with osteoarthritis was estimated to be about $15 per patient (22).

Trained nonmedical personnel made monthly telephone calls to review medications and side effects, to discuss barriers to keeping appointments, and to encourage appropriate questions. Statistically significant improvements were achieved in pain and physical function, at an estimated cost-effectiveness of $31 per 1-unit improvement in pain and $72 per 1-unit change in physical function. Much more research needs to be done to document the economic benefits of patient education in the rheumatic diseases.

TRENDS IN EDUCATIONAL PROJECTS AND RESEARCH

In addition to the need for more cost-benefit studies, four other areas of research are projected to have significant advances in the next decade: theory development and application, design of programs focused on generic disease management (versus treatment-specific) skills, expansion into a broader range of target populations, and testing of new program delivery methods (4).

There is much to learn about the types or combinations of educational interventions that are most effective and which mechanisms contribute to their efficacy. The work on the ASMP and self-efficacy is representative of how a program's theoretic base and theory-based interventions can grow in tandem. More researchers are not only using theoretical constructs such as self-efficacy, coping, and social support in their intervention studies, but they are also publishing descriptions of how to integrate these theory-based intervention strategies into patient education programs and clinical practice (6,20,37,38).

To address the multiple problems associated with chronic conditions, more studies are shifting from treatment-specific content to development of generic skills. Examples include research on ways to improve doctor–patient communication (37) and problem-solving skills (18,39). Some researchers have conducted long-term follow-up studies of their programs, but there has been minimal evidence of long-term changes in pain relief and physical disability. Various types of relapse prevention strategies are being studied to help ensure long-term maintenance of pain coping skills (6), stress management techniques (30) and physical activity (20).

Programs are being targeted to a broader range of people with rheumatic disease, including people with fibromyalgia, osteoporosis, back pain, rarer forms of rheumatic disease, and culturally diverse populations. The Arthritis Foundation disseminates self-management programs specifically designed for people with systemic lupus erythematosus (16) and fibromyalgia. Community-based education and support programs have been developed for rural (27,28) and inner city low-literacy populations (17,23). Programs targeted to African-Americans and Latinos, the First Nations population in Canada, and a Chinese-speaking population have been developed. These projects underscore the necessity of basing programs on the unique needs of these populations, delivering them in community sites familiar to the target audience, and using peer educators representative of the target group.

The need to reach broader audiences and maximize program cost-effectiveness has led to the pilot testing of many alternative methods for program delivery. Telephone intervention was effective in reducing pain and physical disability and/or improving psychological function in a state-wide sample of people with rheumatoid arthritis or osteoarthritis (24) and in an inner city population (21–23). The Bone Up on Arthritis Program, developed for lower-literacy rural residents was originally tested in a small group versus a home study format. In the home study format, participants used audiocassettes and illustrated print materials and received periodic phone contacts from trained "community coordinators" (27). Both formats achieved positive changes in self-care behaviors, pain level, function, helplessness, and depression. However, a stand-alone version of the Bone Up program, in which participants did not receive any supportive phone calls, achieved behavioral changes but not changes in health outcomes.

The effectiveness of ASMP courses taught simultaneously in a studio and transmitted to three remote sites using interactive television was compared to a traditional non-TV control group class that utilized the same curriculum and course leaders (40). Improvement was best within the studio group and was minimal within the remote populations. These studies demonstrate the value of evaluating any changes in delivery mechanisms so that the educational processes can be refined to increase their effectiveness. A 3-week version of the ASMP is currently being evaluated in an effort to make this program more accessible. Alternatively, a computer-tailored self-management program can be delivered through the mail (29).

Efforts have been made to develop computer-assisted education programs. Such programs were found to be effective in producing behavioral changes and improving some health outcomes in people with rheumatoid arthritis (25) and patients undergoing total joint arthroplasty (26). It has also been effective when used to teach stress management techniques (30).

REFERENCES

1. Lorig K, Konkol L, Gonzalez V: Arthritis patient education: a review of the literature. Patient Educ Couns 10:207–252, 1987
2. Mullen PD, Laville EA, Biddle AK, Lorig K: Efficacy of psychoeducational interventions on pain, depression, and disability in people with arthritis: a meta-analysis. J Rheumatol 14 (Suppl 15):33–39, 1987
3. Tucker M, Kirwan JR: Does patient education in rheumatoid arthritis have therapeutic potential? Ann Rheum Dis 50 (suppl 3):422–428, 1991
4. Daltroy LH, Liang MH: Arthritis education: opportunities and state of the art. Health Educ Q 20:3–16, 1993
5. DeVellis RF, Blalock SJ: Psychological and educational interventions to reduce arthritis disability. Baillieres Clin Rheumatol 7:397–416, 1993
6. Keefe FJ, Van Horn Y: Cognitive-behavioral treatment of rheumatoid arthritis pain: maintaining treatment gains. Arthritis Care Res 6:213–222, 1993
7. Parker JC, Iverson GL, Smarr KL, Stucky-Ropp RC: Cognitive-behavioral approaches to pain management in rheumatoid arthritis. Arthritis Care Res 6:207–212, 1993
8. Hirano PC, Laurent DD, Lorig K: Arthritis patient education studies, 1987–1991: a review of the literature. Patient Educ Couns 24:9–54, 1994
9. Mazzuca SA: Economic evaluation of arthritis patient education. Bull Rheum Dis 43:6–8, 1994
10. Hawley DJ: Psycho-educational interventions in the treatment of arthritis. Baillieres Clin Rheumatol 9:803–823, 1995
11. Burckhardt CS: Arthritis and musculoskeletal patient education standards. Arthritis Care Res 7:1–4, 1994
12. Lorig K, Gonzalez V: The integration of theory with practice: a 12-year case study. Health Educ Q 19:355–368, 1992
13. Lorig K, Holman H: Arthritis self-management studies: a twelve-year review. Health Educ Q 20:17–28, 1993
14. Taal E, Riemsma RP, Brus HL, Seydel ER, Rasker JJ, Wiegman O: Group education for patients with rheumatoid arthritis. Patient Educ Couns 20:177–187, 1993
15. Lindroth Y, Bauman A, Brooks PM, Priestley D: A 5-year follow-up of a

16. Braden CJ: Patterns of change over time in learned response to chronic illness among participants in a systemic lupus erythematosus self-help course. Arthritis Care Res 4:158–167, 1991
17. Bill-Harvey D, Rippey R, Abeles M, et al: Outcome of an osteoarthritis education program for low-literacy patients taught by indigenous instructors. Patient Educ Couns 20:167–175, 1989
18. Perlman SG, Connell KJ, Clark A, et al: Dance-based aerobic exercise for rheumatoid arthritis. Arthritis Care Res 3:29–35, 1990
19. Minor MA, Brown JD: Exercise maintenance of persons with arthritis after participation in a class experience. Health Educ Q 20:83–95, 1993
20. Allegrante JP, Kovar PA, MacKenzie CR, Peterson MG, Gutin B: A walking education program for patients with osteoarthritis of the knee: theory and intervention strategies. Health Educ Q 20:63–81, 1993
21. René J, Weinberger M, Mazzuca SA, Brandt KD, Katz BP: Reduction of joint pain in patients with knee osteoarthritis who have received monthly telephone calls from lay personnel and whose medical treatment regimens have remained stable. Arthritis Rheum 35:511–515, 1992
22. Weinberger M, Tierney WM, Cowper PA, Katz BP, Booher PA: Cost-effectiveness of increased telephone contact for patients with osteoarthritis: a randomized, controlled trial. Arthritis Rheum 36:243–246, 1993
23. Mazzuca SA, Brandt KD, Katz BP, Chambers M, Stewart KD, Byrd DJ, Hanna M: Self-care education improves the health status of inner-city patients with osteoarthritis of the knee (abstract). Arthritis Rheum 38 (suppl 9):S269, 1995
24. Maisiak RS, Austin JS, Heck L: A controlled comparison of the effect of two interventions on the health status of rheumatoid arthritis or osteoarthritis patients (abstract). Arthritis Rheum 38 (suppl 9):S383, 1995
25. Wetstone SL, Sheehan TJ, Votaw RG, et al: Evaluation of a computer based education lesson for patients with rheumatoid arthritis. J Psychol 12:907–912, 1985
26. Reisine S, Lewis C: Impact of a structured computer assisted patient education program in total joint arthroplasty (abstract). Arthritis Care Res 6:S3, 1993
27. Goeppinger J, Arthur MW, Baglioni AJ Jr, et al: A reexamination of the effectiveness of self-care education for persons with arthritis. Arthritis Rheum 32:706–716, 1989
28. Goeppinger J, Macnee C, Anderson MK, Boutaugh ML, Stewart K: From research to practice: the effects of the jointly sponsored dissemination of an arthritis self-care nursing intervention. Appl Nurs Res 8:106–113, 1995
29. Gale FM, Kirk JC, Davis R: Patient education and self-management: randomized study of effects on health status of a mail-delivered program (abstract). Arthritis Rheum 37 (suppl 9):S197, 1994
30. Parker JC, Smarr KL, Buckelew SP, Stucky-Ropp RC, Hewett JE, Johnson JC, Wright GE, Irvin WS, Walker SE: Effects of stress management on clinical outcomes in rheumatoid arthritis. Arthritis Rheum 38:1807–1818, 1995
31. Lanza AF, Revenson RA: Social support interventions for rheumatoid arthritis patients: the cart before the horse? Health Educ Q 20:97–117, 1993
32. Green LW, Kreuter MW: Health Education Planning: A Diagnostic Approach. Mountain View, CA, Mayfield Publishing Co., 1991
33. Corbin J, Strauss A: Unending Work and Care. San Francisco, Jossey-Bass Publishers, 1988
34. Falvo DR: Effective Patient Education: A Guide to Increased Compliance. Rockville, MD, Aspen Publications, 1985
35. Lorig K, et al: Patient Education: A Practical Approach. Second edition. Thousand Oaks, CA, Sage Publications, 1996
36. Jensen GM, Lorish CD: Promoting patient cooperation with exercise programs: linking research, theory, and practice. Arthritis Care Res 7:181–189, 1994
37. Daltroy LH: Doctor-patient communication in rheumatological disorders. Baillieres Clin Rheumatol 7:221–239, 1993
38. Gonzalez VM, Goeppinger J, Lorig K: Four psychosocial theories and their application to patient education and clinical practice. Arthritis Care Res 3:132–143, 1990
39. DeVellis RF, Blalock SJ, Hahn PM, et al: Evaluation of a problem-solving intervention for patients with arthritis. Patient Educ Couns 11:29–42, 1988
40. Hawley D: Increasing the dissemination of the Arthritis Self-Management Course: a controlled experiment with interactive television: follow-up results at 1 year (abstract). Arthritis Care Res 7:S11, 1994

controlled trial of an arthritis education programme. Br J Rheumatol 34:647–652, 1995

Cognitive Behavioral Interventions

FRANCIS J. KEEFE, PhD; and DAVID S. CALDWELL, MD

Persons with rheumatic diseases may be similar in disease severity yet vary substantially in their pain, physical disability, and psychological disability. A rheumatoid arthritis (RA) patient, for example, who feels unable to cope with their disease and who has little social support from friends or family may report severe pain and become quite disabled in the face of mild to moderate disease. Another patient with the same degree of disease severity may complain little of pain and lead an active and productive life. Such variations in response to rheumatic disease cannot be explained by biomedical models which tend to view arthritis pain and disability as primarily due to disease activity. Newly developed cognitive-behavioral models maintain that cognitive factors (that is, beliefs, coping strategies, or appraisals) and behavioral factors (home or work environment) may be just as important as biomedical factors in understanding how individuals adjust to chronic diseases. These models have led to innovative treatments that have been shown in recent controlled studies to be effective in managing pain and disability in individuals with rheumatic disease (1,2).

ELEMENTS OF COGNITIVE BEHAVIORAL THERAPY

Cognitive behavioral therapy for rheumatic disease patients has three basic elements: a rationale for treatment, coping skills training, and training in methods for maintenance of coping skills in order to prevent setbacks in coping efforts.

Rationale for Treatment

The rationale for cognitive behavioral therapy should be introduced at the start of treatment, prior to any training in pain coping skills. The rationale is designed to educate patients about the influence that cognitive and behavioral factors can have on pain and other arthritis symptoms. It emphasizes the role that coping skills can play in managing symptoms and reducing physical and psychological disability. Finally, it enhances a sense of control over the disease.

Most cognitive behavioral therapy programs use an adaptation model to help patients understand the interrelationships between arthritis symptoms and patterns of adjustment. To introduce this model, patients are typically asked to describe how the symptoms of their rheumatic disease, such as pain, stiffness, or fatigue, have affected the behavioral, cognitive, and affective areas of functioning. Patients often can identify a variety of problematic behaviors (e.g., reduced tolerance for activities, decreased involvement in pleasurable activities, and increased dependence on others), cognitions (negative thoughts about self, others, and the future), and affective responses (depression, guilt, or anxiety). In discussions with patients, the emphasis is on increasing awareness of how problematic pat-

terns develop and are learned over time, as well as on helping patients recognize the connections between their thoughts, feelings, and behaviors.

An important tenet of the cognitive-behavioral model is that learned patterns of adjustment can be changed by learning new cognitive and behavioral coping skills. Patients are systematically trained to use a variety of cognitive coping skills such as imagery and cognitive restructuring, and behavioral coping skills such as activity-pacing and goal setting. Cognitive behavioral therapy thus encourages patients to take an active role in managing and controlling their symptoms and disease. While this type of therapy is effective in reducing pain and related symptoms, it will not allow patients to achieve total control over a rheumatic disease such as RA. In providing a treatment rationale, the therapist helps patients understand that they can increase their ability to control symptoms while acknowledging that, at times, there may be disease flares and symptoms that are beyond their control.

Coping Skills Training

In cognitive behavioral therapy, each treatment session is structured to maximize the learning of cognitive and behavioral coping skills. The individual is first instructed in a coping skill and is guided by the therapist through a brief practice session. After the practice session, the therapist provides corrective feedback and suggestions for applying the skill in controlling arthritis symptoms. Coping skills are practiced in order of difficulty, starting with the least difficult (e.g., relaxation training) and proceeding to the more difficult and complex (cognitive restructuring).

A hallmark of cognitive behavioral therapy is that it provides training in a variety of coping skills. The skills are grouped together on a list or "menu" to highlight the fact that patients have multiple coping options and can mix and match skills to deal with different problems.

Relaxation Training. Relaxation training is one of the most important and basic coping skills for rheumatic disease patients. Relaxation training is typically introduced early, because it is easy to learn and is effective in controlling patients' symptoms. Training in relaxation methods provides several benefits. First, it can reduce muscle tension that may contribute to pain or tension. Second, it helps make people more aware of increases in their level of tension so that they can intervene early before tension causes increased pain or fatigue. Third, when patients relax they are able to shift their attention away from arthritis symptoms, which often reduces pain. Finally, learning to relax can improve patients' abilities to rest and sleep.

Although there are a variety of methods for teaching relaxation, including meditation, autogenic training, and biofeedback, most cognitive behavioral training programs use a progressive relaxation method similar to that of Bernstein and Borkovec (3). Progressive relaxation involves a series of exercises in which individuals are asked to alternately tense and relax major muscle groups throughout the body. The exercises focus on muscles in the legs, arms, trunk, shoulders, neck, and face. The patient repeats each exercise slowly while attending to the sensations that accompany tension and relaxation. Instructions are often recorded, and patients are encouraged to listen to the 15 to 20 minute audiotape twice a day. After 2 to 3 weeks of daily practice, most arthritis patients show an excellent ability to relax when in a quiet and comfortable environment. Training then shifts to the application of learned relaxation skills to more physically demanding activities such as walking or climbing stairs. Patients can be taught abbreviated relaxation methods in which they briefly (for 30 seconds) scan major muscle groups, identifying and then relaxing any areas of excessive tension. These abbreviated methods can be done while the patient is engaged in other activities such as eating, talking on the phone, or driving, and they provide an excellent means of generalizing the benefits of relaxation to a variety of home and work activities.

Imagery Training. Imagery is a useful method of diverting attention away from pain and other rheumatic disease symptoms. Imagery is often introduced early in cognitive behavioral therapy as an adjunct to relaxation training. Many types of imagery are used, but probably the most common is pleasant imagery, for example, imagining oneself reclining on a sunny beach. The instructions for pleasant imagery emphasize the need to focus on the imagined scene for a specific period of time (usually a few minutes) and encourage the individual to involve as many sensory modalities as possible. For example, the patient would try to imagine feeling the warmth of the sand on the beach, seeing the blue sky, hearing the sounds of the waves breaking and seagulls flying overhead, and even tasting the slight salty taste that might be on one's lips after a brief swim. It is important to emphasize that the patient is in control of the image. He or she can select an appropriate scene and can switch to a new scene or stop focusing on the image whenever they want. This reduces patients' concerns that the therapist is controlling their thoughts or hypnotizing them. Asking patients to close their eyes and relax deeply usually helps them concentrate more fully on the imagery.

Activity–Rest Cycling. Patients with rheumatic diseases often have difficulty pacing their activities. Many patients report a cycle in which they overdo daily activities, experience increased pain and fatigue, and then require a prolonged period of rest to recover. When this cycle is repeated over the course of months and years, it has many negative consequences, including a decreased tolerance for activity, a belief that one is incapable of being active, and a tendency towards a restricted lifestyle that provides few diversions from pain or other symptoms. Activity–rest cycling is designed to break this maladaptive pattern by teaching patients to plan their daily schedule so that moderate periods of activity are followed by limited periods of rest (see Chapter 12, Rest and Exercise, and Chapter 15, Enhancing Functional Ability). For example, a patient with RA who experiences severe joint pain after 2 hours of working at a computer terminal can plan to type no longer than 30 minutes before taking a 5-minute break. Over a period of weeks the duration of the activity phase of the cycle is gradually increased (e.g., from 30 to 40 and then 50 minutes of typing) and the rest phase of the cycle is decreased (from 5 to 2 to 1 minutes). This enables patients to gradually increase their

Table 1. Recording form: three column method.

Situation	Automatic Thoughts	Feelings
Flare in my arthritis	It is hopeless, I am never going to get better	Depressed and discouraged

activity without increasing their symptoms. Benefits of using the activity–rest cycle include a reduction in pain and fatigue, increased tolerance for activities of daily living, and an enhanced sense of control over rheumatic disease symptoms.

Cognitive Restructuring. In cognitive restructuring, patients are taught to identify, challenge, and modify negative automatic thoughts that may contribute to increased pain or emotional distress. Individuals with rheumatic disease who are depressed, anxious, or have severe pain typically have negative thoughts about themselves, others, and the future. These negative thoughts represent how persons view their situation, and do not reflect the actual situation. When erroneous and distorted, these thoughts can trigger emotional responses such as depression or anxiety. The goal of cognitive restructuring is to help patients become aware of negative thoughts and to restructure their underlying attitudes and beliefs. Because the negative thoughts occur spontaneously for brief periods of time, patients need to systematically monitor them. A common form of monitoring is the three-column method that asks patients to record the situation, their thoughts, and feelings (Table 1). Patients are encouraged to recognize the connection between the situations, their automatic thoughts, and their feelings. The therapist works with the patient to examine the evidence for negative thoughts and to develop alternative ways of appraising the situation, such as "I've been through flares in the past. They are difficult, but I know my symptoms will improve with time." When patients change their negative automatic thoughts, they report substantial improvements in mood. They are also better able to adhere to and maintain the use of other cognitive and behavioral coping skills.

Training in Maintenance Enhancement Methods

The daily use of coping strategies appears to be an important mediator of the long-term outcome of cognitive behavioral therapy. Patients with RA who use coping skills frequently have had much better outcomes 12 months after completing cognitive behavioral training than those who did not (4). However, individuals who are faced with flares in disease activity or other stressful life events may question the effectiveness of their coping abilities and may reduce or curtail their coping efforts. To prevent such setbacks, most cognitive behavioral programs include some training in maintenance enhancement methods. Comprehensive training in maintenance enhancement has been used to prevent relapse from disorders such as smoking, obesity, and alcoholism and has recently been extended to rheumatic disease patients (5).

These programs have several important features. First, they use cognitive therapy methods to increase patient awareness of potential relapse situations. These methods include developing a list of high-risk situations likely to lead to setbacks, identifying early warning signs of relapse, and cognitively rehearsing how one might cope with different relapse situations. Second, maintenance enhancement programs use behavioral rehearsal to develop a sense of self-efficacy in managing arthritis symptoms. In behavioral rehearsal, the patient identifies a high-risk situation that might lead to a setback or relapse, such as a stressful life event. The therapist models coping strategies that could be used, has the patient rehearse these strategies, and then provides feedback. Finally, maintenance enhancement emphasizes training in self-control skills in order to maintain frequent practice of coping skills. Patients may be taught how to use diaries and calendars to monitor important target behaviors, such as the frequency of relaxation practice or early warning signs of a setback. They are also trained to use self-reinforcement to reward the appropriate use and practice of coping skills.

OUTCOMES OF COGNITIVE BEHAVIORAL THERAPY

Controlled studies have evaluated the efficacy of cognitive behavioral therapy in rheumatic disease patients. The design of most of these studies is similar. Patients are randomly assigned to cognitive behavioral training or one or more control conditions. The cognitive behavioral interventions are typically carried out in group sessions that last from 1.5 to 2 hours for 6 to 10 weeks. Outcome is evaluated using a comprehensive set of pain, physical disability, and psychological disability measures administered before and after treatment. Many studies have included a long-term follow-up assessment in order to evaluate the maintenance of therapeutic improvements.

Several controlled studies have documented the efficacy of cognitive behavioral training in the management of RA. Patients receiving this training have shown significant reductions in pain, pain behavior, anxiety, and depression compared to patients in a social support control condition (6). Persons with RA undergoing cognitive behavioral therapy have also been found to improve significantly in terms of pain relief, coping, and function (4,7). Long-term follow-up studies (4,8) have revealed that many patients are able to maintain these gains over 12 months. Long-term improvements in pain and functional status are most apparent in patients who continued to practice coping skills on a frequent basis (4).

Controlled research has also examined effects of cognitive behavioral interventions in osteoarthritis (OA) patients. Research conducted in our lab has demonstrated that cognitive behavioral training is more effective than an arthritis education condition and standard care control condition in reducing pain and psychological disability in patients with OA of the knees (9). An intervention that combined cognitive behavioral training with educational information about arthritis has been tested in a large sample of patients, 85% of whom had OA (10). Results indicated significant reductions in pain and psychological disability. A follow-up study of these patients found that they were able to maintain improvements in pain and depression up to 4 years after completing treatment (11).

The effects of cognitive behavioral training on fibromyalgia have only recently been evaluated in controlled studies. The most recent and most rigorously controlled study compared the separate and combined effects of a cognitive behavioral intervention (biofeedback and relaxation training) and exercise training program (12). At the end of treatment, subjects in the cognitive behavioral, exercise, and combined cognitive behavioral/exercise groups showed improvements in one or more outcomes relative to an educational control condition. However, at follow-up, only the combined cognitive behavioral/exercise group maintained key improvements relative to the control group. This study suggests that, for certain pain conditions, combining cognitive behavioral therapy with other pain management interventions such as exercise may enhance the long-term effects of treatment.

PATIENT REFERRAL

Cognitive behavioral therapists are typically clinical psychologists who have graduate training in cognitive and behavioral psychology and who are experienced in working with medical patients. Cognitive behavioral therapy is one of the most popular techniques, thus, many teaching hospitals have trained therapists on their faculty or staff. Many of the psychologists listed in the membership directory of the Association of Rheumatology Health Professionals, a division of the American College of Rheumatology, have experience in and accept referrals for cognitive behavioral training. The directory is available by writing to the American College of Rheumatology. The Association for the Advancement of Behavior Therapy (305 Seventh Avenue, New York, NY 10001-6008, (212) 647-1890) also maintains a referral service for the general public that can provide the names of cognitive behavioral therapists in the patient's area along with a pamphlet offering guidelines on choosing a therapist.

Many patients with rheumatic disease are reluctant to accept a referral to a psychologist or mental health professional, because they view this as a sign that their symptoms are not being taken seriously. Thus, it is important to prepare the patient before making the referral. Individuals should be reassured about the reality of their diagnosis and symptoms and told that cognitive behavioral training is designed to help them cope with their disease. It may be helpful to emphasize that cognitive behavioral therapy focuses on coping in the "here and now" and does not dwell on early childhood conflicts or underlying unconscious conflicts. We usually encourage patients who are skeptical or otherwise concerned about the therapy to pursue treatment on a three-session trial basis. At the end of the trial, most patients have become quite involved in treatment and choose to continue.

Several skills used in cognitive behavioral training are also taught at an introductory level in the Arthritis Self-Help Course developed by the Arthritis Foundation, which may provide another option for referral. After completing the course, patients who require additional intervention can be referred to a therapist who has more extensive formal training in cognitive behavioral therapy.

COGNITIVE BEHAVIORAL THERAPY AND ONGOING MEDICAL TREATMENT

Cognitive behavioral therapy is designed to complement the medical treatment of rheumatic diseases, not replace it. Although some patients may reduce their use of pain medications during treatment, most patients continue with important components of their treatment regimen such as the use of medications or physical therapy.

Cognitive behavioral training methods may actually be useful in enhancing rheumatic disease patients' adherence to medical regimens. Consider, for example, the RA patient who becomes depressed during a major disease flare and decides to stop taking medicine. By applying coping methods such as cognitive restructuring and relaxation, the patient may be able to calm himself or herself, reduce emotional distress, and make a more rational choice about the need for arthritis medication.

Some rheumatic disease patients tend to consider their symptoms from either a purely medical or purely psychological viewpoint. Patients who see their disease as simply a medical problem are willing to pursue medical treatment options, but view psychological treatments as irrelevant. Conversely, patients who respond quite well to psychologically based treatments may downplay the significance of medical treatments. To circumvent this problem it is important to help patients adopt a biobehavioral model of their disease. Such a model acknowledges the relevance of both biological and behavioral factors in the understanding and treatment of disease.

Gate Control Theory

In our work on arthritis pain management, we have used a simplified version of the gate control theory (13) to help patients adopt a more biobehavioral perspective. We begin by drawing a schematic diagram that illustrates basic elements of the traditional pain pathway, such as pain receptors in a joint, a neural pathway through the spinal cord, and sensory centers in the brain. We then discuss how this traditional model of pain sensation fails to account for many clinical phenomena such as the persistence of pain after amputation, the absence of pain during sports or wartime injuries, or the fact that surgical interruption of the pathway often fails to abolish persistent pain.

The gate control theory is then introduced as an alternative explanation. This theory maintains that there is a gating mechanism in the spinal cord, which regulates the flow of neural impulses from the site of disease or injury to the brain. When the gate is closed, pain signals are blocked at the level of the spinal cord and thus do not reach the brain. When the gate is open, however, the signals are free to pass through to centers of the brain responsible for pain sensation. Research findings indicate that centers of the brain responsible for cognition (e.g., thoughts, memories, and expectations) and emotions (e.g., depression, anxiety) can influence whether the gate is open or closed. (Basic research examining the influence of psychological factors on pain physiology has been reviewed recently in 14.) The role of the patient's own coping efforts in controlling problematic cognitive and emotional responses is then discussed. Arthritis patients respond quite positively to the gate control theory and report that it helps them better understand the connections between cognitive behavioral interventions and their own disease symptoms.

INVOLVEMENT OF FAMILY

It is important to remember that patients have symptoms that occur in a social context. The way that a spouse or family member responds to the individual can have an important impact on treatment outcome. There has been growing interest in involving spouses or significant others in cognitive behavioral treatment programs. Involving these individuals may help

the patient acquire coping skills, increase the frequency of coping skills practice, and enhance treatment outcome.

When the patient's spouse or family is included in treatment, it is important to have them actively participate rather than passively observe the treatment process. The spouse, for example, can be taught relaxation techniques along with the patient, and the couple then can be encouraged to practice together at least once a week. Family members can also be encouraged to prompt and reinforce the use of coping skills. A family member could accompany the patient to an exercise session and encourage the patient to use activity–rest cycling to pace their exercise or to use imagery techniques to reduce pain or stiffness following vigorous exercise. Training in communication skills can be provided to help patients and family members communicate more effectively about newly learned coping techniques.

Although there are few controlled studies on the effects of involving spouses or family members in cognitive behavioral training programs for arthritis, available evidence suggests that this approach may be quite effective. For example, some of the greatest effects of cognitive behavioral training on pain and pain behavior were obtained in a study (8) that incorporated spouses or family members in the treatment program. Only one published study (15) has directly compared a spouse/family assisted cognitive behavioral intervention with an arthritis information control condition that involved a spouse or family member. Results indicated that the spouse/family assisted cognitive behavioral intervention was significantly more effective in reducing the severity of pain and number of swollen joints.

USE AS AN EARLY INTERVENTION

Patients are usually referred for cognitive behavioral therapy late in the course of their disease. Most published studies have been conducted with patients with disease duration of 6 to 12 years. This therapy need not, and probably should not, be reserved as a treatment of last resort. Early intervention with cognitive behavioral training could have many benefits in the management of rheumatic disease patients, such as reducing pain and emotional distress, enhancing the effects of ongoing treatment, improving treatment adherence, and possibly altering disease course.

Although cognitive behavioral therapy is relatively new, it represents an important addition to the list of therapeutic strategies for managing rheumatic diseases.

REFERENCES

1. Keefe, FJ, Dunsmore J, Burnett R: Behavioral and cognitive-behavioral approaches to chronic pain: recent advances and future directions. J Consult Clin Psychol 60:528–536, 1992
2. Young LD: Psychological factors in rheumatoid arthritis. J Consult Clin Psychol 60:619–627, 1992
3. Bernstein DA, Borkovec TD: Progressive Relaxation Training: A Manual for the Helping Professions. Champaign, IL, Research Press, 1973
4. Parker JC, Frank RG, Beck NC, et al: Pain management in rheumatoid arthritis patients: a cognitive-behavioral approach. Arthritis Rheum 31: 593–601, 1988
5. Keefe FJ, Van Horn Y: Cognitive-behavioral treatment of rheumatoid arthritis pain: maintaining treatment gains. Arthritis Care Res 6:213–222, 1993
6. Bradley LA, Young LD, Anderson KO, et al: Effects of psychological

therapy on pain behavior of rheumatoid arthritis patients: treatment outcome and six-month followup. Arthritis Rheum 30:1105–1114, 1987

7. Applebaum KA, Blanchard EB, Hickling EJ, Alfonso M: Cognitive behavioral treatment of a veteran population with moderate to severe rheumatoid arthritis. Behav Ther 19:489–502, 1988

8. Bradley LA, Young LD, Anderson KO, Turner RA, Agudelo CA, McDaniel LK, Semple E: Effects of cognitive-behavior therapy on rheumatoid arthritis pain behavior: one year follow-up. In, Pain Research and Clinical Management, 3 (Proceedings of the Vth World Congress on Pain). Edited by R Dubner, G Gebhart, M Bond. Amsterdam, Elsevier, 1988, pp. 310–314

9. Keefe FJ, Caldwell DS, Williams DA, Gil KM, Mitchell D, Robertson D, Roberston C, Martinez S, Nunley J, Beckham JC, Helms M: Pain coping skills training in the management of osteoarthritic knee pain: a comparative study. Behav Ther 21:49–62, 1990

10. Lorig K, Lubeck D, Kraines RG, Seleznick M, Holman HR: Outcomes of self-help education for patients with arthritis. Arthritis Rheum 28:680–685, 1985

11. Holman H, Mazonson P, Lorig K: Health education for self-management has significant early and sustained benefits in chronic arthritis. Trans Assoc Am Phys 102:204–208, 1989

12. Buckelew SP, Parker JC, Conway R, Kay DR, Minor MA, Hewett JE, Johnson J, Peterson J: The effects of biofeedback and exercise on fibromyalgia: a controlled trial. Arch Phys Med Rehabil 73:P-980, 1992

13. Melzack R, Wall P: Pain mechanisms: a new theory. Science 50:971–979, 1965

14. Melzack R: The Challenge of Pain. London, Penguin Press, 1996

15. Radjovec V, Nicassio PM, Weisman MH: Behavioral intervention with and without family support for rheumatoid arthritis. Behav Ther 23:13–30, 1992

Pharmacologic Interventions

DONALD R. MILLER, PharmD

There are many drugs available to treat rheumatic disease; often several are used concurrently. These drugs provide varying degrees of symptomatic benefit, but none provide a cure or permanent alteration in disease. In recent years, the toxicity of nonsteroidal anti-inflammatory drugs (NSAIDs) and the long-term ineffectiveness of "disease-modifying" drugs have been recognized, leading to confusion about, and reassessment of, the proper use of antirheumatic drugs. Consequently, their use may vary from physician to physician, depending on their experience and comfort with the various drugs (1). Health care professionals should recognize the expected therapeutic and adverse effects of antirheumatic drugs so they can participate in patient assessment and monitoring. Medications are only part of the management of rheumatic disease; nonpharmacologic interventions also play a critical role.

All medications have potential benefits as well as potential adverse effects. The decision to use any drug is based on the expected ratio of risk versus benefit in a specific patient. In general, the safest possible drug should be used, unless the desired benefit can only be obtained by using a riskier therapy. Drugs should be used in adequate doses and for a long enough time to see benefits before changing or adding another. Some drugs require 3 to 6 months to show full efficacy. Successful therapy may involve a combination of drugs with different mechanisms of action and toxicities. Finally, the intensity of treatment should reflect the type and severity of arthritis. It is inappropriate to use corticosteroids in osteoarthritis (OA), for example, but they may be essential in dealing with life-threatening complications of systemic lupus erythematosus (SLE).

Traditionally, drug therapy in rheumatoid arthritis (RA) began with NSAIDs, and additional drugs were added one at a time, based on their apparent risk/benefit ratio (the "pyramid" approach). More recently, many authors have advocated more aggressive strategies, such as early use of multiple drugs, aimed at halting the disease process as early as possible (2). It has yet to be determined whether these more aggressive strategies will be superior to the old.

ANALGESICS

Because a cardinal manifestation of all types of arthritis is pain, analgesic drugs play a central role in therapy. Analgesics alone are the therapeutic mainstay in noninflammatory arthritis such as OA, but they are insufficient when inflammation is prominent. Only a limited number of pure analgesic drugs are available.

Acetaminophen

One of the safest drugs available, acetaminophen is known by several nonprescription brand names, including Tylenol®, Panadol® and Anacin-3®. The usual dose is 650 to 975 mg up to 4 times daily. Higher doses are usually well tolerated, but may increase risk of liver toxicity with no increase in benefit. Acetaminophen does not cause gastrointestinal bleeding and has almost no toxicity in recommended doses. It can be used alone to treat OA or can be used as an adjunct to NSAIDs and other drugs. Unfortunately, there is a ceiling to its analgesic effect. Also, acetaminophen has no anti-inflammatory effect.

Narcotics

Weak narcotic drugs such as propoxyphene (Darvon®), codeine, and oxycodone (Percodan®, Percocet®), are frequently used as adjunct therapy. They reduce the perception of pain in the central nervous system. Thus, their mechanism of action is different from, and complementary to, the peripheral mechanism of other analgesics. Occasional doses may induce sleepiness, dizziness, or constipation but otherwise are safe for short-term use. Regular narcotic use is controversial due to the potential for physical and psychological dependence. Regular use of these drugs should be based on the severity of pain, lack of effect of other drugs, and a clear understanding by the patient of permissible maximum daily doses. With careful supervision, use of these drugs sometimes may be a reasonable option.

Capsaicin

Capsaicin, available in a topical cream in 0.025%, 0.075% and 0.25% concentrations (Zostrix®, Dolorac® and others), is a derivative of red chili peppers that depletes peripheral sensory nerves of a neurotransmitter called substance P. Initially capsaicin causes stinging or burning sensations as it displaces substance P. After a few days, however, pain perception is reduced. Studies in patients with OA have shown that capsaicin can decrease pain by about 40% when applied to specific joints four times daily for a month (3).

NONSTEROIDAL ANTI-INFLAMMATORY DRUGS

The NSAIDs are a large group of drugs that have peripheral analgesic and anti-inflammatory effects. These drugs are often divided into several classes based on chemical category, but such classification is arbitrary and is not helpful in choosing a specific drug. The similarities between drugs far outweigh the minor differences. The prototype NSAID is aspirin (acetylsalicylic acid), which is converted to salicylic acid shortly after absorption. Several other nonacetylated, salicylate derivatives are also available. These differ from aspirin in their inability to

Table 1. Nonsteroidal anti-inflammatory drugs.

	Daily Dose Range (mg)	Doses/Day
Salicylates (Brand Name)		
Aspirin	2400–6000	3 to 4
Salsalate (Disalcid)	1500–3000	2 to 3
Choline salicylate (Arthropan)	2600–4350	3 to 5
Magnesium salicylate (Magan)	2400–4800	3 to 4
Choline magnesium trisalicylate (Trilisate)	1500–3000	2 to 3
Other NSAIDs (Brand Name)		
Diclofenac (Voltaren)	100–150	2 to 3
Diflunisal (Dolobid)	500–1000	2
Etodolac (Lodine)	600–1200	2 to 4
Fenoprofen (Nalfon)	1200–3200	3 to 4
Flurbiprofen (Ansaid)	200–300	2 to 3
Ibuprofen (Motrin)	1200–3200	3 to 4
Indomethacin (Indocin)	50–150	3 to 4
Ketoprofen (Orudis, Oruvail)	150–300	3 to 4
Meclofenamic Acid (Meclomen)	200–400	3 to 4
Nabumetone (Relafen)	1000–2000	1
Naproxen (Naprosyn)	500–1500	2 to 3
Oxaprozin (Daypro)	1200–1800	1
Phenylbutazone (Butazolidin)	200–400	2 to 4
Piroxicam (Feldene)	20	1
Sulindac (Clinoril)	200–300	2
Tolmetin (Tolectin)	1200–2400	3 to 4

inhibit prostaglandin synthesis. A complete list of NSAIDs currently available in the U.S. is provided in Table 1.

Most NSAIDs inhibit the enzyme cyclo-oxygenase, which converts a precursor molecule into various prostaglandins. Prostaglandins are ubiquitous, locally synthesized chemicals that have a role in inflammation as well as numerous other body processes. The nonspecific inhibition of prostaglandin synthesis throughout the body explains the wide range of adverse effects caused by NSAIDs. However, the nonacetylated salicylates are very weak inhibitors of prostaglandin synthesis.

The analgesic action of NSAIDs occurs at lower doses than anti-inflammatory effects. Thus, low doses may be adequate in OA. The analgesia occurs peripherally by inhibition of prostaglandin synthesis. Prostaglandins sensitize afferent sensory nerves to the effect of pain-inducing chemical stimuli. Anti-inflammatory effects of NSAIDs occur near the high end of their dosage range. The anti-inflammatory mechanism may be due to several effects. In addition to inhibiting prostaglandin synthesis, NSAIDs have multiple independent effects such as altering macrophage and neutrophil function (4). Although NSAIDs provide symptomatic relief of arthritis, they have no effect on underlying disease processes. This is one reason why many physicians start additional drug therapy at early stages of rheumatic disease.

When NSAIDs are compared in clinical trials, there is little difference between them in effectiveness or tolerance. None is superior to aspirin in efficacy. However, patient response is variable and highly individual. A patient may respond to one drug in the class despite no benefit from another. This unpredictability means that drug selection is essentially a trial and error process. To prevent patients from becoming discouraged, they may be told at the onset that several drugs may have to be tried before finding one that is effective. Although pain relief is obtained quickly with NSAIDs, it may take 2 to 4 weeks before full anti-inflammatory effect is achieved. Thus, patients

are usually given a 1-month trial before deciding to alter therapy.

Two areas in which NSAIDs differ are duration of action and frequency of dosing. Longer-acting drugs may be useful for patients who have difficulty remembering to take frequent doses. All NSAIDs are well absorbed. Taking with food may delay, but does not reduce absorption. Normally, NSAIDs are taken with meals to reduce gastrointestinal (GI) distress. Another area in which these drugs differ significantly is cost (4). Because they are comparably effective, it is reasonable to try a lower cost NSAID or a generic version before moving to more expensive drugs.

Gastrointestinal complaints are the most common problem with NSAIDs. Nausea and abdominal complaints may be reduced by taking medication with food. These drugs also cause gastric and duodenal bleeding, but objective signs of bleeding do not correlate with subjective patient complaints. All NSAIDs may cause GI bleeding and ulcers. This may be due to two separate effects. First, almost all NSAIDs are weak acids capable of disrupting GI mucosa by direct topical actions. This effect may be reduced by putting an enteric (delayed release) coating on the drug tablet, or by giving nonacidic NSAIDs. Second, NSAIDs inhibit synthesis of prostaglandins in the GI tract, rendering it less able to protect and repair itself.

Some NSAIDs may cause ulcers less commonly than others. In large population-based surveillance studies, nonacetylated salicylates, ibuprofen, and enteric-coated forms of aspirin appear safer (5). In theory, sulindac and nabumetone, which are nonacidic "pro-drugs" (not in pharmacologically active form when swallowed) should be safer. However, this has not been shown to be true for sulindac. Additional epidemiologic data are needed with nabumetone, which may selectively inhibit prostaglandin synthesis in inflammatory tissues more than it does in the GI tract (6).

Patients at high risk of GI ulcers include the elderly, those with a previous history of ulcers, smokers, those taking concurrent corticosteroids, and those with severe arthritis (5). Some type of prophylactic therapy should be considered for patients with multiple risk factors. Misoprostol, an orally active prostaglandin analog, has been shown to prevent both gastric and duodenal ulcers. Histamine-2 receptor antagonists like cimetidine and ranitidine prevent development of duodenal ulcers but not gastric. When an ulcer does develop from NSAID use, it will heal with normal ulcer therapies. If the NSAID must be continued, omeprazole has been shown to heal most ulcers even during concomitant NSAID therapy.

Central nervous system toxicities may also occur with NSAID use. Dizziness, headache, drowsiness, or ringing in the ears will sometimes occur. Indomethacin is particularly likely to cause headaches.

Use of NSAIDs may affect kidney function in patients who already have some intrinsic renal dysfunction or who have reduced renal blood flow (e.g., patients with congestive heart failure, and the elderly). The kidneys synthesize prostaglandins to help maintain blood flow in situations where perfusion is reduced. Some patients develop retention of sodium and water, resulting in weight gain or mild leg edema; others develop worsening of hypertension. Occasionally, NSAIDs may cause acute renal failure. These drugs can also cause an interstitial nephritis that is unpredictable and allergic in nature. Safer alternatives for patients at risk of renal toxicity include nonacetylated salicylates, which are very weak prostaglandin inhibitors, and sulindac, which is not excreted by the kidney in active form.

Some patients develop pseudo-allergic reactions to NSAIDs. A syndrome of wheezing, nasal rhinitis, and laryngeal edema has been described. This syndrome is prostaglandin mediated, so patients who react to one NSAID may react to others. A nonacetylated salicylate may be cautiously tried. A second type of reaction to aspirin involves urticaria and angioedema, and patients are more likely to cross-react to other salicylates as well as NSAIDs.

Nonsteroidal drugs cause minor elevations of liver enzyme levels in up to 15% of patients. Serious liver toxicity is rare, but both hepatocellular and cholestatic reactions, with occasional deaths, have been reported. Cases of agranulocytosis and aplastic anemia have been reported rarely, mostly with phenylbutazone and indomethacin use. All NSAIDs except nonacetylated salicylates inhibit platelet aggregation. Aspirin irreversibly acetylates platelets, while other NSAIDs inhibit platelet function only while they are in the bloodstream.

Patients taking NSAIDs should be monitored regularly for efficacy and safety. If little or no benefit is obtained within 1 month, it is reasonable to try an alternative NSAID. Combining two or more NSAIDs is not beneficial and adds to the risk of toxicity. Monitoring for safety usually includes complete blood counts to watch for anemia as a sign of GI bleeding, serum creatinine and potassium to watch for renal impairment, and possibly liver enzyme tests to watch for liver problems.

CORTICOSTEROIDS

Corticosteroids are analogs of cortisone, a natural anti-inflammatory hormone first isolated in the 1940s. They were heavily used as "wonder drugs" during the 1950s, until their adverse effects became apparent. Corticosteroids are still recognized as the most powerful anti-inflammatory drugs available. However, they should be used judiciously in the lowest dose for the shortest possible time in order to avoid long-term adverse effects. Corticosteroids are used only in conditions where inflammation is prominent and not responsive to NSAIDs. Corticosteroids do not alter the course of RA (7). In certain cases of organ inflammation complicating SLE or rheumatoid vasculitis, however, large doses may be life saving.

The mechanism of action of corticosteroids is complex (8). They alter the distribution and function of white blood cells, suppress both humoral and cell-mediated immune function, and inhibit phospholipase, an enzyme in cell membranes that generates a prostaglandin precursor. A list and comparison of corticosteroids is shown in Table 2.

A "physiologic" dose of systemic corticosteroid is considered to be the equivalent of the body's normal daily secretion of 20 to 30 mg of hydrocortisone. Thus, a physiologic dose of prednisone is 5 to 7.5 mg/day. Doses lower than this cause few adverse effects, whereas larger doses are likely to cause significant adverse effects of the type listed in Table 3 (9). Prednisone is usually the steroid of choice in rheumatic disease because of its intermediate duration of action, which allows once-daily dosing. However, if given in the morning, prednisone's effect will have diminished by the time the body's endogenous hydrocortisone secretion peaks early the next morning. To further minimize adrenal suppression, prednisone is sometimes given only on alternate days. However, alternate

day therapy is not maximally effective and is not suitable for initiating therapy or for controlling highly active disease. Steroids with a long duration of action may suppress the adrenal gland even on alternate day therapy.

Corticosteroids may be given orally, intravenously, or intraarticularly. Local injection into a joint, tendon sheath, or bursa may be used when inflammation is localized, whereas systemic administration is used for generalized inflammation. Intraarticular injections should not be repeated more than 3 to 4 times per year because of a risk of osteonecrosis (8).

Indications for systemic steroids are controversial but usually include short-term treatment of RA while waiting for slow-acting drugs to work, severe synovitis that impairs functional ability, and extra-articular inflammation. Low doses of prednisone (less than 7.5 mg/day) are sufficient for articular inflammation, modest doses (10–15 mg/day) are used in polymyalgia rheumatica, and high doses (40–60 mg/day) may be used in SLE or vasculitis. Occasionally, large intravenous boluses (up to 1 g/day methylprednisolone for 3 days) may be used in severe or refractory extra-articular disease.

Clinical benefit from corticosteroids occurs rapidly. Patients usually notice improvement within 24 hours. Once improvement has stabilized, the dose is tapered to the minimum effective dose. Monitoring of corticosteroid therapy should include blood counts, serum potassium level, and glucose and clinical observation for the side effects listed in Table 3.

SLOW-ACTING ANTIRHEUMATIC DRUGS

This heterogenous group of drugs has a delayed onset of action, ranging from 3 weeks to 3 months. They are sometimes

Table 2. Comparison of oral corticosteroids.

DRUG (Trade Name)	Equivalent Dose (mg)	Relative Anti-inflammatory Potency
Short Acting		
Hydrocortisone (Cortef)	20	1
Cortisone (Cortone)	25	0.8
Intermediate Acting		
Prednisone (Deltasone)	5	4
Prednisolone (Delta-Cortef)	5	4
Methylprednisolone (Medrol)	4	5
Triamcinolone (Kenacort)	4	5
Long Acting		
Betamethasone (Celestone)	0.6	25
Dexamethasone (Decadron)	0.75	30

Table 3. Adverse effects of corticosteroids.

Endocrine	**Central Nervous System**
Hypothalmic-Pituitary-Adrenal axis suppression	Euphoria
Growth retardation	Depression
Amenorrhea	**Cutaneous**
Musculoskeletal	Acne
Osteoporosis	Hirsutism
Aseptic bone necrosis	Impaired wound healing
Myopathy	Striae
Metabolic	**Ocular**
Glucose intolerance	Cataracts
Hyperlipidemia	Glaucoma
Cardiovascular	**Immunological**
Sodium and water retention	Susceptibility to infection
Hypertension	
Hypokalemic Alkalosis	

referred to as "second-line drugs," because they have traditionally been used only after a trial of several NSAIDs. They may work at an earlier stage in the inflammatory process than NSAIDs; however, their ability to slow radiologic changes and functional disability is less than optimal. Once they were believed to alter the underlying course of disease and were called "remission-inducing" or "disease-modifying" drugs. However, they seldom improve disease enough to cause true remission. Furthermore, beneficial effects are often short-lived, with disease activity returning to baseline shortly after drug discontinuation. Even with continued treatment, only one-half of all patients stay on individual drugs longer than 2 years (10). It has been suggested that the disappointing long-term efficacy of these drugs is due to the fact that they are usually started too late in the disease course (11). One reason for this delay has been fear of severe organ toxicity, but data suggest that adverse effects of these drugs are no more severe than those of NSAIDs (12). The current approach is to start the drugs earlier, sometimes in combination.

Gold Compounds

Gold compounds were the first slow-acting drugs to be used, and they remain a standard for comparison of new drugs. There are two compounds (gold sodium thiomalate and gold thioglucose) administered only by intramuscular injection, and one (auranofin) given orally. The parenteral and orally administered drugs are not interchangeable, as they have different profiles of safety and efficacy.

Intramuscular compounds were accidentally discovered to have activity in RA during the 1930s. Their dosage protocols developed empirically. The standard regimen is a 50 mg injection once a week. Lower doses are often given at first to test for tolerance, and less frequent doses (50 mg every 2 to 4 weeks) are used for maintenance. Injectable gold compounds produce clinical improvement in about 70% of patients. However, it may take 3 to 6 months for improvement to occur.

A major drawback to the use of these compounds are the adverse effects, which occur in approximately 30% of patients. The most common reactions are mucocutaneous. A dermatitis may occur in the first weeks of therapy, but resolves on drug discontinuation. Less frequent reactions include stomatitis, generalized pruritus, gray-blue discoloration of mucous membranes, alopecia, and exfoliative dermatitis. Proteinuria occurs in 2% to 10% of patients. It may be mild and transient and not require discontinuation. Nephrotic syndrome may occur. Therapy is usually stopped if urinary protein is greater than 1 g per 24 hours. Blood dyscrasias are another serious adverse effect. Leukopenia, thrombocytopenia, and aplastic anemia have all been reported. Monitoring of injectable gold therapy should include blood counts and urinalysis every 1 to 2 weeks prior to the next scheduled injection.

Auranofin is the orally active gold compound. It is given twice daily in 3 mg capsules. Its effectiveness is less than injectable gold, which offsets its convenience (13). Adverse effects are similar to injectable gold except that diarrhea is very common with auranofin, while the incidence of renal and hematologic effects may be somewhat lower.

Penicillamine

Penicillamine was first used as a heavy metal chelator and was discovered to have antirheumatic activity in the 1960s. Its mechanism of action is unknown. It is taken orally, starting at 250 mg once daily and increasing to 250 mg three times daily if necessary. Because penicillamine is a metal chelator, it must be taken on an empty stomach, and 2 hours apart from iron salts or antacids, to assure adequate absorption. The effectiveness of penicillamine is similar to injectable gold, but adverse effects may be more common.

Many side effects of penicillamine are similar to those seen with gold compounds. Blood counts and urinalysis need to be monitored regularly. Additional effects caused by penicillamine include nausea, changes in taste that may resolve with continued therapy, and rarely, autoimmune syndromes. Most side effects are believed to be dose-related, so attempts should be made to keep the dose as low as possible.

Antimalarial Drugs

Chloroquine and hydroxychloroquine were used as antimalarial compounds before their antirheumatic activity was discovered. They are believed to work by raising the pH of cytoplasmic compartments in antigen-processing cells like macrophages, thus diminishing immune response. These drugs are slightly less effective in RA than injectable gold or penicillamine (13), but their safety is far greater (12,13). They are also very useful in treating joint and skin symptoms in SLE.

Antimalarial drugs are well tolerated, occasionally causing significant nausea or dizziness. The major concern is ocular toxicity. The drugs have a high affinity for the retina, and if early signs of retinal damage are not detected they can become irreversible and lead to blindness. If regular ophthalmic exams are done every 6 months, damage is easily detected at an early stage. Patients may report poor distance vision, difficulty reading, night blindness, and small areas of vision loss. The drugs may also deposit in the cornea, but this does not cause serious problems.

Ocular toxicity is dose related. Consequently, dosage is limited to less than 4 mg/kg/day (typically 250 mg/day) for chloroquine and 6.5 mg/kg/day (400 mg/day) for hydroxychloroquine. Overall, the safety and minimal monitoring required make antimalarial drugs a good choice in early RA and SLE.

Sulfasalazine

Sulfasalazine is better known for its role in treating inflammatory bowel disease. Although it is not FDA-approved for use in rheumatic disease, it has been used effectively in RA, ankylosing spondylitis, and other spondylarthropathies (14). Antibacterial, anti-inflammatory, and immunomodulatory effects may all contribute to its efficacy but no predominate mechanism has been established. Like other slow-acting drugs, improvement requires at least 8 to 12 weeks of treatment. The dose is 2–3 g/day in divided doses, although the starting dose is usually smaller to avoid side effects.

Common side effects are nausea, vomiting, headache, or fever. Other potential adverse reactions may include rash, hemolysis, blood dyscrasias, and male infertility. Compared to other slow-acting drugs it is equally efficacious, but has a high frequency of side effects (13). It is a useful alternative for patients who fail other drugs in this category.

Methotrexate

Methotrexate, an analog of folic acid, is currently the most promising treatment for RA, although its mechanism of action is unclear. It was originally believed to inhibit dihydrofolate reductase, an enzyme critical to synthesis of DNA in actively dividing cells. However, other mechanisms such as adenosine release are probably important, as small doses of supplemental folic acid do not interfere with methotrexate's efficacy. Methotrexate has both anti-inflammatory and immunosuppressive properties, but anti-inflammatory activity predominates at the low doses used in RA.

Methotrexate can be given orally or parenterally in a once weekly dose. The unusual dosing regimen was developed to minimize the drug's liver toxicity. The typical starting dose is 7.5 mg/week with a maximum of 25 mg/week. It is available in specially designed reminder cards as Rheumatrex®. Methotrexate's effectiveness is at least equal to other slow-acting antirheumatic drugs (13), and some studies find that patients are likely to stay on methotrexate longer (10). Another advantage is the relatively fast onset of action (3 to 6 weeks). Many rheumatologists now use methotrexate before other slow-acting drugs.

The adverse effects of methotrexate are usually well tolerated, although some may be life-threatening. Common side effects are nausea, vomiting, diarrhea, mouth ulcers, decreased white blood cell counts, and megaloblastic anemia. Hepatotoxicity is the most worrisome long-term effect. An increase in liver enzymes occurs commonly after a methotrexate dose. A small number of patients develop significant liver fibrosis or cirrhosis, and periodic liver biopsies are advocated by some authors. Patients taking methotrexate should be warned to avoid alcoholic beverages, which increase liver toxicity. Other risk factors are obesity, diabetes, and impaired renal function. Another potentially fatal toxicity of methotrexate is the unpredictable development of pulmonary interstitial inflammation. Methotrexate is teratogenic but is not known to cause malignancy.

Although folate antagonism may not account for methotrexate's therapeutic efficacy, it does cause much of the toxicity. Several investigations have shown that low-dose folic acid supplements (5 to 27.5 mg/week) lessen adverse effects without altering efficacy (15). On the other hand, the antibiotic trimethoprim, found in Proloprim®, Septra®, and Bactrim®, is also a human folate antagonist and should be avoided.

Azathioprine

Azathioprine (Imuran®) is an immunosuppressive or cytotoxic drug believed to interfere with cell division by inhibiting metabolism and synthesis of proteins and DNA. It has been used in doses of 0.75 to 2.5 mg/kg/day for rheumatic diseases. Dosage is started at the low end and is gradually increased as needed. Allopurinol interferes with azathioprine metabolism, necessitating a 50% reduction in dose.

Azathioprine is similar in effectiveness to other slow-acting drugs in the treatment of RA (13). The usual lag period is required to see an effect. Side effects include GI intolerance, reduced white blood cell counts with risk of infection, pancreatitis, hepatotoxicity, and long-term risk of malignancy.

Cyclophosphamide

Cyclophosphamide (Cytoxan®) is an alkylating agent, which nonspecifically kills cells by chemically reacting with DNA and RNA molecules. It suppresses the immune system by killing lymphocytes. Oral dosage begins at 50–75 mg/day, and may be cautiously increased after 8 weeks if poor response is seen. Large intravenous doses may be used for lupus nephritis.

This drug is infrequently used in RA because of its considerable toxicity. However, it has an important role in treatment of lupus nephritis and various forms of vasculitis. Nausea, mouth sores, alopecia, and low white blood counts are common. Suppression of ovarian and testicular function may occur with chronic therapy. A unique problem with cyclophosphamide is hemorrhagic inflammation of the urinary bladder, due to accumulation of an irritating drug metabolite. Patients may complain of painful urination and/or blood in the urine. Bladder cancer can be a long-term adverse effect. These problems are reduced by drinking plenty of fluids, and frequently emptying the bladder, especially before bedtime.

Cyclosporine

Cyclosporine (Sandimmune®) is an immunosuppressive drug used to prevent organ rejection. It inhibits production and utilization of interleukin-2, a growth factor for lymphocytes. Though not FDA-approved in rheumatology, numerous studies have documented benefit in RA. It has a 6- to 12-week lag period before producing benefit. Renal damage, hypertension, and increased body hair are the most common adverse effects. Research has focused on low-dose (3–5 mg/kg/day) regimens to reduce toxicity, but adverse effects are still seen at these levels (16). Currently, cyclosporine is reserved for severe, progressive disease that is unresponsive to other drugs.

Combination Therapy

Because patient outcomes with single drug therapies have been disappointing, it was hoped that combinations might yield additive or synergistic effects by utilizing different mechanisms. Unfortunately, in several studies combinations of slow-acting drugs have yielded greater increases in toxicity than efficacy. However, work continues and useful combinations may one day be used routinely.

INVESTIGATIONAL TREATMENTS

Minocycline

Two recent double-blinded trials have shown minocycline to have a modest, slow-acting effect in RA (17). However, because minocycline is already marketed as an antibiotic and is well tolerated except for nausea and dizziness, it may be an attractive addition to the drug arsenal.

Biologic Agents

A new and exciting approach to RA therapy is to target specific parts of the immune system. Antibodies have been produced against helper T-lymphocytes with some short-term therapeutic success (16). One could also target chemical messengers that coordinate the autoimmune process. Two of these chemicals are interleukin-1 (IL-1) and tumor necrosis factor-alpha (TNF-α). A monoclonal antibody to TNF-α and an IL-1 receptor antagonist have been used in early clinical trials with promising results (18).

MEDICATIONS FOR GOUT

Medications used in gout can be divided into two groups: those used for treating acute gouty arthritis and those used to prevent long-term complications by lowering uric acid blood levels. The first group includes NSAIDs and corticosteroids, which have been discussed already, and colchicine. In the second group are probenecid, sulphinpyrazone, and allopurinol.

Colchicine

Colchicine has been used in plant form for centuries, but it is less often used today because of its toxicities. It inhibits neutrophil function by an effect on microtubules. The traditional regimen for acute gouty arthritis has been a 0.5 or 0.6 mg tablet of colchicine given orally every hour until relief is obtained, until intolerable side effects occur, or a maximum dose of 6 mg is reached. Colchicine may also be given on a chronic basis (1–2 tablets daily) to prevent gouty arthritis.

Although effective, most patients complain of significant nausea, vomiting, and diarrhea from colchicine. The side effects can be partly overcome by giving the drug intravenously (up to 3 mg), but administration by this route is more likely to produce organ toxicity such as neuropathy, bone marrow depression, renal and liver toxicity, and shock. The maximum dose should be lowered for the elderly and those with renal or hepatic impairment (19).

Probenecid and Sulphinpyrazone

These two drugs are uricosurics, meaning they increase excretion of uric acid in the urine. The dose range is 500–2,000 mg/day for probenecid and 100–800 mg/day for sulphinpyrazone (19). In both cases, the dose should start at the lower end to avoid precipitation of renal stones, and fluid intake should be increased concomitantly. Both drugs are ineffective in patients with poor renal function and can be antagonized by even low doses of aspirin. In the early weeks of therapy they can actually increase the risk of gouty arthritis, so a prophylactic anti-inflammatory drug should also be prescribed. The drugs are well tolerated, with occasional rashes or GI distress reported.

Allopurinol

Allopurinol works by lowering the formation of uric acid. The usual dose is 300 mg/day; this should be lowered to 100 mg/day in patients with renal impairment. It is more versatile than uricosurics, being effective at all levels of renal function and also in both overproducers and underexcretors of uric acid. However, allopurinol inhibits metabolism of many other drugs and can cause rashes, bone marrow depression, and a multiorgan hypersensitivity syndrome involving fever, severe skin reactions, and renal and hepatic failure. Neither allopurinol nor uricosurics should be used in asymptomatic hyperuricemia.

MUSCLE RELAXANTS

Muscle relaxing drugs such as carisoprodol, cyclobenzaprine, methocarbamol, and chlorzoxazone are used to relieve secondary muscle spasm in back pain and other chronic painful conditions. Cyclobenzaprine (Flexeril®) is widely used in fibromyalgia. Both cyclobenzaprine and a chemically related antidepressant, amitriptyline, have been shown to improve sleep and relieve pain in fibromyalgia (20). Cyclobenzaprine's dose is 10 mg 1 to 3 times daily, while amitriptyline is used in low doses (10 to 50 mg) at bedtime. Both of these drugs frequently cause drowsiness and anticholinergic side effects such as dry mouth, constipation, confusion, and urine retention.

REFERENCES

1. Criswell LA, Henke CJ: What explains the variation among rheumatologists in their use of prednisone and second line agents for the treatment of rheumatoid arthritis? J Rheumatol 22:829–835, 1995
2. Wilske KR, Healey LA: Remodeling the pyramid—a concept whose time has come. J Rheumatol 16:565–567, 1989
3. McCarthy GM, McCarty DJ: Effect of topical capsaicin in the therapy of painful osteoarthritis of the hands. J Rheumatol 19:604–607, 1992
4. Furst DE: Are there differences among nonsteroidal anti-inflammatory drugs? Comparing acetylated salicylates, nonacetylated salicylates, and nonacetylated nonsteroidal anti-inflammatory drugs. Arthritis Rheum 37: 1–9, 1994
5. Miller DR: Treatment of nonsteroidal anti-inflammatory drug gastropathy. Clin Pharmacy 11:690–704, 1992
6. Lichtenstein DR, Syngal S, Wolfe MM: Nonsteroidal antiinflammatory drugs and the gastrointestinal tract. Arthritis Rheum 38:5–18, 1995
7. McDougall R, Sibley J, Haga M, Russell A: Outcome in patients with rheumatoid arthritis receiving prednisone compared to matched controls. J Rheumatol 21:1207–1213, 1994
8. Weiss MM: Corticosteroids in rheumatoid arthritis. Semin Arthritis Rheum 19:9–21, 1989
9. Saag KG, Koehnke R, Caldwell JR, Brasington R, Burmeister LF, Zimmerman B, Kohler JA, Furst DE: Low dose long-term corticosteroid therapy in rheumatoid arthritis: an analysis of serious adverse events. Am J Med 96:115–123, 1994
10. Pincus T, Marcum SB, Callahan LF: Longterm drug therapy for rheumatoid arthritis in seven rheumatology private practices. II. Second line drugs and prednisone. J Rheumatol 19:1885–1894, 1992
11. Fries JF: Reevaluating the therapeutic approach to rheumatoid arthritis: the "sawtooth" strategy. J Rheumatol 17 (Suppl 22):12–15, 1990
12. Fries JF: ARAMIS and toxicity measurement. J Rheumatol 22:995–997, 1995
13. Felson DT, Anderson JJ, Meenan RF: The comparative efficacy and toxicity of second-line drugs in rheumatoid arthritis: results of two meta-analyses. Arthritis Rheum 33:1449–1461, 1990
14. Pinals RS, Kaplan SB, Lawson JG, Hepburn B: Sulfasalazine in rheumatoid arthritis: a double-blind, placebo-controlled trial. Arthritis Rheum 29:1427–1434, 1986
15. Morgan SL, Baggott JE, Vaughn WH, et al: Supplementation with folic acid during methotrexate therapy for rheumatoid arthritis: a double blind, placebo-controlled trial. Ann Intern Med 121:833–841, 1994

16. Klippel JH, Strober S, Wofsky D: New therapies for the rheumatic diseases. Bull Rheum Dis 38:1–8, 1989
17. Paulus HE: Minocycline treatment of rheumatoid arthritis. Ann Intern Med 122:147–148, 1995
18. Arend WP, Dayer J-M: Inhibition of the production and effects of interleukin-1 and tumor necrosis factor α in rheumatoid arthritis. Arthritis Rheum 38:151–160, 1995
19. Star VL, Hochberg MC: Prevention and management of gout. Drugs 45:212–222, 1993
20. Carrette S, Bell MJ, Reynolds WJ, et al: Comparison of amitriptyline, cyclobenzaprine, and placebo in the treatment of fibromyalgia: a randomized, double-blind clinical trial. Arthritis Rheum 37:32–40, 1994

Additional Recommended Reading

1. Dahl SL: Advances and issues in the pharmacotherapy of rheumatoid arthritis. J Clin Pharm Ther 20:131–147, 1995
2. Cash JM, Klippel JH: Second-line drug therapy for rheumatoid arthritis. New Engl J Med 330:1368–1375, 1994
3. Drugs for rheumatoid arthritis. Med Lett Drugs Ther 36:101–106, 1994

Rest and Exercise

MARIAN A. MINOR, PhD, PT

Finding the correct balance of rest and physical activity in the comprehensive management of rheumatic disease is an historic and continuing challenge. The ability of the person with arthritis to effectively combine rest and exercise plays a crucial role in achieving optimal outcomes. Historically, active–resistive and weight-bearing exercises have been discouraged and rest has been recommended when pain, joint swelling, cartilage damage, or active systemic disease were present. Current knowledge of joint physiology and disease etiology provides a basis for more specific recommendations for rest, and more positive recommendations for exercise.

REST

Rest is a key component of rheumatic disease care. It can be divided into two types: whole body (general) rest and rest of specific joints. Adequate general rest, including restorative sleep at night, is necessary for health. During periods of active systemic inflammatory disease, additional rest is recommended to offset the fatigue that may be a physiologic consequence of increased inflammatory activity. Rest also protects involved organs and organ systems (cardiovascular, musculoskeletal, pulmonary, and renal) from pathologic stress that may result from strenuous activity. An adequate prescription of general rest should include instructions for time, place, and proper positioning. Rest is not a benign prescription; unnecessary, prolonged inactivity produces illness and leads to disability (1).

Rest of specific joints is often necessary in both inflammatory conditions and osteoarthritis (OA). The purpose of specific joint rest is to avoid activity-related injury, provide periods of joint unloading, reduce pain and swelling, and encourage maintenance of function and activity in spite of isolated joint swelling or pain. This type of rest includes activity modifications, use of assistive devices, and protective or supportive splinting. Suggestions to limit particular activities; alternate movements to avoid repetitive strain; or avoid certain activities such as stair climbing, lifting, power gripping, or running are examples of activity modifications. Assistive devices such as jar openers and electric can openers can rest particular joints by passing the activity on to another joint. Joints also may be rested by using splints and orthoses to support joints during activity, limit motion, or assure proper positioning during rest. Complete immobilization usually is not recommended.

During periods of active inflammation, joint structures (including capsule, ligaments, tendons, and cartilage) should be protected. However, rest cannot control the ill effects of inflammation. Additional management, including medication, joint aspiration, and injection, is essential to reduce inflammation and swelling quickly. Inflammation of the joint can lead to stretching or rupture of capsule, ligaments, and tendons. Inflamed joints are unstable and vulnerable to activity-related

injuries. Neuromuscular response, muscle strength and endurance, and proprioception—necessary for joint protection—also can be diminished.

Recommendations for Rest

General Body Rest. During periods of acute inflammatory disease, at least 8 to 10 hours of sleep at night and 30- to 60-minute morning and afternoon rest periods are recommended. In some systemic diseases such as polymyositis and polymyalgia rheumatica, acute episodes of muscular inflammation and systemic complications may require total bed rest. Total body rest should be prescribed for specific durations and at specific times to avoid extreme fatigue or exhaustion.

Night rest should start with relaxing activities (warm bath or shower, gentle range-of-motion or relaxation exercise) early in the evening, to provide adequate time for sleep. A regular sleep and wake schedule should be encouraged. Pain, stiffness, anxiety, and depression that often accompany rheumatic diseases may disrupt sleep patterns and lead to additional problems related to inadequate rest. Therefore, attention to good sleep habits is an important part of comprehensive care and effective self-management.

Suggestions for posture and positioning during rest include a firm sleeping surface; egg crate, sheep skin or other mattress covers for comfort; a pillow that supports the head and neck without causing neck flexion and forward shoulders; pillows to maintain body alignment if patient lies on his/her side (supine with hips and knees extended is preferred); and night splints, if needed.

Specific Joint Rest. A number of methods can be used to rest a specific joint or joints during periods of pain or inflammation. Biomechanical stabilization and support is provided by orthoses or splints to decrease motion and/or loading of specific joints. This type of support is usually recommended for specified rest periods or during potentially stressful activities. Examples include functional wrist splints, finger and thumb splints, resting or night splints, rigid foot orthoses to support and stabilize the foot during weight bearing, and shoe modifications or orthoses to eliminate or reduce metacarpal extension.

Joint loading may be controlled by modifying activities with respect to muscular contraction, weight bearing, and impact forces. Suggested modifications may include restricting stair climbing for persons with hip and knee joint involvement; reducing time spent standing; alternating periods of weight bearing with periods of non-weight bearing; or modifying recreational exercise to low-impact or gravity-reduced activities such as swimming, bicycling, or walking.

Repetitive joint motion and loading should be alternated with rest. This can be achieved by a schedule of regular rest breaks during repetitive activities such as using a keyboard,

Table 1. Purpose, components, and recommendations for rest.

Whole Body Rest	Joint Specific Rest
Purpose	
Offset disease-related fatigue	Reduce swelling
Protect involved organs from pathologic stress	Avoid activity-related injury
	Unload joint as needed
	Maintain general function/activity levels
Components	
Nighttime sleep	Activity modification
Daytime rest periods	Assistive devices
	Orthoses/splinting
Recommendations	
8–10 hours nighttime sleep	Modify physical activity to avoid overuse of deforming forces on specific joints
30–60 minute rest periods during day	Provide biomechanical stabilization and support
Use relaxation techniques	Control joint loading and weight bearing
Proper posture, positioning	Alternate rest with dynamic activity
Determine specific times and places	
Establish good sleep practices	

sewing, playing an instrument, production line work, walking, or sitting. Conversely, regular exercise periods should be scheduled during the day for joints that are being immobilized by a splint.

In addition to following the recommendations for rest, some self-monitoring method should be chosen to assess effectiveness of the rest prescription. Appropriate indicators include reduced joint swelling, less fatigue, heightened energy level or mood, or less morning stiffness. The rationale, components, and recommendations for rest in rheumatic disease are summarized in Table 1.

EXERCISE

Persons with arthritis demonstrate limited range of motion, decreased muscle strength and endurance, abnormalities in gait and posture, functional limitations, and general deconditioning (1,2). Appropriate regular exercise can lead to improvement in these areas, as well as reducing pain, fatigue, and depression (1,3,4).

Physical activity can be defined as "any bodily movement produced by skeletal muscles that results in energy expenditure." Regular physical activity is necessary for general health. It also reduces the risk for a number of diseases, and it reduces levels of dysfunction and disability in arthritis. Exercise is further defined as "planned, structured, and repetitive bodily movement done to improve or maintain one or more components of physical fitness." Therapeutic exercise is often prescribed for the person with arthritis to reduce impairment (range of motion/flexibility, muscular function, pain, fatigue) and maintain or improve function (activities of daily living, locomotion, balance). Cardiovascular health and general fitness, also dependent on adequate levels of exercise or physical activity, are addressed in Chapter 23, Deconditioning.

The assumption that exercise causes joint damage has been challenged by a number of research reports. It appears that dynamic exercise, both resisted and non-resisted, can improve range of motion, strength, endurance, function, and gait without exacerbation of disease or increased joint symptoms (3–8). Joint immobilization leads to cartilage and periarticular tissue weakening and pathology, whereas regular joint motion and intermittent weight bearing appear to be protective (9,10). It is true, however, that some forms of exercise or motion can momentarily increase joint pressure. In persons with knee joint effusions, prolonged isometric contraction of the quadriceps and extreme knee flexion can increase intra-articular pressure (9), and maximal contraction of gluteal muscles can increase hip joint contact pressure (11).

Persons with arthritis in hip or knee joints often are cautioned against weight-bearing activities such as walking, running, dancing, and stair climbing. Exercise research and evidence of joint loading and intra-articular pressures in normal and diseased joints provide information to guide exercise and activity recommendations. In addition to aquatic exercise and stationary bicycling, weight-bearing exercise such as walking and low impact aerobic dance can be performed safely by persons with symptomatic joints. Improvements in flexibility, strength, endurance, function, cardiovascular fitness, and general health status have been documented, with no aggravation of symptoms (1,3–7). In persons with rheumatoid arthritis (RA), reduction in joint swelling has been reported from a number of aerobic exercise studies (6,7).

Some weight-bearing activities do increase joint loading and probably should be avoided or minimized. Stair descent and ascent and carrying loads greater than 10% of body weight significantly increase loading of the hip (12); and faster walking speeds increase biomechanical stress at the knee (13). Although walking does not increase intra-articular pressure in a healthy knee joint, it has been shown to increase pressure in effused knees (10). Duration and consequences of this increased pressure have not been studied. However, a recent report of exercise effects on synovial blood flow in effused knees demonstrated that dynamic exercise (cycling and walking) improved circulation, while isometric contraction of the quadriceps did not (10).

Range of Motion and Flexibility Exercise

Exercise can relieve stiffness, increase or maintain joint motion, and increase length and elasticity in muscle and periarticular tissues. In arthritis, active and active/self-assisted exercise is recommended. During acute joint inflammation, joint motion should be maintained with at least one complete range-of-motion exercise daily. It is important not to overstretch inflamed tissues, as tensile strength can be reduced by as much as 50%, and tears and overstretching can occur. Application of cold prior to exercise may reduce pain. When joint symptoms are subacute or chronic, goals can include increasing range of motion with gentle, controlled stretching. The use of heat prior to stretching is useful.

Active range-of-motion exercise can produce benefits in addition to maintaining flexibility and joint motion. Gentle exercise performed in the evening can significantly reduce morning stiffness for persons with RA (14). An exercise program of active exercise and relaxation (the ROM or Range of Motion Dance program) has shown significant improvements in self-reported function and pain (15). Table 2 lists the normal range of motion for the major joints, as well as the range required to perform various activities.

Table 2. Range of motion of major joints: normal range and range required to perform activities in a normal manner (22).

Joint	Joint Motion	Normal Range	Functional Range	
			ADLs	Level Walking
Wrist	Flexion/Extension	85°/75°	10°/35°	–
Elbow	Flexion/Extension	140°/0°	130°/30°	–
	Pronation/Supination	70°/80°	50°/50°	–
Shoulder	Flexion/Extension	170°/60°	100°/30°	–
	Abduction/Adduction	180°/0°	90°	–
	Rotation	90°/90°	30°/70°	–
Hip	Flexion/Extension	140°/15°	120°/5°	40°/5°
	Abduction/Adduction	30°/25°	20°/5°	5°/5°
	Rotation	90°/70°	20°/20°	5°/5°
Knee	Flexion/Extension	140°/0°	117°/0°	67°/0°
Ankle	Plantarflexion/Dorsiflexion	30°/15°	15°/10°	15°/10°
Toes (MTP)	Hallux	30°/90°	5°/65°	5°/65°
	Toes	50°/90°	5°/65°	5°/65°

* ADLs = Activities of daily living; MTP = Metatarsophalangeal joint.

Recommendations for range of motion/flexibility exercise include the following: 1) exercise daily when stiffness and pain are the least; 2) take a warm shower, or apply heat and/or cold prior to or after exercise; 3) perform gentle range-of-motion exercise in the evening to reduce morning stiffness and in the morning to limber up prior to arising; 4) modify exercises (decrease frequency or adapt movement) to avoid increasing joint pain either during or after the exercise; 5) use self-assistive techniques (such as overhead pulleys or wand exercises) to perform gentle stretching; 6) reduce number of repetitions when joint is actively inflamed.

Muscle Conditioning Exercise

Decreased muscle strength, endurance, and power in persons with arthritis may be due to a number of factors. Some of these include intra-articular and extra-articular inflammatory disease processes, side effects of medication, disuse, reflex inhibition in response to pain and joint effusion, impaired proprioception, and loss of mechanical integrity around the joint (3,7,8). Mus-

cle conditioning programs can improve strength, endurance, and function without exacerbation of pain or disease activity (16–18). Table 3 outlines the purpose and recommendations for isometric and dynamic muscle conditioning exercise.

Isometric Exercise. Isometric exercise is often suggested prior to or in conjunction with dynamic resistive and aerobic exercise programs. Initially, isometric exercise may be indicated to improve muscle tone, static endurance, and strength, and to prepare joints for more vigorous activity. This type of exercise involves muscle contraction without joint movement. Isometric contractions performed at 70% of the maximal voluntary contraction, held for 6 seconds and repeated 5 to 10 times daily can increase strength significantly. Successful isometric regimens include contractions at several combinations of muscle length and joint angles (16). Although isometric exercise avoids the concern of joint motion and mechanical irritation, it can produce other unwanted effects. Isometric exercise at more than 40% maximal voluntary contraction constricts blood flow through the exercising muscle, which can produce unnecessary post-exercise muscle soreness. Also, the increased peripheral vascular resistance produces increased blood pressure. In the knee and hip, high intensity isometric contraction has been shown to increase intra-articular pressure (10,11).

Instructions for isometric exercise should include the following cautions: maintain the contraction for no more than 6 seconds; avoid maximal effort, as it is neither necessary nor desirable; exhale during the contraction and inhale during a similar period of relaxation; and avoid contracting more than two muscle groups at a time.

Dynamic Exercise. Dynamic exercise is repetitive muscle contraction and relaxation involving joint motion and changes in muscle length. It includes both shortening (concentric) and lengthening (eccentric) contractions. Dynamic exercise can improve strength and endurance. Resistance (physiologic overload) can be supplied by weight of the body part or external resistance in the form of free weights, elastic bands, or a variety of resistive exercise equipment. A cautious approach to resistance training is recommended to protect unstable or inflamed joints from damage.

Table 3. Purpose and recommendations for isometric and dynamic muscle conditioning exercise.*

Isometric	Dynamic
Purpose	
Minimize atrophy	Maintain/increase dynamic strength and endurance
Improve tone	Increase muscle power
Maintain/increase static strength and endurance	Improve function
Prepare for dynamic and weight bearing activity	Enhance synovial blood flow
	Promote strength of bone and cartilage
Recommendations	
Perform at functional joint angles	Capable of 8–10 repetitions of motion against gravity before additional resistance
Exhale during contraction; avoid valsalva maneuver	Progressive resistive regimen
Intensity: ≤ 70% one MVC	Perform in pain-free range
Duration: 6 second contraction	Use functional activities/movement patterns
Frequency: 5–10 repetitions daily	Intensity: progress to ≤70% one RM
	Duration: progress to 8–10 exercises, 8–10 repetitions
	Frequence: 2–3 times/week on alternate days
Precautions	
Decreased muscle blood flow	May increase biomechanical stress on unstable or malaligned joints
May increase intra-articular pressure	Avoid forces on involved hands and wrists
May increase blood pressure	

* MVC = maximal voluntary contraction; RM = repetition maximum.

Adequate neuromuscular warm up and a cool down with gentle stretching of the exercised muscles enhance safety and comfort. If exercise is painful in the outer range of motion, the exercise should be performed within the pain-free range. Exercise of 8 to 10 anti-gravity repetitions should be well tolerated before additional resistance is added. Maximum benefit and maintenance are achieved by incorporating functional movements and body positions in the recommended exercise routine. The patient should learn to perform exercises rhythmically with well controlled movement toward the outer part of the range. Resistance, repetitions, or frequency can be modified as needed.

Gradual progression of resistance and repetition is recommended. Intensity, frequency, or motion should be reduced if joint swelling or pain occurs. Loads of up to 70% one repetition maximum (1RM), used in a circuit resistance training program of persons with controlled RA, demonstrated significant improvements in strength and function with no exacerbation in joint symptoms (18). In persons with knee OA, 16 weeks of progressive muscular training, including isometric and isotonic exercise of increasing loads and speeds, resulted in improved function, independence, and decreased pain (16).

Researchers have used isokinetic equipment to measure and improve strength; however, this equipment is expensive and not readily available in the context of self-management and community-based care. Therefore, isokinetic training is not generally recommended.

High intensity exercise, discomfort, and injuries are clearly associated with poor adherence to exercise programs. Thus, it is important that people with arthritis—who are often unaccustomed to exercise and are afraid of causing pain and damage—experience success and enjoyment early in the exercise regimen. Physiologic adaptation may take longer in this population.

Implementing an Exercise Routine

The most important requirements for the successful design, implementation, and maintenance of an exercise routine are to: 1) establish reasonable goals, 2) understand how and when to adapt and modify the exercise program, and 3) monitor for effectiveness.

Establish Reasonable Goals. Reasonable goals emerge when patient and professional collaborate to assess and prioritize needs. For persons with few involved joints, mild disease, and recent onset, this process is fairly straightforward. For the person with multiple joint involvement, fluctuating or severe disease, and functional loss, the decision-making process is more complex. An exercise prescription of reasonable length and complexity, designed to reduce impairments and increase functions important to the patient, will more likely be maintained than a complex, time-consuming program.

Each exercise prescription should include a functional assessment, either by patient self-report or through observed performance, and a determination of joint protection needs. Assessment must extend beyond active disease. For example, joint disease in one knee is commonly accompanied by decreased range of motion and strength in hip and ankle on the involved side, and in lower extremity joints on the opposite side. Disturbed gait kinetics and kinematics are also seen. Hand and wrist pain often results in decreased motion and strength in elbows and shoulders and poor head and upper body posture.

Adapt Exercise Program. Self-management skills are essential for exercise maintenance. The person with arthritis must make day-to-day decisions about exercise adaptation and modification. Pain, joint swelling, and fatigue are good markers to use in this decision-making: they are important, well known experiences, and they have clinical relevance. Increases in these markers may indicate increased disease activity, overexertion, or aggravation of symptoms from other daily activities. The appropriate response is modification of current exercise until the problem subsides or additional treatment is undertaken. The person with arthritis should be encouraged to readily discuss changes in pain, swelling, and fatigue with a knowledgeable health care provider.

Monitor for Effectiveness. Both the health care provider and the person with arthritis need to monitor program success. Effectiveness can be evaluated with measures of disease activity such as joint swelling or stiffness; measures of impairment such as range of motion, strength, endurance, pain, or fatigue; or functional assessments such as gait, activities of daily living, or depression. An exercise program may also affect physical activity levels, occupational performance, or social factors. When the exercise recommendation is based on clear goals that are important to both health professional and patient, and the program is designed to achieve those goals, the choice of evaluation tools is relatively simple. When and how often to evaluate are important considerations that should be based on a determination of when changes can be expected.

Simple self-tests can be used to show improvements in strength, endurance, range of motion, or function. For example, a meaningful self-test in an exercise program to increase shoulder motion could be to periodically mark vertical reach on a wall or attempt to reach an object placed on a higher shelf. If increased ankle motion is an exercise goal, the patient could measure ankle dorsiflexion by the thickness of books that can be accommodated under the forefoot. Self-tests provide evidence of progress and success to the exerciser. Therefore, it is important to ensure that the test chosen can be expected to show meaningful improvement. For example, a program to increase walking endurance could include a choice of "measures of success" such as a greater distance walked, less exertion, or time to walk the original distance.

PAIN AND EXERCISE

Pain can be assessed in several ways: 1) as a general experience; 2) with respect to performance of a specific physical activity; or 3) by the impact of pain on performance of daily activities. The apparent effect of exercise on arthritis-related pain depends on the questions used to assess pain. Research in exercise and arthritis has shown conflicting results in general pain improvement following a course of exercise. Studies that assessed pain related to specific activities report significant reductions in pain with exercise. Another study, comparing outcomes from exercise programs for persons with RA who were instructed to use pain as an exercise guide or to set exercise goals and not consider pain, found that the goal-setting group increased exercise performance and reported less pain (19). A consistent finding in exercise research is the improvement in function and physical activity levels without increased pain or arthritis symptoms. It is not necessary to include pain reduction as an exercise goal; however, it is often a side effect.

Of all the physical modalities, exercise appears to be the most consistently effective in reducing pain (20). Pain may indicate tissue damage and should be respected and investigated in the process of prescribing and implementing rest and exercise. However, persons who have previously experienced severe pain or who are depressed or inactive may have a lower threshold for stimuli that are interpreted as pain. Therefore, pain as a guide to exercise should be assessed for specific motions or by musculoskeletal examination for activity-induced injury.

At the beginning of an exercise program, the most common pain reports arise from delayed-onset muscle soreness and overstretching. Both situations can be corrected in subsequent exercise sessions. Overuse of the joint is usually accompanied by swelling, heat, and pain. Immediate treatment consists of ice, elevation, and rest to reduce the swelling; modification of the exercise regimen to avoid re-injury; and implementation of appropriate exercise to condition the joint. Increased joint pain in weight-bearing joints most often follows prolonged standing, fast walking, or walking on uneven ground. Planned periods of non-weight bearing, slower walking speeds, use of shock absorbing footwear, and walking on level surfaces can minimize or eliminate this type of pain.

JOINT PROTECTION AND EXERCISE

Exercise plays an important role in joint protection. Joints can be injured by inflammatory activity, biomechanical stress, pathologic joint loading, immobilization, increased intra-articular pressure, and diminished blood flow (1,10,21). Regular dynamic exercise is associated with improved blood flow and cartilage health, as well as improved range of motion and increased strength and endurance of surrounding muscles (9,10,21). Strong and fatigue-resistant muscles can provide shock attenuation of impact forces crossing a joint. Weak, easily-fatigued muscle cannot provide joint stability or control. An intact neuromuscular mechanism is the most important component of shock attenuation and is vital to adequate proprioception (21). Exercise can protect joints by conditioning muscles surrounding the joint to improve stability, strength, endurance, and power during functional activities. In addition, exercise helps maintain adequate flexibility to allow pain-free, active range of motion and joint alignment.

Joint protection principles must be followed while performing exercise. There are a number of methods to incorporate joint protection strategies into an exercise program. Joint loading should be alternated with periods of unloading. Activities that incur unnecessary or painful joint loading, such as stair climbing, fast walking or running, prolonged standing, or carrying loads should be avoided. Finally, biomechanical stress should be reduced with orthoses and positioning to provide joint support and alignment.

ROLE OF THE HEALTH CARE PROFESSIONAL

Self-efficacy is the degree of confidence that a person feels in his/her ability to perform a particular behavior. Higher self-efficacy is associated with willingness to adopt and maintain a behavior. Strategies that foster self-efficacy include successful

Table 4. Guidelines for evaluating community-based exercise programs or facilities.

Physical Accessibility – Proximity to parking or public transportation. Ability to move easily and safely about within the facility, especially bathrooms and changing areas.

Social Accessibility – Attitude and friendliness of staff and members. Feeling at ease and comfortable. Willingness of instructors to listen and respond to members about special needs or modifications. Ongoing classes of appropriate size, intensity, and activities.

Cost – Possibility of paying only for classes or times attended rather than a prepaid membership fee. Allowances in membership policy to allow for times when participation is medically inadvisable. Able to observe and participate before making a financial commitment.

Qualifications of Staff/Instructors – Current certification by a professional organization and CPR certification. Training or experience in teaching exercise for people with arthritis or other special needs. Demonstrated interest in learning about arthritis and exercise.

experience with the behavior, reinterpretation of signs and symptoms associated with the behavior, encounters with others who have been successful with the behavior, and encouragement and persuasion. Strategies to enhance self-efficacy can be embedded in an exercise recommendation by prescribing exercise that can be successfully performed and that produces a desired result. In addition, the health care provider should help the exerciser recognize sensations such as faster breathing, warmth, or muscular tension as normal and desirable effects of exercise. Referral to an exercise class in which other persons with arthritis are successful exercisers, and providing an encouraging and supportive environment are additional strategies.

With knowledge and support from health care providers, the person with arthritis can use community-based resources for exercise and physical activity. The advantages of community-based exercise include economy, socialization, self-management, wellness focus, and variety in activities, participants, and locations. Communication between community-based providers and health care professionals provides positive, successful exercise experiences and continuity for the client. Exercise programs are available through local YMCA organizations, health clubs, hospital-sponsored fitness facilities, community colleges, parks and recreation departments, senior centers, and cooperative programs between the Arthritis Foundation and local groups.

Not all community-based programs are appropriate for persons with arthritis. Both health care provider and the person with arthritis should keep in mind guidelines for evaluating a facility or program in addition to the usual requirements of safety (Table 4).

REFERENCES

1. Galloway MT, Jokl P: The role of exercise in the treatment of inflammatory arthritis. Bull Rheum Dis 42:1–4, 1993
2. Messier SP, Loeser RF, Hoover JL, Semble EL, Wise CM: Osteoarthritis of the knee: effects on gait, strength, and flexibility. Arch Phys Med Rehabil 73:29–36, 1992
3. Stenström CH: Therapeutic exercise in rheumatoid arthritis. Arthritis Care Res 7:190–197, 1994
4. Bunning RD, Materson RS: A rational program of exercise for patients with osteoarthritis. Semin Arthritis Rheum 21 (suppl 2):33–43, 1991
5. Kovar PA, Allegrante JP, MacKenzie CR, Peterson MGE, Gutin B, Charlson ME: Supervised fitness walking in patients with osteoarthritis of the knee. Ann Intern Med 116:529–534, 1992

6. Perlman SG, Connell KJ, Clark A, et al: Dance-based aerobic exercise for rheumatoid arthritis. Arthritis Care Res 3:29–35, 1990
7. Semble EL, Loeser RF, Wise CM: Therapeutic exercise for rheumatoid arthritis and osteoarthritis. Semin Arthritis Rheum 20:32–40, 1990
8. Hurley MV, Newham DJ: The influence of arthrogenous muscle inhibition on quadriceps rehabilitation of patients with early unilateral osteoarthritic knees. Br J Rheumatol 32:127–131, 1993
9. Michel BA, Fries JF, Bloch DA, Lane NE, Jones HH: Osteophytosis of the knee: association with changes in weight-bearing exercise. Clin Rheumatol 11:235–238, 1992
10. James MJ, Cleland LG, Gaffney RD, Proudman SM, Chatterton BE: Effect of exercise on ^{99m}Tc-DTPA clearance from knees with effusions. J Rheumatol 21:501–504, 1994
11. Krebs DE, Elbaum L, O'Riley P, Hodge WA, Mann RW: Exercise and gait effects on in vivo hip contact pressures. Phys Ther 71:301–309, 1990
12. Neumann DA: Biomechanical analysis of selected principles of hip joint protection. Arthritis Care Res 2:146–155, 1989
13. Schnitzer TJ, Poppovich JM, Andersson GBJ, Andriacchi TP: Effect of piroxicam on gait in patients with osteoarthritis of the knee. Arthritis Rheum 36:1207–1213, 1993
14. Byers PH: Effect of exercise on morning stiffness and mobility in patients with rheumatoid arthritis. Res Nurs Health 8:275–281, 1985
15. Van Deusen J, Harlowe D: The efficacy of the ROM dance program for adults with rheumatoid arthritis. Am J Occup Ther 41:90–95, 1987
16. Fisher NM, Pendergast DR, Gresham GE, Calkins E: Muscle rehabilitation: its effect on muscular and functional performance of patients with knee osteoarthritis. Arch Phys Med Rehabil 72:367–374, 1991
17. Ekdahl C, Andersson SI, Moritz U, Svensson B: Dynamic versus static training in patients with rheumatoid arthritis. Scand J Rheumatol 19:17–26, 1990
18. Rall LC, Lundgren N, Joseph L, Dolinkowski G, Kehayias JJ, Roubenoff R: The metabolic cost of rheumatoid arthritis: reversal with progressive resistance exercise (abstract). Arthritis Rheum 37 (suppl 9):S222, 1994
19. Stenström CH: Home exercise in rheumatoid arthritis functional class II: goal setting versus pain attention. J Rheumatol 21:627–634, 1994
20. Minor MA, Sanford MK: Physical interventions in the management of pain in arthritis: an overview for research and practice. Arthritis Care Res 6:197–206, 1993
21. Bland JH, Cooper SM: Osteoarthritis: a review of the cell biology involved and evidence of reversibility: management rationally related to known genesis and pathophysiology. Semin Arthritis Rheum 14:106–133, 1984
22. Nordin M, Frankel VH: Basic Biomechanics of the Musculoskeletal System. Second edition. Philadelphia, Lea & Febiger, 1989

Additional Recommended Reading

1. Exercise and arthritis. Arthritis Care Res 7(4), 1994
2. Ekdahl C: Muscle function in rheumatoid arthritis: assessment and training. Scand J Rheumatol S86:9–61, 1990
3. Goldstein TS: Geriatric Orthopaedics, Rehabilitative Management of Common Problems. Gaithersburg, MD, Aspen Publications, 1991
4. Hoenig H, Groff G, Pratt K, Goldberg E, Franck W: A randomized controlled trial of home exercise on the rheumatoid hand. J Rheumatol 20:785–789, 1993

Physical Modalities

KAREN W. HAYES, PhD, PT

Physical modalities of heat, cold, and electricity are often used to alleviate the symptoms of rheumatic disease. While no modality is capable of curing arthritis, amelioration of symptoms may lead to improved function. Overall function depends on the freedom from impairments such as weakness, limitation of motion, and pain. Specific treatment goals may include decreasing pain, increasing flexibility, and decreasing swelling. Heat, cold, and electrical stimulation are the modalities most commonly used to produce improvement in these impairments.

SUPERFICIAL AND DEEP HEAT

Superficial and deep heat are used primarily to decrease pain and improve flexibility. Heat contributes to pain relief by increasing the pain threshold, increasing blood flow, and washing out pain-producing metabolites. Heat also decreases muscle guarding through its effects on the muscle spindle and golgi tendon organs (1). Ultrasound, a deep heat produced by the conversion of sound waves into heat, was once thought to produce preferential slowing of nerve conduction in small sensory fibers. However, more recent evidence has shown that sensory conduction usually increases after heating (2). An effect on nerve conduction is therefore unlikely to explain the action of ultrasound in reducing pain.

Heat may improve flexibility by reducing pain or by increasing the extensibility of connective tissue (3). In addition, heat increases the viscous properties of collagen, which could lead to increased range of motion if combined with low load, prolonged stretch (4).

Application Of Superficial Heat

Superficial heat can be applied by using hot packs, paraffin wax baths, Fluidotherapy™ (a bath of small solid particles suspended in a stream of warmed air), infrared radiation (heat lamps), or hydrotherapy. Regardless of the source, superficial heat is in the infrared portion of the electromagnetic spectrum; thus, it penetrates through the skin only a few millimeters. Superficial heat should be applied for about 20 minutes to elevate skin temperature and activate optimal heat loss responses by the body. Physiologic effects occur through these reflex vascular and neural responses. Superficial heat is convenient and safe for home use if patients have received proper instruction on its use.

Application Of Deep Heat

Deep heat is provided through shortwave diathermy and ultrasound. Like superficial heat, deep heat elevates temperature, but it reaches deeper tissues such as muscle and connective tissue. Shortwave diathemy is usually applied for 20 minutes to fairly large areas of the body. Ultrasound, on the other hand, may be focused on very small areas and is applied for shorter periods of time (3 to 10 minutes). The heat from shortwave diathermy and ultrasound is produced by conversion of electrical or sound energy into heat energy below the level of the skin heat receptors. Consequently, people perceive the heat from deep heat sources to be much milder. Because of the mechanisms of heat production and the milder but deceptive heat perception, deep heat sources can be hazardous. With shortwave diathermy, any condition that concentrates the electric field, such as metal or perspiration, can produce a burn. Ultrasound, if focused too long at a particular site, can also produce burning. Deep heat should be used under the supervision of a physical therapist. The deep heat sources are usually not portable, and they are too expensive and dangerous for home use.

Contraindications

Heat applications to large areas of the body, producing systemic heat loss responses, are contraindicated for people with conditions that prevent adequate thermoregulatory responses (such as cardiac insufficiency or impaired peripheral circulation). They are also contraindicated in conditions that could be aggravated or spread, such as swelling, fever, infection, hemorrhage or malignancy (1). Local heat applications to small areas may be used safely in stable cardiac conditions or when applied at a distance from areas of swelling, infection, hemorrhage, and malignancy. Because the amount of heat applied depends on the patient's perception, it should not be used with people who have impaired sensation or impaired judgment or cognition.

In addition to these contraindications, there are several precautions associated with the use of heat in persons with acute, inflammatory arthritis. Heat may increase inflammation, thus increasing edema of the synovial membrane (5). Increasing the intra-articular temperature could damage joint surfaces due to increased activity of collagenolytic enzymes (6). It was previously thought that short applications of superficial heat (less than 10 minutes) cooled the joint and that superficial cooling warmed the joint (7). However, new evidence shows that both joint and skin temperature elevate following superficial heating, especially with treatment times more like those used in clinical practice (20 minutes) (8,9). Shortwave diathermy also heats the interior of the joint along with the skin, although not as much as superficial heat (8). There is no clinical evidence that heat affects progression of rheumatoid arthritis (RA) as evidenced by elevations in erythrocyte sedimentation rate (10), white blood cell count and phagocytosis (11), or radiography (12), but the use of heat for people with acute inflammatory arthritis is best avoided.

People with RA often have unstable vascular reactions in response to heat. They may vasodilate more slowly, causing them to retain heat (13). People with vasculitis associated with RA also may have impaired vasomotor heat loss responses (14). When heat is used in people with RA, they should be monitored carefully to be sure they do not become susceptible to heat stress.

Effectiveness

Investigators have shown that superficial heat can decrease pain and increase range of movement (15–17), but others have found that superficial heat is not effective (10,18). When superficial heat combined with exercises is compared with exercises alone, heat produces no greater effect than exercises alone (15,19).

Many patients report global improvement following superficial heat treatments, despite lack of clinical evidence for improvement (17). If the appropriate contraindications or precautions are observed, patients who feel better or more inclined to be active following heat use should be encouraged to use it. There is little danger or cost associated with using superficial heat, and no apparent negative effects.

Deep heat appears to be capable of increasing range, decreasing pain (20,21), and decreasing functional incapacity, especially with younger patients and those with less severe disease (22). On the other hand, some investigators have found that deep heat is not effective (23,24), and when combined with exercises, deep heat appears to be no more effective than exercise alone (18,25,26). In one study, the only people whose symptoms worsened were those who received shortwave diathermy (26).

Patients who received deep heat treatment have been shown to perceive a more satisfactory outcome than those who received placebo treatments, even when they have persistent disability (20). However, deep heat must be applied in a clinical setting. Such treatments are expensive and may be harmful. When exercise or superficial heat can accomplish the same goals, there is little rationale for using deep heat.

COLD

The primary reasons for using cold applications are to decrease pain, swelling, and inflammation. Pain is decreased by slowing or blocking nerve conduction, decreasing activity of the muscle spindle (1), or releasing endorphins (16). Swelling is decreased through vasoconstriction, which decreases blood flow and capillary pressure. Gentle cold also blocks histamine release, decreasing inflammation. The intra-articular temperature decreases as skin temperature decreases (8), perhaps reducing collagenolytic enzyme activity and inflammation in the joint.

Application

Cold is applied to the skin through ice or cold packs, ice massage, cold baths, or vapocoolant sprays. It is usually applied for 10 to 30 minutes, depending on the intensity of the cold source and the depth of the tissue to be reached. Deeper tissues require longer treatment times. Milder cold sources are more appropriate for swelling; very cold sources, capable of producing skin anesthesia, are more appropriate for pain reduction. Care should be taken not to frost the skin.

Contraindications

Contraindications for the use of cold are essentially the same as those for heat. People must have sufficient vasoconstriction capabilities to conserve heat. In addition, because cold causes vasoconstriction, its use may delay healing. Thus, cold is used only for 24 to 48 hours following acute injury.

As with the use of heat, several precautions must be taken when using cold treatments. Cold produces stiffness in connective tissues in laboratory studies (3), but such stiffness does not necessarily manifest clinically in decreased range of motion. Nonetheless, caution must be exercised to move cooled joints more slowly. Tension production also may be affected by cold treatments. After using a cold treatment that is sufficient to cool the motoneurons and block nerve conduction, entire motor units may temporarily cease to function, with resulting weakness.

Some people are hypersensitive to cold; others actually exhibit cold allergy manifested as urticaria. People with RA have been shown to experience increased pain with cold exposure (27), especially if they smoke (28). Rheumatoid arthritis patients have more vasomotor instability and get colder and stiffer in response to cold exposure. They also have been shown to cool and rewarm more slowly (13). Raynaud's phenomenon, a condition aggravated by cold exposure, is associated with people having a history of joint pain (29) and systemic sclerosis (30).

Effectiveness

Cold treatments can be effective in decreasing pain, improving function, and decreasing stiffness (16,17,31). The effect of cold on swelling in arthritis patients has not been extensively studied, but one study showed that post-surgical hand volume and pain did not change following cold treatments (32). The small sample in this study prevented the observed decreased pain and hand volume from being statistically significant.

Heat and cold appear to be about equally effective for managing pain, stiffness, and limitation of motion (16,17). Cold has been shown to produce earlier decreases in pain and stiffness than shortwave diathermy or placebo treatments (31). Heat appears to be better for improving motion, while cold may be better for reducing pain (17).

TRANSCUTANEOUS ELECTRICAL NERVE STIMULATION

Both decreased pain and inflammation may result from treatment with transcutaneous electrical nerve stimulation (TENS). The use of TENS was originally based on the gate control theory advanced by Melzack and Wall (33). Stimulation of the large sensory fibers is thought to prevent impulses from the smaller pain fibers from being transmitted in the ascending tracks in the spinal cord. Theoretically, impulses from C fibers are blocked better than impulses from other fiber types. Because C fibers innervate the synovium and joint capsule, TENS could prove useful in the treatment of arthritis (34). In addition, forms of TENS may cause the release of endogenous opioids in the midbrain (35).

Use of TENS has been shown to raise intra-articular temperature about 0.5°C in rabbits after a 5-minute treatment, but it also decreased inflammatory exudate and joint pressure and volume (36). The decreased inflammation and joint volume may help relieve pain in inflammatory arthritis.

Application

There are several modes of TENS, but the three most common are high frequency TENS, low frequency or acupuncture-like TENS, and burst mode TENS. High frequency TENS stimulates only the sensory nerve endings, using a continuous train of 100 μsec pulses in a frequency range of 70 to 100 Hz. The usual electrode placement for people with arthritis is around the involved joint. Pain relief is rapidly achieved.

Low frequency TENS stimulates the motor endplates of muscles using wider, 250 μsec pulses at a frequency of 1 to 3 Hz. This mode causes the release of endorphins, which theoretically produces longer lasting pain relief. Electrodes are placed over motor points of muscles in the myotome related to the painful joint.

Burst mode TENS combines elements of both the high and low frequency modes. In burst mode, the carrier frequency of the current is 70 Hz, but it is delivered in small "bursts" at a rate of 3 bursts per second. Burst mode also uses motor level stimulation with electrode placements similar to those used with low frequency TENS. This method produces longer lasting pain relief, apparently through the same mechanisms as low frequency TENS (37). The advantage of burst mode is the greater comfort of the current, as compared with low frequency TENS.

Low frequency and burst mode TENS are usually applied for about 30 minutes. High frequency TENS is often used for several hours, depending on the pain relief achieved. In people with rheumatic disease, pain relief from high frequency and burst mode TENS has been shown to last from 2.5 hours (38) to 18 hours (39), while pain relief from low frequency TENS appears to be several hours shorter (39).

One patient with RA reportedly developed paresthesias and increased pain following heat and TENS. These effects were delayed, so patients should be monitored closely by a qualified therapist (40).

Because TENS is controlled by the patient, it is a good tool for home use when people are properly instructed and monitored. As with all home programs, the treatments are more effective if people adhere to the recommended program.

Contraindications

People with cardiac pacing problems or who use pacemakers should not use TENS near the heart. Electrodes should not be placed over the carotid sinus or the laryngeal or pharyngeal muscles (37). In addition, TENS should not be used during the first trimester of pregnancy, because the effect on the fetus is unknown.

As with other modalities, there are precautions associated with the use of TENS. Persons using TENS should use the joint carefully while being treated. Some people receiving TENS treatments find them uncomfortable. Discomfort may arise from skin irritation from the electrode couplant or adhesion system as much as from the electricity itself.

Effectiveness

Pain relief from TENS has been found to be about 50% in people with arthritis, slightly beyond the relief produced by placebo (38). The usual amount of pain relief attributed to placebo is about 30% to 40%; pain relief beyond that may be attributed to the TENS treatment. Pain relief produced by TENS has been shown to be longer lasting than that produced by painkilling medications (38). Surprisingly, stiffness may decrease as well (34,41).

There is little evidence to favor one mode of TENS over another for patients with rheumatic disease. High frequency and burst modes have been shown to produce more and longer lasting pain relief when compared with low frequency TENS (39). In a comparison of burst mode TENS with high frequency and placebo TENS in persons with osteoarthritis (OA), neither mode produced more pain relief than placebo, but the burst mode produced longer pain relief than placebo. High frequency TENS decreased stiffness better than placebo, and both modes produced longer stiffness relief than placebo. High frequency TENS reduced knee circumference better than burst mode, and burst mode was better than placebo for increasing range of motion (41).

Overall, TENS appears to be useful for decreasing pain and stiffness, and the symptomatic relief may last longer than relief produced by other treatments. The mode should be selected based on the desired goal. Either high frequency or burst mode will provide long lasting relief from pain, but high frequency might be selected if the goal is also to decrease stiffness. Low frequency TENS does not appear to be appropriate for patients with arthritis.

In comparing TENS with other treatments for people with OA of the hip, electrical stimulation alone decreased pain as well as ultrasound, shortwave diathermy, or ibuprofen. Appropriate use of TENS could decrease the need for pharmacologic interventions (26) and would be superior to deep heat, which requires clinic-based application.

SUMMARY

The therapeutic goals for people with arthritis include decreased pain, stiffness, and swelling. Superficial heat is helpful in achieving these goals, but may not be necessary if patients exercise appropriately. However, if patients who do not have acutely inflamed joints feel better after using superficial heat treatments, there appears to be no reason not to use them. Deep heat is costly, potentially hazardous, and requires clinic visits. Because other, safer means such as exercise can meet these goals without aggravating symptoms (especially in inflammatory arthritis), there is little reason to use deep heat in patients with arthritis.

In addition to the goals of symptomatic relief, it may be desirable to cool the joint, thereby decreasing the destructive inflammatory process for patients with inflammatory arthritis. Cold treatments are able to cool the joint as well as promote improvement in pain, motion, and swelling. Cold treatments are not often considered for patients with arthritis, and patients may prefer heat, even when their symptoms are relieved better with cold (16,17). Patients should be encouraged to try cold treatments, especially when they are acutely inflamed.

Use of TENS is effective for decreasing pain and stiffness without the potential hazard to joint surfaces. The high frequency and burst modes appear to work best for patients with arthritis. Patient improvement may be longer lasting, and patients may be able to decrease medication use.

REFERENCES

1. Lehmann JF, DeLateur BJ: Therapeutic heat. In, Therapeutic Heat and Cold. Third edition. Edited by JF Lehmann. Baltimore, Williams & Wilkins, 1982
2. Currier DP, Kramer JF: Sensory nerve conduction: heating effects of ultrasound and infrared. Physiotherapy Canada 34:241–246, 1982
3. Wright V, Johns RJ: Quantitative and qualitative analysis of joint stiffness in normal subjects and in patients with connective tissue diseases. Ann Rheum Dis 20:36–46, 1961
4. Warren CG, Lehmann JF, Koblanski JN: Heat and stretch procedures: an evaluation using rat tail tendon. Arch Phys Med Rehabil 57:122–126, 1976
5. Weinberger A, Fadilah R, Lev A, Levi A, Pinkhas J: Deep heat in the treatment of inflammatory joint disease. Med Hypotheses 25:231–233, 1988
6. Harris ED, McCroskery PA: The influence of temperature and fibril stability on degradation of cartilage collagen by rheumatoid synovial collagenase. New Engl J Med 290:1–6, 1974
7. Hollander JL, Horvath SM: The influence of physical therapy procedures on the intraarticular temperature of normal and arthritic subjects. Am J Med Sci 218:543–548, 1949
8. Oosterveld FGJ, Rasker JJ, Jacobs JWG, Overmars HJA: The effect of local heat and cold therapy on the intraarticular and skin surface temperature of the knee. Arthritis Rheum 35:146–151, 1992
9. Weinberger A, Fadilah R, Lev A, Pinkhas J: Intra-articular temperature measurements after superficial heating. Scand J Rehabil Med 21:55–57, 1989
10. Harris R, Millard JB: Paraffin-wax baths in the treatment of rheumatoid arthritis. Ann Rheum Dis 14:278–282, 1955
11. Dorwart BB, Hansell JR, Schumacher HR Jr: Effects of cold and heat on urate crystal-induced synovitis in the dog. Arthritis Rheum 17:563–571, 1974
12. Mainardi CL, Walter JM, Spiegel PK, Goldkamp OG, Harris ED: Rheumatoid arthritis: failure of daily heat therapy to affect its progression. Arch Phys Med Rehabil 60:390–393, 1979
13. Martin GM, Roth GM, Elkins EC, Krusen FH: Cutaneous temperature of the extremities of normal subjects and of patients with rheumatoid arthritis. Arch Phys Med 27:665–682, 1946
14. Dyck PJ, Conn DL, Okazaki H: Necrotizing angiopathic neuropathy: three-dimensional morphology of fiber degeneration related to sites of occluded vessels. Mayo Clin Proc 47:461–475, 1972
15. Green J, McKenna F, Redfern EJ, Chamberlain MA: Home exercises are as effective as outpatient hydrotherapy for osteoarthritis of the hip. Br J Rheumatol 32:812–815, 1993
16. Utsinger PD, Bonner F, Hogan N: The efficacy of cryotherapy and thermotherapy in the management of rheumatoid arthritis pain: evidence for an endorphin effect (abstract). Arthritis Rheum 25 (suppl 4):S113, 1982
17. Williams J, Harvey J, Tannenbaum H: Use of superficial heat versus ice for the rheumatoid arthritic shoulder: a pilot study. Physiotherapy Canada 38:8–13, 1986
18. Hamilton DE, Bywaters EGL, Please NW: A controlled trial of various forms of physiotherapy in arthritis. BMJ 1:542–544, 1959
19. Hecht PJ, Bachmann S, Booth RE, Rothman RH: Effects of thermal therapy on rehabilitation after total knee arthroplasty. Clin Orthop 178:198–201, 1983
20. Konrad K: Randomized, double blind, placebo-controlled study of ultrasonic treatment of the hands of rheumatoid arthritis patients. Eur J Phys Med Rehabil 5:155–157, 1994
21. Newman MK, Murphy AJ: Application of ultrasonics in chronic rheumatic diseases. Michigan State Med Soc 51:1213–1215, 1232, 1952
22. Jan M, Lai J: The effects of physiotherapy on osteoarthritic knees of females. J Formos Med Assoc 90:1008–1013, 1991
23. Hashish I, Harvey W, Harris M: Anti-inflammatory effects of ultrasound therapy: evidence for a major placebo effect. Br J Rheumatol 25:77–81, 1986
24. Mueller EE, Mead S, Schulz BF, Vaden MR: A placebo-controlled study of ultrasound treatment for periarthritis. Am J Phys Med 33:31–35, 1954
25. Falconer J, Hayes KW, Chang RW: Effect of ultrasound on mobility in osteoarthritis of the knee: a randomized clinical trial. Arthritis Care Res 5:29–35, 1992
26. Svarcová J, Trnavský K, Zvárová J: The influence of ultrasound, galvanic currents and shortwave diathermy on pain intensity in patients with osteoarthritis. Scand J Rheumatol 67 (Suppl):83–85, 1988
27. Jahanshahi M, Pitt P, Williams I: Pain avoidance in rheumatoid arthritis. J Psychosom Res 33:579–589, 1989
28. Helliwell P, Wallace F, Evard F: Smoking and ice therapy in rheumatoid arthritis. Physiotherapy 75:551–552, 1989
29. Leppert J, Åberg H, Ringqvist I, Sörensson S: Raynaud's phenomenon in a female population: prevalence and association with other conditions. Angiology 38:871–877, 1987
30. Medsger TA, Steen V: Systemic sclerosis and related syndromes: clinical features and treatment. In, Primer on the Rheumatic Diseases. Tenth edition. Edited by HR Schumacher, JH Klippel, WJ Koopman. Atlanta, Arthritis Foundation, 1993
31. Clarke GR, Willis LA, Stenner L, Nichols PJR: Evaluation of physiotherapy in the treatment of osteoarthrosis of the knee. Rheumatol Rehabil 13:190–197, 1974
32. Rembe EC: Use of cryotherapy on the postsurgical rheumatoid hand. Phys Ther 50:19–23, 1970
33. Melzack R, Wall PD: Pain mechanisms: a new theory. Science 150:971–979, 1965
34. Kumar VN, Redford JB: Transcutaneous nerve stimulation in rheumatoid arthritis. Arch Phys Med Rehabil 63:595–596, 1982
35. Sjolund BH, Eriksson MBE: Endorphins and analgesia produced by peripheral conditioning stimulation. In, Advances in Pain Research and Therapy. Edited by JJ Bonica, J Liebeskind, DG Albe-Fessard. New York, Raven Press, 1979
36. Levy A, Dalith M, Abramovici A, Pinkhas J, Weinberger A: Transcutaneous electrical nerve stimulation in experimental acute arthritis. Arch Phys Med Rehabil 68:75–78, 1987
37. Foley RA: Transcutaneous electrical nerve stimulation. In, Manual for Physical Agents. Fourth edition. Edited by KW Hayes. Norwalk, CT, Appleton & Lange, 1993
38. Lewis D, Lewis B, Sturrock RD: Transcutaneous electrical nerve stimulation in osteoarthrosis: a therapeutic alternative? Ann Rheum Dis 43:47–49, 1984
39. Mannheimer C, Carlsson A: The analgesic effect of transcutaneous electrical nerve stimulation (TNS) in patients with rheumatoid arthritis: a comparative study of different pulse patterns. Pain 6:329–334, 1979
40. Griffin JW, McClure M: Adverse responses to transcutaneous electrical nerve stimulation in a patient with rheumatoid arthritis. Phys Ther 61:354–355, 1981
41. Grimmer K: A controlled double blind study comparing the effects of strong burst mode TENS and high rate TENS on painful osteoarthritic knees. Aust J Physiotherapy 38:49–56, 1992

Splinting of the Hand

PAMELA B. HARRELL, OTR, CHT

Splints have been used throughout history to protect, immobilize, or mobilize various parts of the body. A splint may be defined as "a rigid or flexible appliance used for the prevention of movement of a joint or for the fixation of displaced or moveable parts." In current practice, splints are used to maintain and enhance motion as well as to prevent it. Splints serve various purposes in the management of the hand with rheumatic disease; however, controversy over the roles and benefits of splinting exists. There are studies that support the use of splints to reduce pain and inflammation. Further studies are indicated to determine the outcome of splinting in prevention and correction of deformity. Indications for and use of splints vary widely among practitioners; however, most agree that splinting does play an important role in the management of rheumatic disease.

The use of splints should be based on knowledge of rheumatic disease, mechanisms of joint inflammation, and pathomechanics of joint deformity. Type of arthritis and stage of joint involvement should influence the treatment program, which may include splinting. How the joint has been affected by arthritis, and more importantly, how joint involvement has affected the person's ability to function should also be considered.

EVALUATION

A complete evaluation is necessary prior to establishing goals for a splinting program. An evaluation should include the following components.

Interview and Subjective Assessment. Obtain a clear history of the disease including duration, medical management, functional performance, and effect of the arthritis on a person's lifestyle. The subjective assessment of pain, stiffness, and fatigue should include information such as intensity, duration, and activities that increase or decrease symptoms.

Objective Measurements. Assessment of range of motion, strength, sensation, and functional abilities will also provide input into splint design. Observe joint function during objective measurements. For example, during grip and pinch strength testing, observe the stability of the metacarpophalangeal (MCP) joints. Is there an increase in ulnar deviation during gripping activities?

Visual Inspection. Through observation of swelling, joint alignment, and tendon and ligamentous integrity, articular and nonarticular manifestations of disease can be identified. These manifestations should be addressed in the splinting process. For example, a splint may be utilized to provide external support for ligamentous laxity of proximal interphalangeal joints, which may reduce pain and improve function.

Establishing Splinting Goals

An individualized approach should be used in establishing splinting program goals, based on problems identified during the evaluation. In the case of a patient with rheumatoid arthritis (RA) who has MCP ulnar drift, goals for splinting should be established as follows: 1) the splint will place the fingers in a more functional position for hand use; and 2) the splint will rest the MCP joints to reduce pain and inflammation. Caution should be utilized in the application of splints. They should only be implemented after fully evaluating the patient's functional ability and establishing goals of splinting. Table 1 lists questions that may help define the parameters of a splinting program.

PURPOSES OF SPLINTING

Reducing Pain

Splints reduce pain by immobilizing or supporting painful joints and periarticular structures (1–4). Immobilization reduces stress on the joint capsule and synovial lining, thereby reducing pain. Supporting a painful joint with a splint allows improved functional use through reduction of pain. By reducing joint pain, reflexive muscle spasm is also reduced, which further reduces joint pain (3). Splints can reduce pain in periarticular structures such as tendons and ligaments by restricting full excursion and overstretching. The benefits of splinting in terms of pain reduction are well documented (2–8). One study found that more than 60% of patients had moderate to great pain relief by using splints (6,9). Another study showed that patients with splints achieved greater relief from pain than relief from morning stiffness (10). The same study also found that patients continued to wear splints because of the benefits of pain reduction.

Decreasing Inflammation

Splints reduce joint and tendon inflammation by restricting motion. Inflammation is also reduced by decreasing external forces on the inflamed tissues. Several studies have demonstrated reduction in joint inflammation through splinting and rest (1,2,4,7,8,10). Consensus has not been reached on how much rest is necessary to reduce inflammation. It has been suggested, however, that splints used for the purpose of reducing inflammation be continued at night for several weeks after acute inflammation has resolved (6,11,12). Patients can be taught to monitor their inflammation and adjust their use of splints accordingly.

Table 1. Questions to aid in establishing the parameters of a splinting program for the hand.

1. What is the goal of the splint? Is the splint being utilized to reduce pain and inflammation or to support an unstable joint? Is the splint being utilized to prevent or possibly correct deformity?

2. What is the best splint design for this particular person? Which joint or joints need to be supported or immobilized to achieve the goal? Should the splint be dorsal or volar? Which materials will best achieve the goals of the splint?

3. When should the splint be worn? Is the splint a resting splint for night wear or a functional daytime splint? How long should the splint be worn?

Preventing Deformity

Splints are often used to support joints in an attempt to prevent deformity. Controversy exists in this area, as there is a lack of outcome data supporting the use of splints for this purpose. Despite this, splints are often prescribed for patients with early signs of deformity to hopefully delay progression, and for patients with more advanced deformity to prevent further deterioration.

Wrist involvement in juvenile arthritis is common, and wrist splints are often prescribed to prevent deformities of subluxation and ulnar deviation (13,14). Wrist splints have been shown to improve writing skills in more than 60% of children with arthritis; however, prevention of deformity has not been documented.

Hand deformity, particularly MCP ulnar deviation, is a common finding in RA (5). Resting hand splints and other ulnar deviation supports are commonly used to prevent or delay progression of deformity. Few studies have addressed the role of splinting in preventing or correcting deformity. The use of a resting splint at night for at least 1 year was not found to delay the progression of ulnar deviation in one controlled study (5). The study also suggested that dynamic splints could reduce ulnar deviation of the MCP joints. Splints used for the purpose of preventing a deformity should be closely monitored.

Correcting Deformity

Splints may be used to correct flexion deformities of the fingers and wrist. Splinting for this purpose can be static (using serial, progressive splinting or casting) or dynamic. Whichever method is used, joint inflammation should be under control, because dynamic forces may exacerbate inflammation. Lateral deformities of the fingers and wrist can also benefit from splinting by providing support to unstable or poorly positioned joints, thereby improving function.

Supporting Function

Hand function can be decreased by painful, inflamed, poorly positioned, or unstable joints. Splinting may improve function by reducing pain and inflammation and by supporting joints in a more stable and functional position. Wrist supports, both commercial and custom-made, reduce forces on the wrist and protect the joint during daily activities, thus allowing for function of the distal joints. Finger and thumb splints place the joints in positions of function and support weakened ligaments,

allowing for pinching and gripping with improved dexterity and/or strength.

Postoperative Management

Dynamic and static splints are used in the postoperative rehabilitation of the hand with rheumatic disease. Dynamic splints allow early postoperative motion in controlled ranges and planes, assist weakened muscles, and protect reconstructed joints and periarticular structures. Dynamic splints also assist in scar formation for stability and motion. Static splints immobilize surgical repairs and stabilize joints in proper alignment. In the case of MCP joint arthroplasty, a dorsal dynamic MCP extension outrigger is utilized continuously for the first 6 to 8 weeks postoperatively to maintain alignment of the joints and to allow exercise in a controlled range of motion. This type of splint may also be used for the same purposes in an extensor tendon repair or transfer. Postoperative splinting for repair of a boutonniere or swan neck deformity is usually static, maintaining the position of the proximal interphalangeal joint while allowing for removal of the splint for periods of exercise. Proper use of splinting postoperatively requires a pre-operative knowledge of the hand, an understanding of operative procedures, established postoperative goals, and a concerted team effort between the surgeon, therapist, and patient.

TYPES OF SPLINTS

Resting Splints

Resting splints are utilized primarily to reduce joint inflammation and pain. They may be used during the day as well as at night. Resting splints may also be used to reduce symptoms of nerve entrapment or tendon irritation, such as triggering and tenosynovitis. Caution should be used when determining the wearing time for resting splints, so that joint motion and muscle strength is not lost due to splint wearing. For this reason, resting splints may be worn at night and intermittently during the day during periods of active synovitis or tenosynovitis, alternating with gentle range of motion and functional activities.

Functional Splints

Functional splints are worn to improve function of the hand by reducing pain, improving joint alignment, or providing stability to weakened ligaments. Functional splints support or immobilize the minimum number of joints, allowing the freedom of movement of all other joints. Functional splints may be *static* (to support weakened or painful joints) or *dynamic* (to gently realign joint deformity).

Corrective Splints

After a complete hand evaluation, it may be determined that joint contracture is the result of a shortening of periarticular structures. If the joint space is preserved, inflammation is at a minimum, and a "soft" end feel is present, splinting may be utilized to gently correct the contracture. Splints used for this

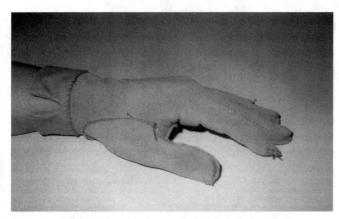

Figure 1. Stretch gloves can be used at night to help decrease morning stiffness and pain.

purpose may be dynamic or static. Dynamic splinting should be approached cautiously in patients with rheumatic disease. Inflammation and pain may be exacerbated by excessive force on the joint. Static splints that are progressively molded to increase range of motion are often better tolerated due to reduced force being placed on the joint.

Soft Splints

Support can be provided to joints with gloves, wraps, and soft splints. Soft splints are often more comfortable to patients and may provide as much symptom relief as rigid splints. Using stretch gloves at night has been shown to decrease morning stiffness and pain, allowing for improved hand function (Figure 1) (16). These gloves work by providing gentle compression and neutral warmth to involved joints. Stretch gloves may be contraindicated if carpal tunnel syndrome is present; there have been reports of exacerbation of paresthesia. Compressive wraps (such as Coban®, Ace®, and Tubigrip®) also provide support and neutral warmth to joints while allowing joint motion.

Circumferential sleeves and tubes (such as Digisleeve®, Digitube®, and Compressogrip®) can be utilized as soft splints for joint support. These splints only slightly limit joint mobility. Individual finger wraps and sleeves also serve as reminders to protect inflamed finger joints and cushion or protect the joint. Soft splints made of neoprene provide joint support and gently assist in realigning joints. Neoprene can be trimmed to fit the patient; however, it does not breathe and may be difficult to put on and wear. Neoprene wraps are often easier for the patient to put on than tubes, especially if there is hand weakness. Another type of soft splint is fabricated from strapping material to support or realign joints (17). Strapping may be used to reposition ulnarly deviated fingers or to block full motion of interphalangeal joints.

FABRICATED VERSUS PREFABRICATED SPLINTS

A multitude of prefabricated splints, custom-ordered splints, and splinting materials exist. It is often difficult to determine whether it is best to custom fabricate a splint or to use a prefabricated design. There are several advantages of custom

fabricated splints. First, the splint is molded to the patient allowing for conformity to joint surfaces. The materials can be selected according to each patient's needs. In addition, a splint can be designed to support certain joints and allow movement of others. Finally, modifications in the fit and design are easily made as needed.

The disadvantage of custom fabricated splints is the cost; custom fabricated splints are usually the most costly type of splint due to fabrication time and materials used. Also, making these splints requires a skill that not all therapists possess. The time needed to fabricate the splint is longer than the fitting time of a prefabricated splint.

Prefabricated splints also have advantages and disadvantages. They are usually less expensive than custom fabricated splints; however, they may not have the desired fit or provide as much support or immobilization. Prefabricated splints are usually available in three or four basic sizes. Achieving a good fit may be problematic due to deformity, size of the forearm in relation to the hand, or general design of the splint. Some prefabricated splints allow for customization by molding of a metal bar or thermoplastic insert, trimming of splint edges, or adjustment of strapping.

PROBLEM IDENTIFICATION AND SPLINT SOLUTION

Identification of the problem through evaluation is the first step toward determining the best type of splint. Some of the more common hand joint problems associated with rheumatic disease are listed in Table 2, along with suggested splinting solutions.

Wrist Splints

A wrist splint provides support for the wrist while allowing motion of the thumb and fingers (Figure 2). Indications for a wrist splint include wrist pain, synovitis, tenosynovitis, subluxation, nerve entrapment, and epicondylitis. A wrist support splint may be *dorsal*, which allows for sensation on the volar surface of the hand but does not support volar subluxation, or *volar*, which supports volar subluxation but is often difficult to wear with activities that involve resting the forearm on a surface. Custom fabricated wrist splints are more likely to restrict motion, while prefabricated wrist supports tend to allow more mid-range motion. A functional position of 20° to 30° of extension is advocated for most conditions; however, in carpal tunnel syndrome 10° of extension maximizes the carpal tunnel. Special care should be taken when fitting a wrist support for a patient with RA. If the MCP joints are involved, restricting the wrist motion may place excess stress on these joints, possibly increasing ulnar deviating or subluxing forces. A position of wrist ulnar deviation is advocated to reduce ulnar deviating force on the MCP joints.

Combination Wrist/Thumb Splints

Indications for combination wrist/thumb splints include synovitis of the wrist and thumb joints, tenosynovitis of the wrist and thumb tendons, deQuervain's tenosynovitis, wrist and thumb pain, and/or instability limiting functional use. Types of

Table 2. Problem identification and suggested splinting solution in the hand with rheumatic disease.*

Problem Identified on Hand Evaluation	Splint Solution
Wrist Joint	**Wrist Support Splint**
Synovitis, tenosynovitis	Dorsal, volar, or combination
Pain	Worn at rest and with activity
Instability, subluxation	Removed for range of motion
Nerve entrapment, carpal tunnel syndrome	Positioned in 10° extension
Wrist/Thumb	**Thumb Spica Splint**
Synovitis of wrist and thumb	Volar design
Tenosynovitis of first dorsal compartment	Radial design to limit thumb motions and allow midrange
Pain in wrist and thumb	wrist motion
	C-bar necessary for CMC joint
Wrist/Hand	**Resting Hand Splint**
Synovitis of multiple joints	Full resting splint for immobilization of multiplejoints/tendons
Flexor/extensor tenosynovitis	Modified resting splint for immobilization of wrist/MCP's
Pain at rest	
Changes in joint alignment	
MCP Joint	**MCP Ulnar Deviation Support**
Synovitis	Built into resting hand splint
Ulnar deviation	Hand-based for functional activities
Ligamentous laxity	
Finger	**Finger Splints**
Boutonniere deformity	PIP extension with DIP free
Swan neck deformity	PIP hyperextension block
Lateral instability	Support for deviation
Flexion deformity	Static progressive or dynamic
Thumb	**Thumb Splints**
CMC osteoarthritis with pain	Hand-based CMC support with C-bar
MCP instability/deformity	
IP hyperextension	Figure-eight MCP support
IP lateral instability	IP hyperextension block
	Support for deviation

*CMC = carpometacarpal, MCP = metacarpophalangeal, PIP = proximal interphalangeal, DIP = distal interphalangeal, IP = interphalangeal.

wrist and thumb supports include a volar wrist support with an added thumb support, a thumb spica with a c-bar for carpometacarpal involvement, a thumb spica without a c-bar, and a radial thumb spica (Figure 3).

Combination Wrist/Hand Splints

Indications for combination wrist/hand splints include pain or synovitis in multiple joints, tenosynovitis in flexor/extensor

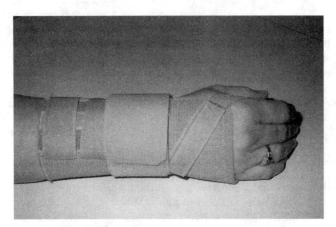

Figure 2. Wrist support splint.

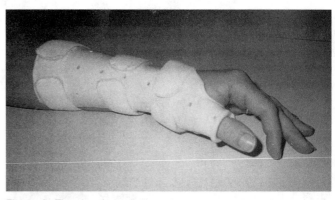

Figure 3. Thumb spica splint.

tendons, pain and/or stiffness at night or in the morning, and complaints of waking with the hand in a fist. A full resting hand splint immobilizes the wrist and fingers to promote relief of pain and inflammation. Studies have shown these splints to be cumbersome to wear, leading to varying rates of use (18). An alternative to a full resting hand splint is the modified resting hand splint, which supports the wrist and MCP joints while allowing interphalangeal movement (Figure 4). The modified resting splint often results in better patient adherence and comfort with less pain and stiffness related to splint wear.

Finger Splints

Splints for ulnar deviation of the MCP joints may be used to place the fingers in a more functional position or to possibly delay progression of deformity (Figure 5). Ulnar deviation splints may also lessen joint pain by supporting weakened ligaments and by resting the joint. Dynamic ulnar deviation splints apply gentle force to realign the joints in a more radial direction. Static splints hold the MCP joint in a more radial direction. These types of splints must be fitted carefully so that they do not interfere with function.

Proximal and Distal Interphalangeal Joint Splints

Splints for the proximal and distal interphalangeal joints are used for synovitis, deformity, instability, pain, and tendon/

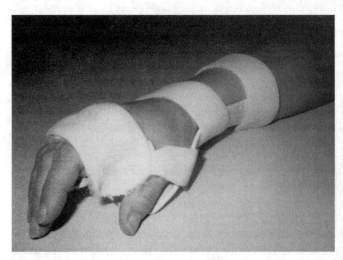

Figure 4. Modified resting hand splint.

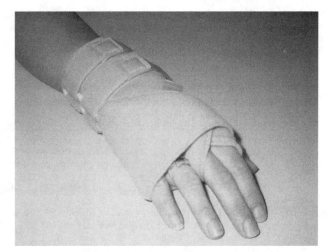

Figure 5. Metacarpophalangeal ulnar deviation splint.

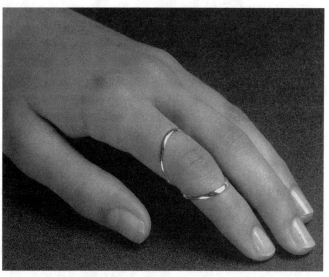

Figure 7. Ring splint for swan neck deformity (photo courtesy of the Silver Ring Splint Company).

ligament involvement. A volar or dorsal resting splint may reduce pain and inflammation. For the distal joint, a volar splint is often more supportive, but it may limit functional use by restricting sensation on the pad of the finger tip. A boutonniere splint (Figure 6) places the proximal interphalangeal joint in extension while allowing flexion of the distal interphalangeal joint. A swan neck splint (Figure 7) supports the volar surface of the proximal interphalangeal joint from hyperextension, but allows flexion of the joint. Lateral instability of the proximal and distal interphalangeal joint limits functional abilities of pinch and fine precision activities. A splint to address lateral instability should provide support in the direction of the instability while allowing the motions necessary to perform daily hand tasks.

Thumb Splints

The thumb accounts for 60% of hand function. When thumb movement is limited by pain, instability, or deformity, hand function is greatly reduced. Osteoarthritis of the carpometacar-

pal joint of the thumb is a common problem encountered in rheumatology. A hand-based thumb support can improve function by reducing pain and supporting ligamentous laxity and joint subluxation (19). The splint should be fitted carefully to address an adequate c-bar. The thumb should be placed in a functional position of opposition to the index finger. In addition, wrist and thumb interphalangeal joint motion should not be restricted.

An unstable, painful, or poorly positioned MCP joint of the thumb can also have a negative influence on hand function. Splints to support the MCP joint of the thumb can improve pinching abilities by providing support and relieving pain. A simple "figure 8" splint for this joint allows movement of the carpometacarpal and interphalangeal joints while providing lateral support and positioning the MCP joint for function. Splints for hyperextension and lateral instability of the interphalangeal joint of the thumb follow the same guidelines as for the proximal interphalangeal joints of the fingers.

SPECIAL CONSIDERATIONS

There are several special considerations in splinting the hand with rheumatic disease to ensure that goals of the splinting program and patient satisfaction are achieved. Patients who become involved in a splinting program should be willing to participate and should be educated as to the benefits of wearing the splint. Patients who are not interested in wearing splints and who do not understand the purposes of splinting are less likely to adhere to this type of intervention.

Materials used to fabricate splints range from rigid to soft and should be selected according to the type and purpose of the splint. Strapping materials can be integral in fitting the splint, ensuring proper support and joint alignment. Different strapping materials, ranging from elastic to cushioned, may help in achieving the best fit. Precautions for joint position, skin integrity, effect on other joints, and wearing times should be communicated clearly to patients in their splinting program. Persons with arthritis may have more fragile skin due to their disease or to medications used to treat the disease. Splint

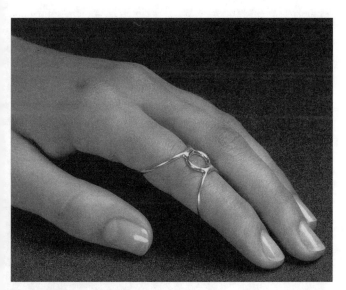

Figure 6. Ring splint for boutonniere deformity (photo courtesy of the Silver Ring Splint Company).

fitting, padding, and lining can address this issue. Effects of immobilization on the targeted joint, as well as adjacent joints, should be considered when developing a schedule for splint wear. Splints should be removed periodically for range of motion exercise and skin care.

PATIENT EDUCATION

Principles of patient education should be applied in teaching patients about their splinting program (see Chapter 9, Patient Education). Patients who learn the purposes of splint use, expectations of splint use, and precautions for splint wear have improved adherence to splint regimes (20). Use of a positive affective tone and encouragement were shown in one study to positively influence splint wearing (20). Results from adherence and splinting studies vary widely, ranging from 25% to 82.5% (10). When patients are better educated about their splinting program, adherence rates should increase. Contracting, written directions, and daily reports are some of the methods used to teach patients about their splints. Regular follow-up visits to ensure proper fit and wearing of the splints are crucial in meeting treatment goals. Partnership among team members—including the patient, therapist, and physician—is crucial in managing the person with arthritis.

REFERENCES

1. Partridge REH, Duthie JJR: Controlled trial of the effect of complete immobilization of the joints in rheumatoid arthritis. Ann Rheum Dis 22:91–99, 1963
2. Gault SJ, Spyker JM: Beneficial effects of immobilization of joints in rheumatoid arthritis and related arthritides: a splint study using sequential analysis. Arthritis Rheum 12:34–44, 1969
3. Melvin JL: Rheumatic Disease in the Adult and Child: Occupational Therapy and Rehabilitation. Third edition. Philadelphia, FA Davis, 1982
4. Feinberg J, Brandt KD: Use of resting splints by patients with rheumatoid arthritis. Am J Occup Ther 35:173–178, 1981
5. Malcus Johnson P, Sandkvist G: The usefulness of nocturnal resting splints in the treatment of ulnar deviation of the rheumatoid hand. Clin Rheumatol 11:72–75, 1992
6. Philips CA: Management of the patient with rheumatoid arthritis: the role of the hand therapist. Hand Clin 5:291–309, 1989
7. Ellis M: Splinting the rheumatoid hand. Clin Rheum Dis 10:673–696, 1984
8. Fred DM: Rest versus activity in arthritis and physical medicine. In, Arthritis and Physical Medicine. Edited by E Licht. Baltimore, Waverly Press, 1969
9. Zoeckler AA: Prenyl hand splints for rheumatoid arthritis. Phys Ther 49:377–379, 1969
10. Nicholas JJ, Gruen H, et al: Splinting in rheumatoid arthritis. I. Factors affecting patient compliance. Arch Phys Med Rehabil 63:92–94, 1982
11. Philips CA: Rehabilitation of the patient with rheumatoid hand involvement. Phys Ther 69:1091–1098, 1989
12. Flatt AE: Care of the Rheumatoid Hand. Third edition. St. Louis, CV Mosby, 1974
13. Eberhard BA, Sylvester KL: A comparative study of orthoplast cock-up splints versus ready-made Droitwich work splints in juvenile chronic arthritis. Disabil Rehabil 15:41–43, 1993
14. Findlay TW, Halper ND: Wrist subluxation in juvenile rheumatoid arthritis: pathophysiology and management. Arch Phys Med Rehabil 64:69–74, 1983
15. Overton EJ, Walcott LE: The role of splints in preventing deformity in the rheumatoid hand and wrist. Missouri Med 6:423–427, 1966
16. Erlich GE, DiPiero AM: Stretch gloves: nocturnal use to ameliorate morning stiffness in arthritic hands. Arch Phys Med Rehabil 51:479–480, 1971
17. Byron P: Splinting the arthritis hand. J Hand Ther 7:29–30, 1994
18. King JW: Splinting the arthritic hand. J Hand Ther 6:46–48, 1993
19. Wolock BS, Moore JR: Arthritis of the basal joint of the thumb. J Arthroplasty 4:65–78, 1989
20. Feinberg J: Effect of the arthritis health professional on compliance with use of resting hand splints by patients with rheumatoid arthritis. Arthritis Care Res 5:17–23, 1992

Enhancing Functional Ability:
Alternative Techniques, Assistive Devices, and Environmental Modification

JILL A. NOAKER, OTR/L, CHT

Rheumatic diseases have a profound and often debilitating effect on an individual's ability to perform normal life activities. These diseases are "cited most often as the principal cause of role limitations by middle-aged and older women, and as the second-ranked cause of limitations (after disease of heart) by men of those ages" (1). Rheumatic diseases affect persons of all ages and can cause numerous symptoms that create impediments to the most routine of daily tasks. The most common symptoms include joint and/or muscle pain, stiffness, fatigue, swelling, limited motion, weakness, and joint instability. The existence, even temporarily, of one or more of these symptoms has the potential to compromise an individual's quality of life.

Health professionals involved with individuals affected by these diseases can identify and recommend appropriate interventions to address their unique functional needs. Most conservative of these interventions is instruction in *alternative techniques*, which are strategies for activity performance that diminish joint stress, reduce vital energy consumption, and allow for greater ease in activities of daily living (ADL). These techniques were developed from the principles of joint protection and energy conservation (2). If the alternative technique is not sufficient to permit independent and safe task performance, an assistive device may be of benefit.

Assistive devices (sometimes known as adaptive devices or assistive technology devices) are aids designed to help an individual perform a selected activity. These devices most often substitute for or accommodate impairments in range of motion, muscular strength, endurance, manual dexterity, and mobility (2). They also may serve to reduce pain and preserve joint integrity by minimizing extraneous stress (3). Assistive devices include aids for personal care (i.e. eating, dressing, grooming, bathing) as well as ambulation and mobility, home management, work, school, and leisure activities.

Environmental modification may be necessary if independent activity cannot be performed with an alternative technique or assistive device alone. Modification of the environment, such as installation of a ramp or stair glide, provides greater accessibility and safety, especially for those individuals who may use an ambulatory device or wheelchair.

ASSESSMENT

Recommendation of interventions designed to enhance an individual's functional abilities should only occur after a thorough assessment of ADL status including home and family situation, work or school situation if applicable, and tasks associated with self-care, mobility, and home management. The assessment is best performed within the environment

relevant to the ADL being addressed (home, work, school, or other location) and at the time of day when those activities occur or are most commonly performed. Often however, the therapist cannot evaluate the person under such ideal conditions and must rely on the results of the ADL assessment performed in the clinical setting. The assessment should be performance-based, allowing the therapist to see exactly which activities are difficult for the individual and to determine the cause of the difficulty.

Critical to any type of ADL assessment process is the therapist's thorough understanding of the disease and its prognosis. The clinician also needs to be aware of and recognize the impact of the current level of disease activity, medications, duration and severity of stiffness, location and type of pain, and level of fatigue (3). Noting the presence of limitations in motion and strength can be instrumental in identifying physical causes for difficulty.

The ADL assessment should answer the following questions: 1) Is the patient performing daily tasks that are causing needless or potentially deforming stresses to involved joints? 2) Is the patient limited in performing daily tasks as a result of a physical impairment? If the response to either question is affirmative, the therapist should determine whether there are adaptive methods or equipment that could minimize or eliminate joint stress or increase the patient's independence or ability to complete these tasks.

The information gathered during the ADL assessment, especially the identified difficulties in activity performance, serves as a foundation on which to proceed when planning the appropriate therapeutic intervention(s).

INTERVENTION

At this juncture, the therapist and the individual with rheumatic disease must collaboratively plan treatment. Treatment recommendations to restore or improve functional abilities include instruction in alternative techniques, provision of assistive devices, and modification of the environment.

Alternative Techniques

If possible, the identified functional limitation(s) should be corrected or minimized by instructing the person in an alternative technique. Individuals with rheumatic diseases most often prefer to do an activity in a modified fashion without the use of a device, rather than with one. Alternative techniques are methods of performing activities that reduce pain, conserve

Table 1. Factors to consider in prescribing assistive devices.

Physical Factors	Does the device reduce pain, stiffness, or joint stress?
	Does the device reduce energy or time expenditure?
	Is the device convenient, easy to use, and if needed, transportable?
	Will the device only be needed at certain times (mornings, bad days)?
	Does the device substitute for an activity that can be done safely without it? Does it promote loss of motion in mobile joint?
Social-Emotional Factors	Does the person desire or value independence in activities of daily living?
	Does the person have a negative response to the appearance or use of the assistive device?
	Is there a fear of failure or low frustration tolerance that may impede learning to use the device?
Environmental Factors	Are the assistive devices or modifications compatible with the architecture and environment of the home/workplace?
	If needed, is there an individual available to install or maintain the equipment?
Financial Factors	Can these devices be made less expensively than purchased?
	Are the devices commercially available rather than available only from medical suppliers?

energy, reduce joint stress, and preserve joint structures. They are the practical application of the principles of joint protection and energy conservation that guide activity performance for persons with arthritis. Some of these principles are reviewed below (3–5).

Respect Pain. Individuals with rheumatic diseases often learn to live with some level of pain in their daily activities. It is important to enable those individuals to recognize the difference between what is a "usual" amount and type of pain versus the pain that is caused by incorrect use or overuse of a joint or muscle. If pain intensity increases or there are overt signs of inflammation, the precipitating activity should be reviewed and strategies to diminish joint stress applied.

Balance Work and Rest. Fatigue can play a significant role in robbing persons with rheumatic diseases of their maximum productivity and ability to accomplish desired activities. Even short rest breaks from activities during the day can help prevent fatigue. Activity scheduling should be "paced" so that heavy tasks like mopping the floor or mowing the lawn are balanced with light ones, such as reading a book.

Conserve Energy. Conservation of energy and reduction of effort in activity can be important for a person with rheumatic disease who may tire quickly and feel exhausted after a few hours of activity. Minimizing excessive or stressful body movements helps conserve limited energy. Suggestions for activity modification may include: 1) prioritizing tasks that are most important, 2) gathering all necessary supplies before beginning a project, 3) limiting the number of trips needed, especially up and down stairs, 4) sitting to perform tasks when able, and 5) using elongated handles on tools to prevent excessive bending or reaching.

Avoid Positions of Deformity. Positions of comfort are often positions of potential deformity. These include neck, elbow, wrist, finger, hip, and knee flexion, all of which can lead to soft tissue contractures if the joints are not moved through the full range or stretched out. Individuals with arthritis should be educated regarding these positions and instructed to avoid them, especially for prolonged periods.

Use Larger/Stronger Joints. Forces applied to larger joints are more efficiently dispersed than when applied to smaller, more vulnerable joints. Use of mechanical advantage in handling or moving objects can effectively reduce joint stress. Recommendations may include using the forearm to carry packages with handles, using both arms to lift and carry packages close to the body, and when possible, sliding objects rather than carrying them.

Use Each Joint in its Most Stable Plane. Joint involvement such as synovitis or bony osteophytes can lead to laxity in the supporting structures and subsequent joint instability and defor-

mity. It is important, therefore, to use each joint in its most stable plane. The patient may be advised to avoid twisting of the fingers to wring a cloth or open a jar (use the flat palm of the hand instead), position work to avoid twisting of the neck or back, and directly face an object when lifting it to avoid twisting of the spine.

Avoid Staying in One Position. Individuals with rheumatic diseases should move and change positions frequently (optimally every 20–30 minutes). Sitting and standing should be alternated in activities to prevent stiffness and possible deformity.

ASSISTIVE DEVICES

Assistive devices can be invaluable tools in preserving functional independence by compensating for physical deficits. Assistive devices can: 1) support weakened joints, 2) provide leverage to increase force while decreasing exertion, 3) maintain joints in the most stable anatomical position, 4) extend reach when joints are limited in motion, and 5) avoid unnecessary use or strain to a joint or muscle (4). However, using an assistive device constitutes a major change for most people. There are many factors to consider before prescribing such an intervention (2,3,6–8) (Table 1). Clinicians should be aware of the impact of these factors on the use (or non-use) of assistive devices.

Once it has been ascertained that an assistive device would be of benefit, the clinician and the patient have a variety of choices. The therapist should determine, based on the individual's unique situation and preferences, which device(s) will work best. Specific instruction and the opportunity to practice enhance adherence and help the patient recognize the benefit and gain a sense of competence and mastery in the use of the device.

Assistive devices can be classified as aids for general daily living; self-care; transfers and mobility; home management; and leisure, work, and school activities. Activities that are commonly difficult within these categories are presented, along with assistive devices that may increase functional independence.

General Daily Living

Activity	Recommended Device or Adaptation
Turning knobs or faucets	Knob turner, faucet turner
	Single lever faucet
	Dycem or non-slip matting to improve grip
Holding/using a key	Key holder (Figure 1)
	Orthotic material built-up handle
Cutting with scissors	Loop scissors or spring-loaded scissors

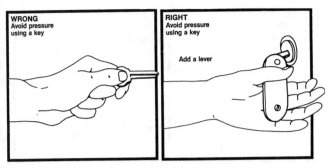

Figure 1. Incorrect and correct ways to avoid pressure to the fingers and hand when using a key (12; reprinted with permission from the author).

Self-Care: Personal Hygiene

Personal hygiene is a very important component in maintaining one's appearance and self-esteem. Most often these activities, such as brushing teeth, hair and nail care, shaving, and toileting, are limited by diminished hand grasp and arm motion. This is often compounded by the presence of morning stiffness when many of these activities are performed.

Activity	Recommended Device or Adaptation
Comb/brush hair	Enlarged handle brush/comb
	Long handled brush/comb
Dental hygiene	Cylindrical foam on toothbrush handle
	Denture brush mounted on suction cup base
	Pump toothpaste dispenser or toothpaste key
Shaving	Enlarged handle razor or cylindrical foam
	Electric razor
	Spray can adapter on shaving cream can
Nail care	Clippers and emery board mounted on suction cup base
	Electric or battery-operated file/buff
Toileting	Toilet tongs to hold paper and extend reach

Self-Care: Bathing

Bathing requires joint mobility, especially in the shoulders, to reach all body parts. In addition, one needs to be able to grasp and hold a washcloth or sponge and apply soap as well as manipulate a towel to dry the body after bathing.

Activity	Recommended Device or Adaptation
Washing/drying	Long handled sponge or brush
	Sponge or wash mitt
	Hand-held shower
	Terry robe after bathing
Using soap or shampoo	Liquid soap in pump or wall-mounted dispenser

Self-Care: Dressing

Dressing can pose a great challenge to a person with rheumatic disease because of its many physical demands. Like grooming, dressing is often performed at times of maximum stiffness. It requires endurance, mobility, strength, and dexterity. Dressing may best be performed after a warm shower to alleviate morning stiffness and in a seated position to reduce energy consumption. In addition to assistive devices for dressing, techniques also exist for adapting clothing. The Guide to Independent Living (5) offers several suggestions.

Activity	Recommended Device or Adaptation
Putting on a bra	Choose front closure style
	Replace hooks with Velcro® closure
Putting on a shirt or jacket	Dressing stick for extended reach
Putting on pants or shorts	Sit to perform task
	Dressing stick to start garment over legs
	Sewn-in loops for easy pull-up
Putting on socks/stockings/shoes	Sock device and/or long-handled shoehorn
	Elastic shoe laces or Velcro® closure shoes
Fasteners (buttons, snaps, zippers)	Button hook, zipper pull, or zipper ring
	Replace snaps with Velcro®

Self-Care: Eating

Eating is an instrumental and often highly social activity. The ability to eat independently is of immeasurable value to most individuals. Rheumatic diseases can make it difficult to prepare food for eating and get the food or drink to the mouth. This is frequently due to limitations in strength and in mobility of the cervical spine, elbow flexion/extension, forearm rotation, and hand grasp.

Activity	Recommended Device or Adaptation
Holding/using utensils	Enlarged handle grips or cylindrical foam
	Utensil cuff
Cutting food	Rocker or angled knife
	Dycem or non-slip matting under plate
	Plate guard or edged scoop dish
Getting food/drink to mouth	Extended handle utensils, swivel utensils
	Extended straws
	Two-handled glass holders, lightweight mugs

Transfers and Mobility

Transfers, or moving from one location to another, are often hampered by limited motion of the hips, knees, ankles, and upper extremities; muscle weakness; joint instability; and pain or stiffness. Independence in transfers is necessary for freedom of normal movement. Safety is of equal importance in preventing falls and reducing the risk of potential injury. Increasing independence and safety in transfers can generally be accomplished by either elevating the seated surface or adding supports for upper extremity assistance.

Activity	Recommended Device or Adaptation
Getting on/off chair	Look for chair with arm supports
	Pillow or elevated cushion on seat
	Lift chair or lift seat insert
Getting in/out of bed	Rope ladder to pull up from supine
	Transfer assist rail
Getting on/off toilet	Elevated toilet seat or frame
	Commode rails
Getting in/out of tub/shower	Tub rails and wall-mounted grab bars
	Shower stool or transfer tub bench (Figure 2)
Getting in/out of car	Elevated or swivel seat cushion

Home Management

Home management encompasses the many activities involved in running a household. Persons with rheumatic diseases can benefit from the recent growth in commercially available power, convenience, and ergonomically designed products for these activities. Not all convenience appliances or products are convenient or easily used by a person with a rheumatic disease, however. Appliance or product use may be difficult due to the weight, force/pressure, or mobility required. Encourage the person to try the product before purchasing to see if it is easily operable for home management tasks. Above all, home management activities are

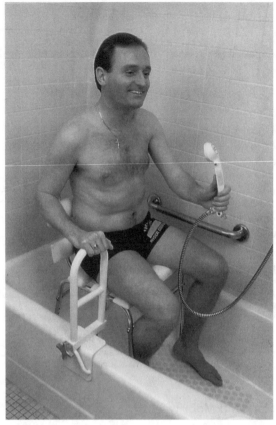

Figure 2. Getting in and out of the bathtub, taking a bath, and standing in the shower can be hazardous when lower extremity function is impaired by arthritis. Methods to improve safety include sitting on a stool or bench, which requires the use of a hand-held shower attachment. A detachable tub rail provides safety while the patient steps in and out of the tub (from the ARHP Arthritis Teaching Slide Collection).

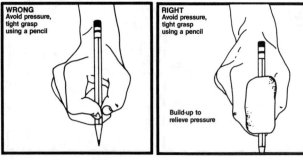

Figure 3. Using enlarged grips for writing relieves pressure on finger and hand joints (12; reprinted with permission from the author).

maintaining normal life roles. Federal legislation, such as the Americans with Disabilities Act, has established regulations promoting the accessibility of public buildings and transportation as well as reasonable accommodations to allow an individual to perform his or her job. Possible accommodations depend on the environment, job, or task and the functional level of the individual. Some common work and/or school activities and recommended devices are listed below.

Activity	Recommended Device or Adaptation
Writing	Large diameter pens, markers, or enlarged grips (Figure 3)
	Writing aids
	Tape Recorder for lectures/meetings, dictating notes
	Laptop computer
Using a computer	Wrist at neutral - cushion in front of keyboard
	Document holder
	Good posture with feet supported on floor
	Stretch frequently
Using a phone	Large number pad phone or phone holder
	Speaker phone or headset
	Lightweight cordless phone
Reading	Book holder or books on tape

Leisure Activities

Leisure activities and hobbies are an important component of a healthy and balanced lifestyle. Individuals with rheumatic diseases may struggle to perform even routine ADLs, leaving little energy to pursue leisure activities. Depression and pain can also prevent people from enjoying valued activities. Health professionals should assess the leisure interests of individuals with arthritis, determine whether they are having any difficulty in the performance of those activities and suggest modifications as needed.

more safely performed by not only using devices, but also by incorporating the principles of joint protection and energy conservation.

Activity	Recommended Device or Adaptation
Opening jars, cans, boxes	Jar openers, electric can opener, box top opener, small kitchen shears or knife
Preparing food	Sit to work when possible
	Utensils with enlarged handles
	Electric food chopper/processor, microwave
Reaching/transporting items	Long handled reacher to retrieve items
	Utility cart
	Lightweight dishes and pans
	Slide objects rather than carry
Cleaning	Long handled non-wringing sponge or mop
	Long broom with attached dust pan, long handled duster
	Lightweight sweeper
	Terry or sponge wash mitt
Maintenance tasks	Tools with enlarged and cushioned handles
	Lightweight power tools
	Spray lubricant or non-slip matting to turn nozzles, valves
	Easy-to-start self-propelled lawnmower or riding mower

Activity	Recommended Device or Adaptation
Gardening	Tools with cushioned handles
	Cushioned kneeler with handles to help get up
	Window box or raised bed gardening
Playing cards	Card holder
	Automatic shuffler
Knitting/crocheting/needlework	Table top clamp-on frame for needlework
	Stretch hands frequently
Woodworking	Light-weight power tools (sander, drill, staple gun)
	Pre-cut kits to assemble and finish
	Cushioned foam handles on tools

Work/School Activities

The ability to perform and sustain one's occupation, whether that be as an employee or student, is crucial in

Table 2. Guidelines for accessible areas within the home.

Outside Entrance	Railings on both sides of stairs (1 1/2" diameter) 32–36" from ground Non-slip surface ramp (portable or permanent) at slope of 1" rise: 12" run
Interior Halls/Doors	Hallways 36" + width, railings at 32–36" adults, 18–24" children Rails 1 1/2" diameter mounted on supports 1 1/2" from wall Doors 32" minimum with lever knobs and push-button locks Light switches at 32–36" from floor
Steps/Stairs	Light switches at either end Railings on both sides—extend past last step to help step up/down Recommended rise of 4" to 11" step (standard 7" rise to 11" tread) Stair glide if needed
Bathroom	Toilet at 17–19" from floor—may add elevated seat to 22" or install elevated toilet; grab bar or commode rails at both sides Walk-in shower with built-in seat or wheel-in version Tub with non-slip surface, vertical grab bars at either end, long grab bar mounted at angle on long wall. May use tub mounted rail as well 30" clearance under sink and 60" turnaround diameter to accommodate wheelchair
Kitchen	U shaped or corridor kitchen design with sink between refrigerator and stove and minimum of 18" counter in between Lazy susan, pull-out shelves, drawer dividers, and baskets for storage Rolling utility cart for transport; pegboard or wire rack with hooks for storage Movable stool or chair to sit when preparing foods
Bedroom	Bedside organization table—phone, remote control, touch lighting Book holder or lap desk Power controls for house lighting and security system

ENVIRONMENTAL MODIFICATION

Environmental modification is another vital component in the total care of the person with rheumatic disease. Environmental modification can create an accessible environment that promotes safety and independence in ADL and other desired activities. Environmental accessibility depends on the nature and extent of the individual's impairment and the limitations posed by his or her specific environment. The clinician must evaluate the individual's ability to function within his or her relevant environment before making suggestion(s) for needed modifications.

Modifications should be carefully planned and discussed with the patient. Cost is usually a concern in environmental modification, as few insurance plans cover such expenses. Additionally, it is important to the individual that the modifications are aesthetically pleasing as well as functional. The trend toward universal and accessible design in building has increased the choices available for home modification. Table 2 outlines general guidelines for creating accessible areas within the home (9–11).

REFERENCES

1. Verbrugge LC, Lepkowski JM, Konkol LL: Levels of disability among U.S. adults with arthritis. J Gerontol 46:S71-S83, 1991
2. Rogers JC, Holm MB: Assistive technology device use in patients with rheumatic disease: literature review. Am J Occup Ther 46:120–127, 1992
3. Melvin JL: Rheumatic Disease in the Adult and Child: Occupational Therapy and Rehabilitation. Third edition. Philadelphia, FA Davis, 1989
4. Sandles L: Occupational Therapy in Rheumatology: An Holistic Approach. London, Chapman and Hall, 1990
5. Guide to Independent Living for People with Arthritis. Revised edition. Atlanta, Arthritis Foundation, 1988
6. Redford JB: Assistive devices. In, Principles of Physical Medicine and Rehabilitation in the Musculoskeletal Diseases. Edited by JC Leek, ME Gershwin, WM Fowler. Orlando, FL, Grune & Stratton, 1986
7. Chamberlain MA: Aids and equipment for the arthritic. Practitioner 224: 65–71, 1980
8. Schweidler H: Assistive devices, aids to daily living. In, Rheumatic Diseases: Rehabilitation and Management. Edited by GK Riggs, EP Gall. Boston, Butterworth, 1984
9. Informed Consumer Guide to Accessible Housing. ABLEDATA Database of Assistive Technology. Silver Spring, MD, Macro International, 1995
10. Woods WL: Architectural and environmental barriers. In, Rheumatic Diseases: Rehabilitation and Management. Edited by GK Riggs, EP Gall. Boston, Butterworth, 1984
11. Salmen JPS: The Doable Renewable Home. Washington, DC, American Association of Retired Persons, 1991
12. Furst GP, Gerber LH, Smith CC: Rehabilitation Through Learning: Energy Conservation and Joint Protection: A Workbook for Persons with Rheumatoid Arthritis. Bethesda, MD, National Institutes of Health, Department of Rehabilitation Medicine, 1987

Additional Recommended Reading

1. Lorig K, Fries JF: The Arthritis Help Book. Second edition. Reading, MA, Addison-Wesley, 1986
2. Axtell LA, Yasuda YL: Assistive devices and home modification in geriatric rehabilitation. Clin Geriatr Med 9:803–821, 1993

Foot Management and Ambulatory Aids

BRUCE M. CLARK, RPT

While the foot is not involved in all of the more than 100 rheumatic diseases, in several diseases it may be significantly impaired, resulting in pain and the inability to walk, stand, and function in the normal activities of daily living. In rheumatoid arthritis (RA), inflammation leads to damage of articular cartilage and supporting ligaments. This produces malalignment of joints, loss of flexibility, and loss of structural integrity of the foot. In ankylosing spondylitis, enthesopathic pain (inflammation of soft tissue attachments to bone) can occur in the sole of the foot or around the achilles tendon. Osteoarthritis (OA) tends to affect three areas of the foot: the metatarsophalangeal (MTP) joint of the great toe, the first metatarsal/cuneiform joint, and the ankle joint.

Some forms of rheumatic disease involve vasculitis, in which small blood vessel flow is compromised, precipitating skin breakdown and poor capacity to heal. In addition, medications such as corticosteroids may affect peripheral blood flow. Soft tissue and nail problems may also be present. For example in psoriatic arthritis, skin and nail problems may co-exist with joint synovitis or damage. Systemic sclerosis or Raynaud's phenomenon may involve the foot. In these cases care should be taken to avoid cold and skin abrasions. Orthoses and special shoes may be necessary.

The foot should not be treated as a separate entity but should be viewed as the base of a dynamic chain that involves the ankle, knee, hip, and spine. Factors that affect the mobility and alignment of the foot and ankle will in turn influence the joints above. The reverse is also true in that joint changes above will affect the alignment and mechanics of the foot and ankle. A pronated foot in RA is commonly seen in association with a valgus deformity at the knee joint.

RHEUMATOID ARTHRITIS

Rheumatoid arthritis affects 1% of the adult population, and approximately 80% to 90% of individuals with RA are reported to have symptoms in the feet (1,2). Problems occur in three distinct areas of the foot, the forefoot, the mid-foot, and the hind foot. While these three areas are related, the problems may be discrete in the early stages of disease.

The Forefoot. The MTP joints are the most commonly affected, with synovitis manifesting as local pain in the joint, swelling and warmth, and difficulty weight bearing through the joint. If early synovitis is controlled, little physical damage will result. More often, however, disease activity persists and chronic inflammation leads to joint changes. If synovitis persists, articular cartilage is progressively lost from the metatarsal head and the base of the proximal phalanx. These erosions progress proportional to the duration and intensity of the synovitis. Cartilage loss leads to loss of smooth motion at the joint, crepitus on movement, and joint disorganization. The supportive ligaments become progressively lax, permitting subluxation of the proximal phalanx dorsally and finally dislocation of the phalanx. As the proximal phalanx migrates upward, the plantar fat pad thins and displaces distally, pulled by dorsal soft tissue contractures of the lesser toes. The metatarsal head is then exposed, separated from the weight-bearing surface only by skin. At this point, all of the weight-bearing forces pass through the metatarsal head. Calluses form over the bony prominences and, in limited instances, the bony metatarsal head takes such pressure that it erodes through the sole of the foot, causing a bony protuberance with skin breakdown. Should this occur, infection and drainage become possible. The most common site of pressure is over the first and second metatarsal head, where greater forces are present (Figure 1).

As dislocation of the MTP joints occur, the forces of weight bearing combine to produce lateral drifting of the toes. The great toe and first metatarsal take a disproportionate share of the load. Unable to carry this force, the great toe begins to develop hallux valgus as the foot rolls over it at toe-off.

Just as painful callosities are prone to develop over the prominent metatarsal heads in the sole of the foot, they are also prone to develop over the dorsum of the interphalangeal joint where the clawed toes produce pressure upward, against the shoe (Figure 2) (3).

The Mid-foot. The weakened ligamentous structures allow the head of the talus and tuberosity of the navicular to rotate forward and downward, creating a flattened medial arch and pronated midfoot. While synovitis and pannus destruction begin the process, rupture of the tibialis posterior tendon that normally passes under the medial side of the foot, acting as a supportive sling, permits the bony arch to collapse further. At heel strike, the jarring force of impact is not absorbed due to loss of mobility in the joints and the loss of articular cartilage. These forces produce further damage.

The mid-foot may be involved with chronic synovitis, loss of joint space, and varying degrees of stiffness or ankylosis. Bony erosions tend not to occur in this part of the foot. The classic deformity is loss of the longitudinal arch. With synovitis there can be a dropping of the metatarsals downward in the foot's bony arch. If the mid-foot remains mobile, this mobile arch can be passively restored. Should joint stiffness occur, conservative methods of elevating the metatarsal heads upward will be less effective (4).

The Hind Foot. The subtalar joint with the talus above, the calcaneum below, and the navicular anteriorly, is often affected in RA. Tenosynovitis may also occur in the tendons and sheaths of the tibialis posterior and flexor hallucis longus. The presence of synovitis in the subtalar joint leads to pannus formation and articular cartilage destruction, and later to bony erosion. In the early stages, the joint is warm and swollen and,

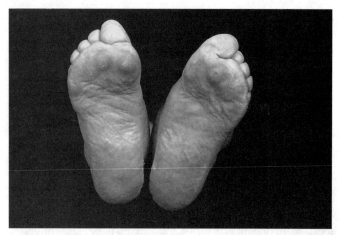

Figure 1. Subluxation/dislocation of the metatarsophalangeal joints, resulting in the toes not participating in weight bearing, has produced points of extreme pressure under each of the metatarsal heads (photo courtesy of the Arthritis Society [B.C. and Yukon Division]).

if chronic, the thick boggy swelling of the persistently inflamed synovium may be palpable.

Initially there may be pain, warmth, and swelling, but no hind foot malalignment. Chronic synovitis produces physical damage to cartilage in the joints, leading to bony erosion. With the high forces of weight bearing imposed, ligaments become extended beyond normal anatomic limits, permitting hypermobility in the affected joints with the hind foot progressively moving into valgus. The heel swings outward from its normal alignment in relation to the achilles tendon as viewed from behind. Once hind foot valgus begins, the shearing forces of weight bearing acting on damaged supporting structures lead to progressive malalignment if unchecked (Figure 3) (5,6).

Assessment of the Foot in RA

Observation should begin as the patient walks into the room. An impression will quickly be formed as to walking speed and ease of motion. Is one side favored? Does the individual follow

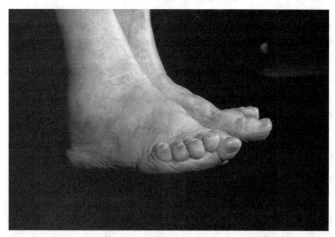

Figure 2. Cocked-up toes from subluxation and dislocation of the metatarsophalangeal joints is seen along with displacement of the heel pad. In walking, the toes will not touch the ground or share in weight-bearing so all pressure is taken directly on the metatarsal heads (photo courtesy of the Arthritis Society [B.C. and Yukon Division]).

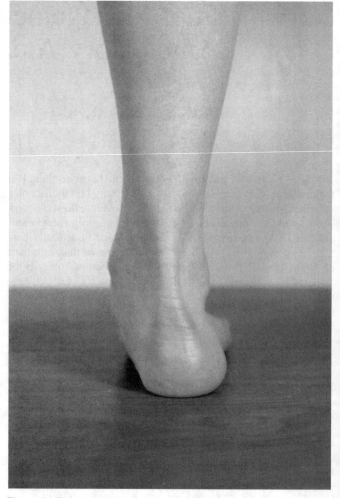

Figure 3. This illustration shows early hind foot valgus. The line of the achilles tendon, instead of being vertical, swings outward toward its attachment to the calcaneum. The mid-foot can also be seen to be pronating, or collapsing downward and inward (photo courtesy of the Arthritis Society [B.C. and Yukon Division]).

the normal pattern of heel strike followed by stance phase, ending with rolling over the metarsals to toe-off? Is the gait pattern symmetric? The rheumatoid foot will often be placed on the ground as one piece, rather than first heel strike, followed by the characteristic rolling forward over the lateral border of the foot and transfer to the medial forefoot for toe-off. The type of shoes being worn should be noted and may themselves be part of the problem, or an attempt at a solution.

Formal gait observation is important and should be done with the shoes removed. The stance phase of gait will reveal the extent of pain and limitation. Observe the individual from a distance to clearly note the gait pattern. The most common problem is likely to be the lack of roll over the metatarsal heads as the weight-bearing leg moves toward toe-off, indicating pain under the metatarsal heads. The individual will tend to lift the whole foot as one piece, possibly compensating for the lack of foot movement with exaggerated motion at the ankle, knee, and hip. Stride length will be shortened, because a normal stride requires rocking over the forefoot as the contralateral leg steps out. Weakened muscles, particularly the plantar flexors, will contribute to these gait changes. Heel strike may occur on the inside of the heel, rather than the customary rear outer aspect of the heel. Because the gait pattern includes no rolling over the toes, knee flexion and hip extension are limited, and the stride length is shortened on the opposite leg (7).

Observation should be made from behind and from the side with shoes removed. From behind, observe the symmetry of the standing position at the ankle and foot. Is the line through the center of the heel in alignment with the leg above, or is it swung outward and, if so, how much? When viewed from directly behind, does the foot extend forward in the mid position, or are there too many toes visible on the lateral side?

From the lateral side, are the toes in contact with the ground or are they "cocked up"? To what degree are they elevated? Are some or all the toes off the ground? Observe the skin over the dorsum of the interphalangeal joints. Examine the skin for corns or obvious areas of pressure or redness. When observed from the medial side or front, is the longitudinal arch evident or is the medial border of the foot in contact with the floor?

Additional problems may include hallux valgus with the great toe drifted outward to possibly overlie or underlie the second toe. A bunion or callosity may overlie the first metatarsal head. The skin may be intact and healthy or may demonstrate areas of thickening or redness, usually over obvious points of pressure. Rheumatoid nodules can occur in the foot, usually at points of pressure such as the back of the heel.

A history will reveal subjective complaints. Ask the patient about the location and severity of any pain. What aggravates or relieves this pain? To what degree does pain limit standing time and walking distance? In the rheumatoid foot the two most common sites of pain are directly under the metatarsal heads and at the subtalar joint. The forefoot pain, under the metatarsal heads, will often be referred to as the sensation of "walking on marbles." Hind foot pain will usually be localized distal to the malleoli. Mid-foot pain may also be present. Pain of joint origin will be aggravated by weight-bearing and alleviated by rest. Vascular pain from circulatory inadequacy may also be aggravated by activity and walking, and alleviated by rest, and will not localize to joints in the feet. The history also will reveal the duration and rate of progression of the symptoms in the foot as well as any previous foot treatment.

Range of motion of the joints should be checked at the hip, knee, and ankle bilaterally. Inversion and eversion, subtalar mobility, and ankle plantarflexion and dorsiflexion are also checked. The mobility of the metatarsals at the tarso-metatarsal joint should be passively tested. Measurement at the tarso-metatarsal joint is made to determine whether this joint will permit sufficient motion to allow the metatarsal to be elevated in the forefoot. If this joint is immobile, an insole intended to lift the metatarsal heads will need to be used in an extra-depth shoe to allow sufficient room to lift the MTP joints without applying pressure to the tops of the toes. The MTP joints should be tested for mobility, both actively and passively.

Treatment

If there is little physical damage, exercise may benefit the patient by increasing mobility, strengthening weakened muscles, and stretching tightened structures (8). Range of motion exercises are useful in maintaining mobility. These exercises should be done bilaterally for the joints of the feet, ankles, knees, and hips. Emphasis on range of motion in RA should focus on the ankle joints, the subtalar joints, inversion/eversion at the mid-tarsal joints, and for flexion at the MTP joints and extension at the interphalangeal joints.

The subtalar joint, if limited, should be mobilized through passive mobilization. The individual cannot actively move this joint through its full range of motion, yet loss of mobility is a problem. When marked loss of mobility at the subtalar joint and valgus deformity are present, treatment should progress from trying to regain mobility to supporting the damaged joint in its present position and preventing further deformity.

The muscles of the feet, particularly the small intrinsic muscles, may become weak. These can be strengthened with exercise, such as increasing the longitudinal arch of the foot and relaxing it. Repetitions can be done using a long strip of fabric, and pulling the fabric in under the feet with each arching movement. Curling the toes down to pick up marbles or small objects, holding them, and then setting them down is useful. This marble exercise can be done in an exercise class. Empty a small jar of marbles onto the floor and have each individual pick them up one at a time and replace them in the jar. Exercises that encourage plantarflexion with inversion will strengthen the posterior tibialis and muscles of the longitudinal arch (9).

When muscle function is very poor, exercises can be taught using the assistance of a faradic foot bath. As active muscle control is achieved, the current is lessened until the individual can do the exercise unassisted. In limited instances, pain relieving modalities may be used. Foot pain in RA is more likely to arise from the pressure of weight bearing, which can be alleviated by appropriate shoes and orthoses. If pain is a particular problem, physical modalities may be helpful (10–13). The major means of alleviating pain and controlling foot deformity in RA is through the use of appropriate footwear combined with the use of commercial or custom-made foot orthotics.

Footwear

Shoes for patients with RA should have a deep and wide toe box to accommodate toes that may be flexed up, and should be wide enough to accommodate the splayed rheumatoid forefoot. It will have a strong medial counter to support the prolapsed medial arch and act as the base upon which the supportive orthosis will rest. This medial arch, while being supportive, should also have sufficient softness and covering to be tolerated. The shoe should be laced or fastened securely on the foot. In addition, shoes should have high heel cups and heel counters that are firm enough to be capable of gripping the calcaneus. The heel of the shoe should be broad based so that the foot is stable on the ground. Removable insoles may be replaced by a custom-made orthosis if necessary. Heel height should be approximately 1 inch. High heels put excessive stress on the MTP joints, while a flat shoe will increase ankle joint strain.

If an orthosis is to be placed inside the shoe or any modification made to the shoe itself, the shoe must grasp the foot firmly. A lace-up shoe is usually preferred, because firm lacing ensures that the foot is held back into the encasing heel. With a non-lacing shoe, the foot may have a tendency to slide forward away from the heel so that the efficacy of any corrective device is lost. Broad Velcro® straps can achieve the same ends. Clearly, a loose slipper, thong, or an ill-fitting shoe will not meet any of these criteria (Figure 4).

Shoes for the individual with foot deformity are primarily of two types: the traditional leather brogue or a modern running shoe. Both forms of shoe may meet all the criteria. The running

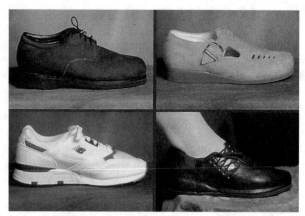

Figure 4. There are many varieties of supportive shoes available for people with arthritis affecting the foot. The extra-depth toe box allows room for the toes, the broad heel provides stability, the high firm heel counter grips the foot firmly, and the laces ensure the foot is held firmly and will not slide forward in the shoe. An athletic shoe may meet all of these criteria and be more acceptable for some people (from the ARHP Arthritis Teaching Slide Collection, 1994 Supplement).

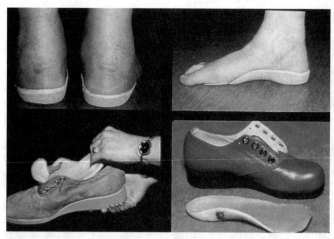

Figure 5. Angulation of the hind foot may be influenced by "posting" applied to the base of the insole. The insole as seen from the side can support the long medial arch and thus relieve pressure from falling directly through the metatarsal heads. An insole must mold to the foot and be held in place by a supportive shoe (from the ARHP Arthritis Teaching Slide Collection).

shoe has very good shock absorption, motion control features, and a removable insole; is breathable and lightweight; and comes in a variety of sizes and styles. Some individuals prefer running shoes, as they are less obtrusive. The orthopedic leather walking shoe meets many of these same criteria but is a formal shoe, equally suited to its purpose of support and control of the foot (14,15). The high-top running shoe, hiking shoe, or work boot are additional options. While meeting the same criteria, these may afford special control over the ankle joint and alignment of the hind foot in some people.

In a limited number of people with arthritis, no ready-made shoe is suitable. They must go to a custom-made shoe or sandal. Heat moldable shoes, such as the Thermold® shoe, may work best for such individuals (16).

Orthoses

Orthoses function in many ways to support the foot and decrease the pressures of weight bearing (Table 1). Prior to fitting an orthosis, it is necessary to ensure that the individual has a suitable shoe into which the device can be placed. Failure to do so means that alterations in alignment or support provided by the device are not transferred to the foot itself. The foot will simply slide off or over the device within the shoe.

It is usually not possible to reverse foot deformity and return the foot to the normal anatomical position in RA. The goal is

Table 1. Function of orthoses.

1. To redistribute weight bearing to a more normal pattern throughout the gait cycle.
2. To control the hindfoot and support the longitudinal arch in order to reduce excessive pronation.
3. To support the transverse arch and provide lift to the metatarsophalangeal joints, reducing weight bearing on these joints.
4. To decrease excessive and/or aggravating interarticular movement during weight bearing.
5. To support bio-mechanical malalignment and reduce associated abnormal compensatory movements.
6. To provide cushioning and shock absorption where a forefoot extension or a full-length liner is used.

to support the foot in a position where no further progression of deformity will occur. In the forefoot/mid-foot, the two major problems are painful metatarsal heads and pronated mid-foot with dropped longitudinal arch. An orthosis can address both of these problems. The patient may be referred to an orthotist, pedorthist, or podiatrist for manufacture of such a device, or a rheumatology physical or occupational therapist may fashion it. Depending on the severity of the problem, the material chosen for fabrication should be sufficiently supportive to relieve the forces and/or hold the corrected position, but it must be soft enough to be comfortable. The softer the orthotic material the more comfortable and less supportive, and the more rigid the material the firmer the support (Figure 5) (17).

Soft Orthoses. The simplest material for correction of a mild problem may be felt, neoprene, or some similar soft, compressible material. Thin leather backed by foam is in this category as well. When the problem becomes more serious, stiffer thermoplastics such as subortholone, polypropylene, or acrylics may be required. As these materials increase in thickness their rigidity increases proportionally. The simplest insole can be made by using a paper outline of the foot and marking the metatarsal heads. The felt or insole material is then cut to follow the outline of the foot from under the heel through the arch of the foot, ending just proximal to the metatarsal heads. This relieves the metatarsal heads of pressure as the foot rocks over the bones in stance phase walking. For greater relief, it is possible to glue an extra thickness of the material and perhaps sand the edge to provide a graduated margin. This insole can be transferred from shoe to shoe as required.

Semi-rigid or Rigid Insoles. Where support is also required of the long arch, the above orthosis will be too soft, and a more rigid material is required. The use of these materials requires first making a cast of the foot, because molding thermoplastics requires high heat and cannot be done on the foot. Negative impression molds are available commercially. These molds contain a soft impression material and the individual simply presses the foot down into the mold, which retains the impression. The negative cast then requires conversion to a positive mold of the foot. The mold is filled with a liquid Plaster of Paris slurry. When this has set, a cast of the foot can be sent away or used for molding thermoplastics. An experienced rheumatology physical therapist or occupational therapist may use this mold to fashion the orthosis, or the clinician may elect to send it to a orthotist, pedorthist, or podiatrist.

Posting the Insole. The curved heel surface of the orthosis, if left, would have a tendency to rotate in the shoe, and the insole itself may slide within the shoe. Posting is the application of additional supportive material to the hind foot aspect of the orthosis. This is done after the insole has been completed. The rear foot post also stiffens the medial longitudinal arch, which greatly enhances the pronation controlling effect. The action of posting also enables some correction of hind foot varus to be made. Posting an insole should only be attempted by someone familiar with the technique. For those not trained it is highly recommended that the cast be sent out for final fashioning and fitting.

A metatarsal bar placed on the external surface of the shoe proximal to the metatarsal heads may provide relief in limited cases where an insole has been inadequate.

Local Pressure. Overlapping toes and resulting pressure points can be dealt with by foam rubber spacers, lamb's wool, or mole skin. The shoe itself may be causing the pressure point, in which case stretching of the shoe leather can be done using leather spray and an internal shoe stretcher. If needed, an extra-depth shoe can be provided.

ANKYLOSING SPONDYLITIS

An *enthesis* is a point of attachment between bone and soft tissue such as ligament or tendon. In ankylosing spondylitis these points may become inflamed (enthesitis). Two common sites for enthesitis are under the heel where the plantar fascia attaches and behind the heel at the achilles tendon insertion. Heel pain can also occur due to plantar fasciitis, subcalcaneal spurs, or rheumatoid nodules. Rest and anti-inflammatory medications are first interventions, but local measures may be of assistance. Rubber or plastic heel cups can alleviate this problem. These devices simply slip over the heel and are worn inside the shoe, molding the soft tissues to provide greater protection between the tender point and the shoe during weight bearing. While not always successful, they are a simple, inexpensive, initial intervention. Sponge inserts with a hole cut like a doughnut can be useful in relieving localized pressure. Because the sponge takes up room in the shoe, it may be necessary to go to a shoe with greater depth.

OSTEOARTHRITIS

Hallux Rigidus

The most common site of involvement in the osteoarthritic foot is the first MTP joint. While common in older individuals with OA, this condition is often seen in younger people, and is seen more often in women than men. Examination reveals restricted mobility of the joint, particularly in extension, resulting in loss of the ability to roll over the toe while moving from stance phase to toe-off in the gait cycle. This results in shortened stance phase on the affected side and a tendency to compensate with external rotation of the leg at the hip and knee, and a turning out of the foot during stance phase and toe-off.

Surgery is often indicated and may include arthrodesis or arthroplasty along with a bunionectomy. However, for those individuals with milder problems, conservative measures should be attempted initially. Heat can be effective at alleviating pain preparatory to exercise. Active mobilizing exercises and passive stretches should be done on individuals with mild to moderate mobility. A rocker bar applied to the sole of the shoe at the level just proximal to the metatarsal head will enable the individual to roll over the bar, thus removing the need for the great toe to extend during toe-off. A rigid rocker concave sole will also help reduce extension force at the first toe. Care must be taken to ensure that a leg-length discrepancy is not introduced with the rocker bar. It may be necessary to build up the opposite shoe to compensate for the bar height.

Ankle Joint Involvement

While not common, OA of the ankle joint does occur. In the early stages, physical modalities may be used to alleviate pain. Bracing can provide support from the lateral forces induced from walking on rough surfaces. If mobility is good, attempts to maintain mobility should include active exercises and possibly passive mobilizing techniques. The use of a cane or crutches may be necessary, and attention to keeping body weight down is important.

Arthroplasty of the ankle is less common than hip or knee surgery; when surgery is performed at this joint, it is usually a fusion. Therefore, when stiffness is marked it is possibly counterproductive to attempt to mobilize the joint. Bracing is important, in conjunction with local pain relieving measures, to facilitate the natural tendency of the joint to fuse. Many individuals with ankle arthritis find that a high-top running shoe or boot affords greater support. The individual should be advised to avoid walking on rough surfaces, which imposes lateral force on the ankle joint.

SKIN CARE

Individuals with rheumatic disease may also have vasculitis. Vasculitis can cause small blood vessels to become occluded, and the foot is the most common site for this to occur. Individuals with active disease may also be taking medications that compromise the peripheral circulation, such as corticosteroids. Shoes should be fitted well, areas of pressure should be alleviated, and no orthotic device should compromise the skin of the foot. Patients should be instructed to be observant about their skin condition and to report any skin breakdown or open areas.

Simple pedicure tasks such as nail clipping can be difficult and potentially dangerous for some individuals. With compromised hand and upper limb function, attempts to cut toenails can result in skin cuts or inadvertent abrasions. It is therefore reasonable for individuals with upper extremity impairment to seek professional assistance from a podiatrist or nurse for basic toenail care (18).

Table 2. Ambulatory aids.

Canes	Crutches	Walkers
Regular round-handle	Axillary	Standard
T-top handle	Forearm	Folding
Straight	Gutter/Platform	Wheeled
Cone-shaped handle		Gutter/Platform
Multi-footed cane		Rolling with seat

AMBULATORY AIDS

Ambulatory aids are often necessary for individuals with rheumatic disease. They may be prescribed to increase stability, to supplement motion where muscles are weak, or to reduce or unload weight-bearing joint surfaces. They may be used in the short term (such as following arthroplasty of a lower limb joint) or they may be in regular use (such as in chronic RA).

Stability depends on the base on which one stands. When standing on one leg, the base is marked by the outer dimensions of the single foot. Standing on two legs, the base extends to include not only the area of the two feet, but the area between the feet. With the addition of a cane or two crutches, the area of the base now becomes that bounded by the two feet, and the points of floor contact of the aids. This may triple and quadruple the base area. Many individuals with rheumatic diseases who are older and possibly frail will benefit from any increase in stability that can be provided.

Weakness is usually not due to any primary muscle pathology but is secondary to pain from articular structures and secondary disuse. For example, hip abductor weakness in OA leads to the "lurching" or Trendelenburg gait seen in individuals with weak or painful hip pathology. When a person stands on one leg, body weight wants to rotate the pelvis downwards around that hip. It requires muscle pull to maintain horizontal alignment. The result of these two forces places more than three times body weight through the hip joint. This excess force can be more than halved by using a cane in the opposite hand. The principle of leverage is at work, and the upward force of the cane and decreased hip force assists walking and alleviates pain. A similar mechanism is at work in the knee joint when a cane is held in the opposite hand.

Canes, Crutches, and Walkers

There are three main forms of assistive aid: canes, crutches, and walkers (Table 2). Many forms of rheumatic disease involve the joints of the upper limb in addition to the lower limb, making it difficult to handle a cane, crutch, or walker. The benefit to the lower limb joint by reducing force is contrasted with the added stress imposed on damaged hands, wrists, elbows, and shoulders.

Canes. Canes are available with a variety of handle shapes, may be adjustable or rigid, may be straight with the curved top, or may be offset so that the weight is taken over the point of contact at the base. Individuals with RA or other inflammatory rheumatic diseases will usually find larger-size hand grips easier to manage. The cone-shaped or spade handle cane provides a counteracting force to ulnar drift by having a wider grip on the ulnar side. The straight-handled cane is also preferable to the traditional curved grip for individuals with hand involvement. Adjustable metal canes are more expensive and are usually not recommended. A simple wooden cane is adequate for most individuals and may be lighter, cheaper, and more stable than the metal alternative.

A good quality rubber tip must be maintained on the base of the cane. These are inexpensive to replace and ensure safety. The preferred form is the inverted cone-shaped tip that extends beyond the wood and provides a flexible grip on all surfaces. Metal tips or spike tips are available for individuals in colder climates where ice is possible. These may be useful in the winter for outdoor use.

With the individual standing erect, in usual walking shoes and with hands hanging by the sides, the top curve of the cane should come to the proximal wrist crease, giving about a 15° bend at the elbow when the cane is held.

Crutches. Crutches come in three major forms: axillary or traditional crutches, forearm crutches that are shorter and have a forward facing handgrip with a metal clasp to grasp the forearm, and gutter or platform crutches that have a horizontal trough for resting the forearm. The standard crutch is appropriate for short-term use, such as following a total hip or knee arthroplasty. Excellent hand function, wrist mobility (extension), and elbow and shoulder strength are required to use these crutches. Body weight is taken through the arms. The padded top support is not for bearing weight but for stability when pulled in against the sides of the chest. Weight bearing through the axilla may result in damage to nerves entering the arm at this level. A space of 2.5 to 3 inches should be left between the top of the crutch and the axilla.

The forearm crutch is more comfortable because there is no pressure against the side of the chest. However, it requires more strength and stability to use. This crutch is most often used by individuals requiring long-term crutch use, as in hip resection arthroplasties. The platform or gutter crutch may be the best choice for individuals with involvement of the lower limbs requiring weight relief who have concurrent poor hand, wrist, and elbow function. The padded support and strap fix the forearm to the crutch. It is possible to take considerable weight through the crutch when ambulating. It is important that this crutch be the correct height, giving a 90° bend at the elbow with the individual in the erect position.

Walkers. Walkers have a wide base of support and thus provide the most stability, but do so at the expense of easy mobility. Stairs are not possible with a walker, ambulation is slow, and distances are usually limited. They are more cumbersome to move, but they are a good choice for individuals requiring the greatest stability.

The standard walker has four legs, is adjustable in height, and requires lifting forward with each step. It is stable when leaned on. An alternative is a walker with wheels on the front two legs. These wheels make it possible to roll the walker forward; stability is achieved by pressure applied to the rear legs on stepping forward. Each of these walkers requires good hand and arm function and good coordination to move the walker forward safely and independently. They are used primarily by individuals in the home or institution and are not practical for outdoor use.

For individuals who have poor upper limb function, particularly in the hands, a walker can be obtained with forearm rests and posts in front to grasp. Weight can thus be taken through the forearms and applied through the gutter rests. This type of walker can benefit patients following joint replacement, when considerable support is required.

A walker with four wheels that is adjustable in height is also available. It may or may not have a brake, and it has a platform across it that can be used as a seat for resting. A basket for carrying objects is optional. This walker is useful for providing an added measure of balance and support in the relatively strong individual who is fairly mobile.

REFERENCES

 1. Vainio K: The rheumatoid foot, a clinical study with pathological roentgenological comments. Am Clin Gynaecol 45 (suppl):1–107, 1956
 2. Spiegel TM, Spiegel JS: Rheumatoid arthritis in the foot and ankle: diagnosis, pathology, and treatment: the relationship between foot and ankle deformity and disease duration in 50 patients. Foot Ankle Int 2:318–324, 1982
 3. Moncur C: Characteristics of rheumatoid arthritis in the forefoot. In, Rheumatic Conditions and Aging. Physical Therapy of the Foot and Ankle. Second edition. Edited by GC Hart, TG McPoil. New York, Churchill Livingstone, pp. 119–121
 4. Moncur C: Characteristics of rheumatoid arthritis in the midfoot. In, Rheumatic Conditions and Aging. Physical Therapy of the Foot and Ankle. Second edition. Edited by GC Hart, TG McPoil. New York, Churchill Livingstone, p. 121
 5. Moncur C: Characteristics of rheumatoid arthritis in the hindfoot. In, Rheumatic Conditions and Aging. Physical Therapy of the Foot and Ankle. Second edition. Edited by GC Hart, TG McPoil. New York, Churchill Livingstone, p. 122
 6. Smidt L: The subtalar joint and rheumatoid arthritis. Baillieres Clin Rheumatol 1:275–287, 1987
 7. Mann RA, Roger A: Principles of examination of the foot and ankle. In, Surgery of the Foot. Sixth edition. Edited by RA Mann. CV Mosby Co., 1986, p. 3142
 8. Melvin JL: Rheumatic Disease: Occupational Therapy and Rehabilitation. Second edition. Philadelphia, FA Davis, 1982, pp. 383–390
 9. Frieberg Richard A, Moncur C: Arthritis of the foot. Bull Rheum Dis 40:1–8, 1991
10. Lehman JL: Therapeutic heat. In, Therapeutic Hot and Cold. Third edition. Baltimore, Williams & Wilkins Co., 1982, pp. 404–562
11. Swezey RL: Therapeutic modalities for pain relief. In, Arthritis: Rational Therapy and Rehabilitation. First edition. Philadelphia, WB Saunders Co., 1978, pp. 133–148
12. Mannheimer C, Carlsson CA: The analgesic effect of transcutaneous nerve stimulation (TENS) in patients with rheumatoid arthritis: a comparative study of different pulse patterns. Pain 6:329–334, 1979
13. Mannheimer JS: Electrode placement for transcutaneous electrical nerve stimulation. Phys Ther 58:1455–1462, 1978
14. McKenzie DC, Clement D, Taunton JE: Running shoes, orthotics, and injuries. Sports Med 2:334–347, 1985
15. Schuster R: Point of purchase: 10 points. The Runner 66–67, 1980
16. Collyer MI: Shoes for the arthritic foot: the foot in arthritis. Baillieres Clin Rheumatol 1:403–412, 1987
17. Tinley P: Appliances for the rheumatic foot. Baillieres Clin Rheumatol 1:383–402, 1987
18. Gilkes JJ: Skin and nail changes in the arthritic foot. Baillieres Clin Rheumatol 1:335–353, 1987

Pre and Post Surgical
Management of the Hip and Knee

SANDY B. GANZ, PT, MSCHE; and GIGI VIELLION, RN, ONC

Total joint arthroplasty (TJA) of the lower extremity is a highly successful surgical procedure that has revolutionized the outlook of patients with arthritis (1). Over 258,000 total hip and 230,000 total knee arthroplasties are performed annually in the U.S. (2). While the majority of TJAs are performed for osteoarthritis, other rheumatic diseases also cause joint destruction and may result in the need for surgery (3). In the early years of TJA, incapacitating pain was the sole indication for surgery. Today, relief of pain is still the primary indication for most arthroplasties; however, quality of life issues such as limited function or joint instability that limit activities of daily living (ADLs) are also considerations (1,2).

Members of the surgical health care team should work closely with those responsible for the medical management of the patients' disease. Total joint arthroplasty of the lower extremity is a highly successful surgical procedure with an excellent outcome. As with any major surgery, there are inherent risks that must be carefully weighed. The patient must be willing to prepare for the surgery and be an active participant in rehabilitation.

PREOPERATIVE EVALUATION

Total joint arthroplasty is an elective procedure and therefore allows for preoperative education and evaluation of the patient. Once it is decided that the patient will benefit from a TJA, the health care team begins the evaluation process. It is important to determine what the patient expects to achieve following TJA. Because some outcomes of surgery are more predictable than others, the health care team can assist the patient in determining if these goals are realistic.

Disease management issues must be considered for all patients, but are especially critical for persons with one of the more complex rheumatic diseases. Assessment of the patient's disease activity and the systems involved, as well as any physical and psychosocial limitations, is essential to developing a plan of care. Special consideration should be given to the routines, medications, and modalities utilized by the individual to manage their disease. Patients are advised to stop taking aspirin and nonsteroidal anti-inflammatory drugs (NSAIDs) approximately 1 day to 1 month before surgery to avoid the risk of increased bleeding (4). The time frame for stopping these drugs varies according to drug half-life.

Most patients will be placed on anticoagulant therapy for several weeks postoperatively. During this time, methods other than aspirin or NSAIDs (except in low doses and with close monitoring of prothrombin times) may be used to manage pain. Analgesics that can be used in place of NSAIDs include acetaminophen, non-acetylated salicylates, tramadol, and mild narcotics. Increased disease activity for those with inflamma-

tory rheumatic disease may be managed using larger doses with very careful titration of prothrombin times. Patients with ankylosing spondylitis, rheumatoid arthritis (RA), and juvenile rheumatoid arthritis, must be evaluated for cervical spine involvement to avoid potentially dangerous manipulation of the neck during anesthesia (1,5). Preoperative cervical spine x-rays should include a lateral flexion view.

Patients should be made aware of factors that could increase their risk of postoperative complications. Smoking, a history of heart or lung disease, use of steroids and/or other immunosuppressive drugs, diabetes, RA, and obesity are factors that can affect rehabilitation and delay wound healing (5). Sources of infection must be eliminated preoperatively to prevent hematogenous seeding at the site of the joint replacement. The most common sources of infection are the teeth, the genitourinary tract, and open areas on the skin (1,5). A dental check-up is recommended within 6 months before surgery is scheduled. A preoperative urine culture is necessary as symptomatic bacteriuria is common in women and prostatic hypertrophy can present increased risk of infection in men. Known medical problems should be treated prior to TJA.

A preoperative physical therapy evaluation should be performed to identify and address areas that may be problematic postoperatively. Early identification of potential problems will expedite rehabilitation and enable the team to plan for appropriate home care. The evaluation should include assessment of gait, range of motion of all joints, strength of all extremities, respiratory status, and functional assessment. This is especially important in patients with multiple joint involvement or one of the more complex rheumatic diseases (5). An observational gait analysis is performed to determine the patient's weight-bearing ability and any abnormal loading on the affected/unaffected limbs. This provides a baseline measure to compare to the postoperative gait status. The preoperative session provides the opportunity to instruct the patient on proper use of the assistive device(s) that they will be using postoperatively. Measurement of range of motion of joints and gross manual muscle testing of the upper extremities and uninvolved lower extremity are performed to determine the type of ambulatory aids that may be needed during the postoperative period. A respiratory evaluation should include auscultation and a measurement of the number of cubic centimeters a patient inspires and expires utilizing an incentive spirometer (5). Pain assessment, using a visual analogue scale or pain disability index scale, should be performed. Finally, each patient should be assessed preoperatively using a functional rating scale in order to determine if there is a change in functional status following surgery. Indices that may be utilized in both the pre- and postoperative evaluation include the Hospital for Special Surgery (HSS) Knee Rating Scale (6), HSS Total Hip Arthroplasty Functional Milestone Form (7), Medical Outcomes Survey

Short Form-36 (8), Western Ontario and MacMaster University Osteoarthritis Index (9), Harris Hip Score (10), Functional Status Index (11), and Tinetti Assessment Tool (12). Additional functional assessments are described in Chapter 5, Health Status Assessment.

Consideration must be given to the support that will be available to the patient after discharge from the hospital. With ever-decreasing length of hospital stays, it is important to evaluate the discharge environment. The home environment should be assessed to ensure patient safety and ability to function. Upon discharge from the hospital, most arthroplasty patients can expect to perform self-care and manage at home with minimal assistance and decreased pain. The patient should be informed prior to surgery of their expected length of hospitalization and their postoperative abilities and limitations. This will allow the social worker or discharge planner, patient, and family the opportunity to make appropriate arrangements for home care before entering the hospital. Preoperative preparation of the home should include removal of scatter rugs, provision of clear pathways for ambulation, and advance meal preparation. Arranging for someone to assist with errands and transportation should be made prior to hospitalization.

PREADMISSION EDUCATION

Preoperative patient education is crucial in the management of the TJA patient (13–15). Studies have shown that preoperative interventions, in the form of patient education classes, enhance the postoperative course. Education may be provided individually or in a group session and should include the patient's family and/or significant other. For every surgical procedure, there are routine events that occur. A *clinical pathway* is a multidisciplinary chart/table that depicts these events. This allows the patient and the health care providers to be aware of what should occur on each postoperative day. Reviewing a clinical pathway that outlines the course of treatment can help the patient to prepare preoperatively for surgery, hospitalization, and recuperation. The expected length of stay should be made clear. Realistic goals should be set, including appropriate time frames.

Explain to patients that their active participation is necessary for an optimal recovery. Description of hospital routines, stressing what will be expected of the patient, gives people a sense of control over their recovery. Patients and their families may benefit from a visit to the inpatient unit and the opportunity to meet the staff. It is helpful to have an anesthesiologist discuss with the patient the type of anesthesia to be used, and the impact of anesthesia on recovery. Instruction and demonstration of postoperative exercises and any precautions the patient will be required to follow should be included. Additionally, if time allows, patients should be taught and encouraged to do exercises to improve muscle strength and tone. This will accelerate the recovery process.

The greatest concern of most patients is how they will manage after surgery. With the rapid decrease in length of stay, patients who cannot manage at home alone, or with home care, may need to be discharged to a subacute facility or rehabilitation center. Patients may need reassurance about their postoperative functional abilities and the discharge setting. Attention must be paid to the patient's other comorbid conditions and current medical management.

POSTOPERATIVE MANAGEMENT

General anesthesia is the standard of care in many hospitals. For patients who are given epidural anesthesia, they will be alert but insensate below the level of the epidural when they arrive in the post-anesthesia care unit. Regardless of the type of anesthesia used, special care must be taken when moving the patient who has had a total hip arthroplasty to avoid dislocating the hip. In most cases, patients having TJA of the lower extremity will have a foley catheter to prevent urinary retention or incontinence while the epidural is in effect.

As the effects of the anesthesia wear off, the pain experience will vary. In some cases, epidural analgesia will be used. Intravenous patient-controlled analgesia may be used, allowing the patient to control the frequency and quantity of pain medication. However, patients must understand the importance of using enough medication to promote early ambulation and deep breathing (to avoid pulmonary complications). Patients with ankylosing spondylitis may be more susceptible to pulmonary problems due to diminished chest expansion.

Both anesthesia and pain medication can slow down the gastrointestinal tract. The patient's abdomen must be auscultated for missing or hyperactive bowel sounds and observed for distention. Waiting until the patient reports being hungry before starting oral intake may prevent an ileus from occurring. The stress of surgery may cause other gastrointestinal problems such as ulcers. Patients who have been taking aspirin or NSAIDs are at increased risk for gastrointestinal bleeding, which may have serious consequences for patients who are already anemic secondary to their chronic disease.

Other known complications of TJA are deep vein thrombosis and subsequent pulmonary embolus. One of the available methods of prophylaxis to prevent deep vein thrombosis should be used for patients with total hip or total knee arthroplasty. Mechanical devices such as the pneumatic sequential compression device or venous foot pump anti-embolism socks are often used in conjunction with a pharmacologic method such as warfarin or low molecular weight heparin (6). While this is important in the postoperative period, it may present problems for patients who depend on aspirin or NSAIDs to manage their rheumatic disease, because these drugs cannot be used without careful monitoring of anticoagulant therapy. In addition to these methods of preventing deep vein thrombosis, active ankle pump exercises and early ambulation are essential.

Infection is a potential complication of TJA. Measures to protect the patient from infection include Laminar Flow in the operating room, prophylactic antibiotics, and educating the patient about the importance of constant vigilance in preventing and recognizing signs of infection (5,6). There is controversy about the need for prophylactic antibiotics before any dental work, including cleaning, and any or all invasive medical procedures. Immediate attention to early infection can protect the joint and avoid a long and costly hospitalization. Patients with inflammatory arthritis who have been treated with immunosuppressive therapy tend to be at increased risk for intraoperative and postoperative complications (1,5). In the postoperative period, patients who are treated with corticosteroids are at increased risk for many complications including friable skin, delayed wound healing, and infection. The risk of infection is also increased in patients with enteropathic arthritis through hematogenous seeding from the bowel and in patients with psoriatic arthritis.

Table 1. Positions to avoid following total hip arthroplasty.

- Knees higher than hips, such as sitting in a low chair or on a low toilet
- Crossing legs while sitting, standing, or lying down
- Bending down to tie shoes or pick up an object from the floor
- Twisting from the trunk while seated or standing with the operative leg planted on the floor
- Leaning forward from the waist while seated
- Any other activity in which hip flexion is greater than 90°, hip is adducted past neutral, and/or hip is internally rotated past neutral

REHABILITATION

In the three decades since the first TJA was performed, methods and philosophies of rehabilitation have changed but the goals of rehabilitation have remained the same. The primary goals following TJA are to restore function, decrease pain, and gain muscle control so that individuals can return to previous levels of functioning.

Total Hip Arthroplasty

Rehabilitation following cemented and cementless total hip arthroplasty is influenced by many factors including surgical technique and approach. The most common approach used is the posterior/posterior lateral. When this approach is used, precautions during rehabilitation should be taken to avoid extremes of hip flexion, adduction, and internal rotation. When an anterior approach is used, extremes of external rotation, extension, and abduction should be avoided. Dislocation may occur during any one or a combination of these movements. If hip arthroplasty is performed in conjunction with a trochanteric osteotomy, additional dislocation precautions include protecting weight bearing and avoiding active hip abduction for 8-12 weeks postoperatively or until the osteotomy site is well healed. The most common maneuvers in which dislocations occur following a posterior lateral approach are: 1) rising off a low surface such as a toilet or recliner; 2) twisting the trunk toward the operated side in either a standing or seated position with feet planted on the floor; 3) bending down to tie shoes from a seated position; and 4) rolling over in bed. There is controversy regarding the length of time patients should adhere to postoperative TJA precautions. Opinions range from 4 weeks to life. Positions to avoid are listed in Table 1.

Regardless of the institution, the postoperative rehabilitation routine may consist of therapeutic exercise, transfer training, gait training, and instruction in ADLs. Therapeutic exercises are performed in order to increase muscle strength and gain control of the limb for various necessary activities. Lower extremity exercises consist of supine ankle circles, quadriceps sets, gluteal sets, hip internal rotation to neutral, and hip and knee flexion to 45°. Transfer training consists of bed to standing, chair to standing, and toilet transfers. The surgeon determines whether the patient will be non-weightbearing, toe-touch weightbearing, partial weightbearing, or full weightbearing. Prior to discharge, patients should be instructed in managing stairs, ramps, and curbs. Patients often have the sensation that their operated limb is longer in the early postoperative period, because temporary abduction contractures may result from enforced abduction in bed or from distal advancement of the trochanter. Unless there is a true leg-length discrepancy, shoe lifts should not be applied for at least 4–6 weeks until the temporary hip abduction contracture resolves.

Following discharge from the hospital, the long-term goal is to improve ambulation to a normal gait without abductor weakness or lurch. It is important to include abductor strengthening in patients' home exercise programs (16). Prolonged weakness in the hip abductors causes abnormal stress on the hip joint; over time, these abnormal forces can lead to implant loosening. A cane should be used until abductor weakness is resolved. Patients should be advised to carry loads on the side that underwent arthroplasty. Research has shown that loads carried on the contralateral side significantly increase force demands placed on the arthroplasty side, while loads as large as 20% of body weight carried on the same side as the hip replacement produce no more hip abductor muscle EMG than that produced while walking without a load (16). Patients must be cognizant of the fact that although the artificial joint causes little or no pain, it is in fact not a normal joint.

There is no consensus regarding which sporting activities persons with hip replacements should be allowed to participate in following surgery. Non-impact loading activities such as bicycle riding, swimming, dancing, golf, and doubles tennis may safely be encouraged in most cases (17). Impact loading activities result in increased stress on the bone-cement interface and may lead to loosening of the prosthesis. Studies have shown that intelligent participation in activities such as walking, golf, bowling, and swimming—where there is no excess load (≥20 lb) placed on the hip—has no influence on the outcome of the total hip arthroplasty (16,17). In general, high activity levels are associated with increased failure rates in conventional cemented hip arthroplasty. Patients must be told that no type of hip replacement can withstand the forces of strenuous loads on the hip without possible loosening (17).

Patients may resume sexual activity as soon as they feel comfortable doing so, as long as they adhere to the precautions to avoid hip dislocation. Studies have shown that patients usually resume sexual activity 4–6 weeks postoperatively (18).

Total Knee Arthroplasty

Rehabilitation following total knee arthroplasty has dramatically changed over the past two decades; however, the goals have remained the same. Whether referring to a unicondylar or bicondylar knee replacement that is constrained, semi constrained or unconstrained; cemented or cementless; the primary goal is to provide a stable joint with a functional range of motion. Patients who underwent knee arthroplasty 20 years ago remained in the hospital for 3 weeks and were placed in a cylinder cast for 7 to 10 days before flexion was initiated. Today, mechanical flexion is initiated within 24 hours after surgery, and the average length of stay for an uncomplicated total knee arthroplasty is 4 to 6 days.

Continuous passive motion (CPM) is a method of mechanical flexion. A machine is applied to the lower extremity to passively flex the knee at a designated speed and degree of flexion, as programmed by the physical therapist or nurse. The efficacy of CPM is controversial. Some studies indicate that it may be beneficial in counteracting the effect of joint immobilization (19); other studies indicate the opposite (20). Contraindications to use of CPM are: 1) sensory deficits excluding epidural anesthesia; 2) excessive wound drainage; 3) postoperative confusion; and 4) a significant knee flexion contracture.

Patients who are having difficulty with flexion and who have a concomitant knee flexion contracture should have limited time in the CPM. A dynamic knee brace may be indicated in these patients. Factors to consider when placing a knee arthroplasty patient in the CPM machine include the type of anesthesia, type of dressing, pain tolerance, and presence of deformity. Continuous passive motion is usually increased to the patient's tolerance, which should be equal to or more than what is achieved with active bending. Care should be taken to increase the amount of flexion slowly to preserve oxygenation of the skin tissue (6). Initiation of transfer activities, gait training, and active range of motion usually occurs on the first postoperative day. Weight bearing status will be determined by the surgeon and depends on the type of implant used. Patients may be discharged with crutches and protected weight bearing for 4 to 6 weeks postoperatively or with a cane and full weight bearing. There have been no prospective, randomized, controlled trials that studied implant loosening in patients who received different weight bearing instructions in the immediate postoperative period.

Important factors that influence postoperative range of motion in the knee are the type of prosthesis, preoperative deformity, and intraoperative bone resection. An exercise program that incorporates flexibility and strengthening may consist of active range of motion, active assisted range of motion, passive range of motion, isometrics (quadriceps and hamstring), straight leg raising, short arc quadriceps, patellar mobilization, and use of a stationary bicycle. Cryotherapy is often used concomitantly with exercise sessions. Aggressive quadriceps strengthening exercises should not be performed during the immediate postoperative period (1–2 weeks) for fear of damaging the capsular closure (6). Historically patients have been discharged from the hospital when they achieve 90° of knee flexion, are able to transfer in and out of bed independently, and can ambulate with a cane unassisted on level surfaces and stairs. With the current emphasis on managing patients in the home, patients are being discharged 4 to 6 days after surgery with varying degrees of flexion. Patients are more frequently managed in their home with home health services or are placed in short-term rehabilitation centers.

The most common type of failure in total knee arthroplasty is mechanical loosening. By placing undue forces on the knee joint, the patient increases the chance of prosthetic loosening and endangers the overall success of the knee replacement. Patients are often instructed prior to and after surgery to avoid sports that place excessive force on the prosthetic knee joint, such as running, jumping, or singles tennis. Most orthopedic surgeons allow patients to play golf. Reports of pain severity during and after golf have been found to be significantly higher in golfers with left knee versus right knee arthroplasty. This may be a direct result of increased torque on the left knee in right-handed golfers (21). The effect of total knee arthroplasty on driving reaction time was studied in 40 patients (22). Results indicated that reaction time returned to normal approximately 8 weeks after surgery for patients with right knee arthroplasty. Thus, driving reaction time, range of motion, and strength should be considered when advising patients to resume driving.

REFERENCES

1. Schumacher HR, Klippel JH, Robinson DR, editors: Primer on the Rheumatic Diseases. Tenth Edition. Atlanta, Arthritis Foundation, 1993
2. NIH Consensus Development Panel: Total hip replacement. JAMA 273: 1950–1956, 1995
3. Laskin RS, editor: Total Knee Replacement. London, Springer-Verlag, 1991
4. Connelly CS, Panush RS: Should nonsteroidal anti-inflammatory drugs be stopped before elective surgery? J Intern Med 151:1963–1966, 1991
5. Sculco TP, editor: Surgical Treatment of Rheumatoid Arthritis. St. Louis, Mosby Year Book, Inc., 1992
6. Insall JN, Windsor RE, Scott WN, Kelly MA, Aglietti P, editors: Surgery of the Knee. Second edition. New York, Churchill Livingstone Inc., 1993
7. Kroll M, Ganz S, Backus S, et al: A tool for measuring functional outcomes after total hip arthroplasty. Arthritis Care Res 7:78–84, 1994
8. Ware J, Sherbourne C: The MOS 36 item short form health survey (SF-36). Med Care 30:473–483, 1992
9. Jette AM: The functional status index: reliability of a chronic disease evaluation instrument. Arch Phys Med Rehabil 61:395–401, 1980
10. Laupacis A, Bourne R, Rorabeck C: The effect of elective total hip replacement on health related quality of life. J Bone Joint Surg Am 75:1619–1626, 1993
11. Jette AM: Health status indicators: their utility in chronic disease evaluation research. J Chronic Dis 33:567–579, 1980
12. Tinetti ME: Performance oriented assessment of mobility problems in elderly patients. J Am Geriatr Soc 34:119–126, 1986
13. Haines N, Viellion G: A successful combination: preadmission testing and preoperative education. Orthop Nurs 9:53–57, 1990
14. Roach JA, Tremblay LM, Bowers DL: A preoperative assessment and education program: implementation and outcomes. Patient Educ Counsel 25:83–88, 1995
15. Lichtenstein R, Semaan S: Development and impact of a hospital based perioperative patient education program in a joint replacement center. Orthop Nurs 12:17–25, 1993
16. Neumann DA, Cook TM: Effect of load and carrying position on the electromyographic activity of the gluteus medius muscles during walking. Phys Ther 65:305–311, 1985
17. Ritter MA, Gandolf VS, Holston KS: Continuous passive motion versus physical therapy in total knee replacements. Clin Orthop 244:239–243, 1989
18. Stern SH, Ganz SB, Sculco TP, et al: Sexual function following total hip arthroplasty. Clin Orthop 228–235, 1991
19. Coutts RD, Kaita J, Barr R, et al: The role of continuous passive motion in the postoperative rehabilitation of the total knee patient. Orthop Trans 6:277–278, 1982
20. Ritter MA, Meding JB: Total hip arthroplasty: can the patient play sports again? Orthopedics 10:1447–1452, 1987
21. Mallon WJ, Callaghan JJ: Total knee arthroplasty in active golfers. J Arthroplasty 8:299–306, 1993
22. Spalding TJW, Kiss J, Kyberd P, et al: Driver reaction times after total knee arthroplasty. J Bone Joint Surg Br 76B:754–756, 1994

Questionable Interventions

RICHARD S. PANUSH, MD

Is there a role for diet or other questionable remedies in the routine therapy of patients with rheumatic diseases? Ten or 15 years ago I, and most of my colleagues, would have responded with a resounding "no." Today, my answer is still "no," but it is softer (1–6). My interest in questionable remedies began in the late 1970s when I began to study diet and arthritis (7). My original expectation was that we would definitively prove no value of diet therapy for arthritis. Surprisingly—at the time, but perhaps not in retrospect—that is not quite what we found (7–9). As we and others made increasingly serious efforts to study nutrition and other questionable remedies for rheumatic disease, my views slowly changed. I have become more tolerant of nontraditional ideas and more charitable to patients seeking them (4).

It behooves us to be familiar with some of these questionable remedies for arthritis. *Alternative* medicine has gained much public attention and now enjoys governmental endorsement, including the new National Institutes of Health Office of Alternative Medicine (3). This chapter will offer a brief perspective for clinicians on the growing curiosity about diets and other questionable remedies. It will emphasize scientific rationale(s) for these, present general considerations and principles pertaining to questionable remedies, and selectively summarize certain available information about them.

DEFINITION OF QUESTIONABLE REMEDIES

There are but three types of therapies: genuine (those proven acceptably safe and effective), questionable, and fraudulent. Questionable remedies are widely used and widely publicized in the U.S. In 1993 the American College of Rheumatology established a committee on questionable remedies to address certain pertinent issues. The committee deliberately selected the term "questionable," thus following the approaches of the National Council Against Health Fraud and the American Cancer Society in not using terms that euphemize questionable remedies. This is preferable to terms like "unapproved" (i.e., by the Food and Drug Administration), "false" (disproven), "unproven" (experimental), "dubious" (very doubtful), "nonstandard" (falling short of practice standards), "irregular" (not used by mainstream medicine), or "alternative" or "complementary" (reflecting various questionable or conventional treatment options) remedies.

THE APPEAL OF QUESTIONABLE REMEDIES

What is the appeal of questionable medicine? It offers hope. Many patients with rheumatic disease experience unpredictable pain and disability. Many struggle to cope with their illness and with the constraints imposed by the limitations of medical

knowledge. The essence of medicine is the reduction of uncertainty (3); health care providers and patients must learn to live with considerable uncertainty, and it is not always easy. Patients may turn from science and seek understanding and relief —indeed empowerment—from questionable sources. We can understand this, and sympathize. (Have not many of us or our family members or friends sipped chicken soup for a cold, or used a rub for an ache?)

How should we view "questionable" remedies, and how should we respond to those who seek them (3–5)? We can dismiss, disdain, and sometimes ridicule questionable remedies. There are repositories of information on questionable remedies where we can inform ourselves, which we are doing. We can try to communicate with patients and the public through the media. But "Doctor's Diet Cures Arthritis" makes instant headlines in the lay press, while "Doctor's Diet Doesn't Cure Arthritis" takes years of research, writing, and revision before appearing in the rheumatology literature, and ultimately impacts minimally on physician and patient practices. We can more aggressively combat public perceptions in the press and in the courts, as does the National Council Against Health Fraud (3–5); however, the success of such initiatives is limited.

The contemporary intellectual view of science is that human problems can be understood and solved by science, that science epitomizes rationality, integrity, progress, and open-mindedness. But science also includes superstition (our tonsillectomies and adenoidectomies of the recent past, and perhaps some practices of coronary artery bypass surgery), fraud, errors, conservatism, pigheadedness, fashion, and trends (3–5). This description seems to fit practitioners of questionable or fraudulent remedies better than it fits health care providers; but some of the accusations with which we discredit others may also apply to us.

There are several explanations for our dismissal of questionable remedies from legitimate study. "Quackery" evokes discomfort and prejudice, seeming to defy rational explanation. It is purveyed by practitioners whom we sometimes consider unsavory and perceive as our intellectual inferiors; they do not share our belief system, and we rarely condescend to consider their notions. Does it not seem absurd to propose, for example, that diet, or antibiotics, or red peppers might (in some circumstances) help arthritis?

HAZARDS OF QUESTIONABLE REMEDIES

Is there harm in permitting patients to try questionable therapies? Are they not usually at least innocuous? Yes, and no. It is not responsible to use therapies that are not generally considered safe and effective. In addition, some questionable therapies are not innocuous but occasionally are harmful. There are documented instances of patients receiving drugs other than those promised, with adverse results including marrow aplasia, serious infections from contaminants, and death (3–5,10,11). Patients seeking questionable remedies may inappropriately neglect their illness. It also has been argued that expenditures on questionable remedies divert scarce health care resources from more appropriate areas.

EXAMPLES OF QUESTIONABLE REMEDIES

Prominent questionable remedies include diet, vitamins and minerals, nutritional supplements, fish oils, antimicrobials (nitroimidazole, rifamycin, ceftriaxone, ampicillin, and amantadine), biologic agents (thymopoietin, transfer factor, placenta-derived factors, venoms, and herbal remedies), certain other pharmacologic agents (cis-retinoic acid, isoprinoside, amiprolose, thalidomide, and dapsone), topical agents (dimethyl sulfoxide), mechanical/instrumental (hyperbaric oxygen, laser irradiation, acupuncture, photophoresis, electromagnetic radiation), chiropractic manipulation, homeopathy, biofeedback, exercise, and many others (i.e., sitting in abandoned uranium mines). Let us consider selective, illustrative questionable remedies. Detailed discussion of these can be found elsewhere (2,12,13), but comments will be offered for several.

Antimicrobial Agents

Several intriguing observations about antimicrobial agents have been made. A microbial etiology for rheumatoid arthritis (RA) has long been an attractive but unproven hypothesis. If true, then antimicrobials could be useful in treatment. There have been several instructive experiences. Nitroimidazole antimicrobial drugs were tried for treatment of RA because of the efficacy of levamisole, another imidazole derivative, and because of claims that RA was caused by _Amoeba limax_. Results were not impressive (1,12,13). Rifamycin, an antibiotic that blocks DNA-dependent RNA polymerase and inhibits cellular protein synthesis, was beneficial for rheumatoid knee synovitis (14).

Tetracycline therapy was tried in RA, based on a putative mycoplasma etiology, and was ineffective. Recent work has found that tetracyclines, particularly minocycline, reduced collagenase activity, limited bone resorption, affected T-cell function, perturbed neutrophil function, and were antiproliferative, anti-inflammatory, and anti-arthritic in animal and possibly human arthritis. Two prospective randomized, double-blind, placebo-controlled trials showed statistically significant but clinically modest benefits of minocycline for RA (15–17). Other antimicrobial agents have been considered for arthritis therapy. Patients with chronic inflammatory arthritis and antibody titers to _Borrelia burgdorferi_ of 1:64 or greater have shown encouraging responses to ceftriaxone (18). Ampicillin was beneficial to RA patients under certain conditions (19). Amantadine, an antiviral agent, was useful to a group of patients with teenage-onset juvenile RA who had elevated antibody titers to influenza A and who were born during an influenza epidemic (20). These are provocative observations. If confirmed, they could be interpreted to mean that chronic arthritis in some patients results from bacterial, spirochete, or viral infection and/or that antimicrobials are antirheumatic.

Exercise

Exercise exemplifies an intervention that was once questionable and is now increasingly credible. Information is still limited about the long-term consequences of exercise on the musculoskeletal system (21–23). Several studies examined a possible relationship between running and osteoarthritis. Most found that runners without underlying biomechanical problems do not develop arthritis at a rate detectably different from non-runners, and also have reduced disability and mortality (22,23). These observations seem to be valid for many other sports activities as well (21). A variety of exercise programs (aerobic dance, water aerobics, treadmill exercise, stationary cycling, and Nautilus-type training)—all previously eschewed—are now utilized for arthritis patients (see Chapter 12, Rest and Exercise).

Diet and Nutritional Supplements

For years we relegated special diets for arthritis to quackery. It was not long ago that the rheumatologic community categorically stated, "If there was a relationship between diet and arthritis it would have been discovered long ago. The simple fact is: there is no scientific evidence that any food has anything to do with causing arthritis and no evidence that any food is effective in treating or 'curing' it" (21). We and others have now re-examined this notion. How might food affect arthritis? First, some patients with rheumatic disease have symptoms that might be a manifestation of food allergy. Second, certain types of diets with particular amounts of calories, protein, and fatty acids might affect the immunologically mediated inflammation that occurs with arthritis (24).

There is no compelling evidence that any diet other than a healthy, balanced one is consistently helpful to arthritis patients. My colleagues and I studied a popular diet for arthritis patients (eliminating red meat, additives, preservatives, fruit, dairy products, herbs, spices, and alcohol) and found no consistent effect on disease (7). Physicians and patients are intrigued that arthritis may occasionally be the result of hypersensitivity to foods. Palindromic rheumatism has been associated with sodium nitrate; Behçet's syndrome with black walnuts; systemic lupus erythematosus (SLE) with canavanine in alfalfa (which may cross-react with native DNA or activate B lymphocytes) and with hydrazine; and RA with many substances including house dust, tobacco, smoke, petrochemicals, tartrazine, dairy products, wheat, corn, and beef. In addition, rheumatoid-like synovitis in rabbits can be induced by dietary cows' milk (1–9,24). Recent prospective, placebo-controlled, double-blind studies confirmed that for selected patients, inflammatory arthritis may be associated with foods. Some of these patients had evidence of immunologic reactivity to food antigens (8).

Fish (or Plant) Oils. Nutritional status exerts a profound influence on immune responsiveness and disease expression. For example, mice with SLE or arthritic rats fed diets rich in eicosapentaenoic acid (a naturally occurring, substituted, polyunsaturated fatty acid analog) fared better than control animals. Clinical trials for patients with RA but not SLE indicated modest decreases in certain symptoms. These observations suggest that dietary factors which modify arachidonic acid-derived prostaglandin affect inflammatory and immunologic responses and may ameliorate symptoms of rheumatic diseases (1,2,5,24).

Nutritional Supplements. A number of substances, including copper, zinc, and vitamin B, are claimed to be helpful for arthritis patients. However, the evidence in support of such claims is scant. Copper salts were antirheumatic in clinical trials, but they were associated with many adverse effects and have never evolved as important therapeutic agents. In one study, some patients with RA benefited from oral zinc; however, improvement was not great, was inconsistent, and was not confirmed in other studies. L-histidine helped a small subgroup of patents with RA but is not an important therapeutic agent. Evidence to support efficacy of vitamin C for arthritis patients is lacking (1,2,5,24).

PERSPECTIVE

There is still no role for diet or other questionable therapies in routine management of rheumatic diseases. By definition, these do not yet have established roles in treating arthritis patients and are best termed questionable remedies (1).

Diet therapy and other questionable remedies reflect our perspectives and outlook in rheumatology. Their prevalence should be considered a reminder of the limitations of our understanding of rheumatic disease and of our abilities to satisfactorily alleviate the suffering of our patients. Educating colleagues, patients, and the public as to proper or inappropriate use of such remedies poses a difficult challenge. Although we need understanding and sympathy for our patients, we also must protect them from unnecessary hazards, maximize available health care resources, and ultimately provide better care. We must strive to maintain a balance between healthy skepticism and willingness to consider new concepts. For antimicrobial agents, diet, exercise, and perhaps others, this has led to new insights about pathogenesis and therapy of rheumatic diseases. Ultimately our hope is to provide better care for our patients' illnesses. As Bertrand Russell wrote, "What science cannot tell us mankind cannot know."

"I have no data yet. It is a capital mistake to theorize before one has data. Insensibly one begins to twist facts to suit theories, instead of theories to suit fact."

Arthur Conan Doyle
The Illustrated Sherlock Holmes Treasury—
The Adventures of Sherlock Holmes.

REFERENCES

1. Panush RS: Is there a role for diet or other questionable therapies in managing rheumatic diseases? Bull Rheum Dis 42:1–4, 1993

2. Panush RS: Non-traditional remedies. In, Primer on the Rheumatic Diseases. Tenth edition. Edited by HR Schumacher. Atlanta, Arthritis Foundation, 1993, pp. 323–327

3. Panush RS: Alternative medicine: science or superstition (editorial)? J Rheumatol 21:8–9, 1994

4. Panush RS: Reflections on unproven remedies. Rheum Dis Clin North Am 19:201–206, 1993

5. Panush RS: Arthritis, food allergy, diets, and nutrition. In, Arthritis and Allied Conditions—A Textbook of Rheumatology. Thirteenth edition. Edited by WJ Koopman. Philadelphia, Lea and Febiger (in press)

6. Panush RS: Food for thought, but not for arthritis. Prim Care Rheumatol 2:1–5, 1992

7. Panush RS, Carter RL, Katz P, et al: Diet therapy for rheumatoid arthritis. Arthritis Rheum 26:462–471, 1983

8. Panush RS, Stroud RM, Webster EM: Food-induced (allergic arthritis): inflammatory arthritis exacerbated by milk. Arthritis Rheum 29:220–226, 1986

9. Panush RS: Food induced ("allergic") arthritis: clinical and serologic studies. J Rheumatol 17:291–294, 1990

10. Dlesk A, Ettinger MP, Longley S, et al: Unconventional arthritis therapies (letter). Arthritis Rheum 25:1145–1147, 1982

11. Kraus A, Guerra-Bautista G, Alarcón-Segovia D: Salmonella arizona arthritis and septicemia associated with rattlesnake ingestion by patients with connective tissue diseases. A dangerous complication of folk medicine. J Rheumatol 18:1328–1331, 1991

12. Panush RS, Katz P: Remedies of unlikely benefit. In, Rheumatoid Arthritis. Edited by PD Utsinger, NJ Zvaifler, GE Ehrlich. Philadelphia, Lippincott, 1985, pp. 819–823

13. Panush RS, Longley S: Therapies of potential but unproven benefit. In, Rheumatoid Arthritis. Edited by PD Utsinger, NJ Zvaifler, GE Ehrlich. Philadelphia, Lippincott, 1985, pp. 695–709

14. Gabriel SE, Conn DL, Luthra H: Rifampin therapy in rheumatoid arthritis. J Rheumatol 17:163–166, 1990

15. Kloppenburg M, Breedveld FC, Terwiel JP, Mallee C, Dijkmans BAC: Minocycline in active rheumatoid arthritis: a double-blind, placebo-controlled trial. Arthritis Rheum 37:629–636, 1994

16. Tilley BC, Alarcon GS, Heyse SP, Trentham DE, Neuner R, Kaplan DA, Clegg DO, Leisen JCC, Buckley L, Cooper SM, Duncan H, Pillemer SR, Tuttleman M, Fowler SE: For the MIRA trial group: minocycline in rheumatoid arthritis: a 48 week, double-blind, placebo-controlled trial. Ann Intern Med 122:81–89, 1995

17. Panush RS: Should minocycline be used to treat rheumatoid arthritis? Bull Rheum Dis 45(2)2–5, 1996

18. Caperton EM, Heim-Duthoy K, Matzke GR, et al: Ceftriazone therapy of chronic inflammatory arthritis. Arch Intern Med 150:1677–1682, 1990

19. Wawrzynska-Pagowska J, Brzezinska B: A trial of ampicillin in the treatment of rheumatoid arthritis: results of long-term observations indicating the possibility of inhibiting the progression of bone deformity. Rheumatologia 22:1–10, 1984

20. Pritchard MH, Munro J: Preliminary report: successful treatment of juvenile chronic arthritis with a specific antiviral agent. Br J Rheumatol 28:521–524, 1989

21. Panush RS, Lane N: Exercise and rheumatic disease. Ballieres Clin Rheumatol 8:1–239, 1994

22. Panush RS, Hanson CS, Caldwell JR, Longley S, Stork J, Thoburn R: Is running associated with osteoarthritis? An eight-year follow up study. J Clin Rheumatol 1:35–39, 1995

23. Fries JF, Singh G, Morfeld D, Hubert HB, Lane NE, Brown BW: Running: the development of disability with age. Ann Intern Med 121:502–509, 1994

24. Panush RS: Nutrition and rheumatic disease. Rheum Dis Clin North Am 17:197–447, 1991

SECTION D. PROBLEM-FOCUSED MANAGEMENT

<table>
<tr><td>CHAPTER
19</td><td># Pain Management</td></tr>
</table>

LAURENCE A. BRADLEY, PhD

Patients with rheumatic diseases regard pain as a major challenge and one of the most important consequences of their illnesses (1). Indeed, pain is a major determinant of patients' health behaviors. It has been found that pain is more important than physical or psychological disability in explaining medication usage among patients with rheumatoid arthritis (RA) (2). Pain is also a significant predictor of patient and physician assessments of the patients' general health status as well as future levels of pain and disability (2). Moreover, despite the advances that have been made in the management of the rheumatic diseases, it is unusual for patients to experience complete pain relief in response to their medication and other treatment regimens.

Pain also presents challenges to health care providers. Because pain is a subjective experience, it cannot be measured directly or assessed in reference to a physiologic gold standard. Health care providers must make inferences regarding patients' subjective pain experiences on the basis of their verbal reports, overt motor behaviors (e.g., grimacing), or responses to various rating scales. Patients' pain experiences are influenced by numerous psychosocial factors (e.g., mood and cultural background) as well as by disease processes. Thus, effective treatment of pain usually requires the efforts of interdisciplinary teams with expertise in medicine, psychology, pharmacology, physical modalities, and exercise. Pain should be evaluated within the context of a full medical and psychosocial assessment (3). A treatment plan then may be developed that will integrate appropriate interventions.

PAIN MEASUREMENT

Pain measurement entails the assignment of numbers to events that are commonly thought to represent the sensory, emotional, or intensity dimensions of the pain experience (4). These events may include patients' ratings of their pain experiences, displays of overt motor behavior, or psychophysiologic responses.

Pain is a complex sensory and emotional experience that cannot be measured directly. Instead, investigators and clinicians must attempt to measure events that are thought to represent various dimensions of the pain experience. All pain measurement methods have strengths as well as weaknesses. Therefore, at least two pain rating measures should be employed to evaluate the consistency of patients' reports of their pain experiences. If possible, it is desirable to complement these pain ratings with observations of patients' pain behav-

iors. Conclusions regarding patients' responses to treatment interventions may be made with greater confidence if similar outcomes are found across measures of subjective pain experience and behavior (4).

Pain Ratings

Pain ratings are subjective estimates of pain intensity or unpleasantness. Intensity refers to the severity of the pain experience, whereas unpleasantness refers to the emotional arousal produced by this experience (4). The three methods used most frequently to measure these dimensions of pain include *numerical* and *verbal rating scales*, *visual analogue scales*, and the *McGill Pain Questionnaire*.

Numerical rating scales consist of a series of numbers placed on a horizontal or vertical line in ascending order of intensity (e.g., 0–10). These scales usually are anchored by verbal descriptors at the endpoints such as "No Pain At All" and "Unbearable Pain." Verbal rating scales are similar to numerical scales except that they consist of a series of words aligned in ascending order of intensity (Table 1). Thus, both the numbers and the words represent rank-ordered categories that form *ordinal scales*. Although individuals generally find it easy to understand and respond to these scales, the meanings of the intervals between the scale categories are unknown.

There are drawbacks associated with the use of numerical and verbal rating scales. First, the nonparametric statistical procedures that should be used with these ordinal scales are limited in power relative to parametric procedures. Second, these rating scales have limited sensitivity for treatment-induced effects (4). Another weakness is associated with the verbal rating scales. The structure of these scales may force patients to choose categories that do not actually represent their pain experiences. For example, a patient may not have a good understanding of the English language and, thus, may have difficulty matching her or his pain experiences with any of the available categories. This individual may erroneously endorse a category primarily to comply with the demands of the measurement procedure. This problem highlights the need to develop reliable and valid pain measurement procedures for persons from Hispanic, Asian, and other non-Anglo cultures (5).

An alternative to ordinal rating scales is the *visual analogue scale* or VAS (Table 1). The VAS consists of a 100-mm horizontal line with endpoints that are anchored by verbal descriptors such as "No Pain" and "Unbearable Pain." Patients

Table 1. Numerical and verbal rating scales of pain intensity (adapted from 4) and a visual analogue scale.

Numerical Rating Scale						
0	1	2	3	4	5	6
No pain at all						Unbearable pain

Verbal Rating Scale
Extremely weak
Weak
Mild
Moderate
Strong
Intense
Extremely intense

Visual Analogue Scale
No Pain┠────────────────────────────────┨Unbearable Pain

respond to the VAS by placing a mark at the point along the scale that best represents the intensity or unpleasantness of their pain experience. Response is scored by measuring the distance from the left endpoint to the individual's mark; this distance represents a quantitative measure of the patient's subjective pain experience.

Compared to numerical and verbal category scales, the VAS has several advantages. First, the VAS has a large number of possible response points, which makes it sensitive to treatment-induced changes. Second, the meanings of the intervals between the response points of the VAS are known; therefore, parametric statistical procedures may be used to analyze responses to this *interval scale* with good power. Finally, children as well as adults may use the VAS to describe their pain experiences (6); however, it usually is necessary to provide patients with more detailed instructions for reliably responding to a VAS (4).

The *McGill Pain Questionnaire* (MPQ) (7) consists of 20 verbal category rating scales that evaluate the sensory, emotional, and intensity dimensions of the pain experience. The verbal descriptors within each scale are rank ordered by pain intensity. A patient must examine each of the 20 scales and choose from each relevant scale one descriptor that best represents her or his pain experience. The questionnaire is scored by summing the number of words from among the 20 category scales or by summing the rank values of these words to form a Pain Rating Index. There is also a short form of the MPQ that includes only 15 verbal descriptors which may be used with patients who are easily tired due to their illnesses (8).

Studies have been performed that document the sensitivity, reliability, and validity of this measure. However, two limitations are associated with its use. First, patients must be given precise instructions in the use of the MPQ, and they often require definitions for some of the words (such as "lancinating"). Second, persons who do not possess good understanding of the English language will not be able to respond to the MPQ in a reliable manner. Fortunately, there are many translated versions of the MPQ that may be used with persons from some non-English speaking cultures.

Pain Behaviors

Investigators have developed observation methods for recording overt motor behaviors that communicate the subjective experience of pain among patients with osteoarthritis (OA) (9) as well as adults and children with RA (10,11). These observation methods require patients to perform a standardized, 10-minute sequence of physical maneuvers for video recording, including sitting, standing, walking, and reclining. Trained observers then view the video recordings and count the frequencies of specific, operationally defined, pain behaviors (Table 2). It has been shown that pain behaviors may be observed in a reliable manner and that counts of these behaviors are characterized by good construct and discriminant validity (4,11).

There are several benefits associated with the measurement of pain behavior. First, it provides quantifiable observational data regarding patients' functional limitations in activities that are directly related to vocational, social, and leisure endeavors (4). Second, in contrast to the significant relationships that are found between patients' pain ratings and their emotional distress levels, measures of pain behavior generally are independent of patients' affective states (4). Finally, measurement of pain behavior in addition to pain ratings allows one to determine whether there are differences between patients' reports of subjective pain experiences and their behavior.

The major disadvantage to the observation of pain behavior is that it entails a large amount of training, professional time, and expense. There have been attempts to develop "live" observation methods of patients' pain behaviors during physical examinations (12). Although these methods are reliable and valid, pain behaviors observed during physical examinations tend to be significantly associated with emotional distress. Thus, observation methods are used infrequently in clinical and research settings.

Table 2. Pain behavior associated with osteoarthritis and with rheumatoid arthritis in adults and children.*

Osteoarthritis	Adult Rheumatoid Arthritis	Juvenile Rheumatoid Arthritis
Guarding	Guarding	Guarding
Active Rubbing	Bracing	Bracing
Unloading Joint	Grimacing	Rigidity
Rigidity	Sighing	Active Rubbing
Joint Flexing	Rigidity	Single Flexing
	Passive Rubbing	Multiple Flexing
	Active Rubbing	

* These behaviors were identified by Keefe et al (9), McDaniel et al (10), and Jaworski et al (11).

Psychophysiologic Responses

Psychophysiologic assessment methods are used primarily to examine the relationships among psychological and environmental factors and the initiation or maintenance of pain and other symptoms (4). These methods have been primarily used for research purposes with arthritis patients. It has been shown that daily stresses among patients with RA are associated with mood disturbances which, in turn, are related to decreases in soluble interleukin-2 receptor levels and increases in joint pain (13). In addition, persons with fibromyalgia exhibit alpha intrusion during non-rapid eye movement sleep and this sleep disturbance is associated with pain and fatigue (14). These patients also show abnormal cerebrospinal fluid levels of substance P and abnormal functional brain activity during resting conditions as well as abnormal cerebral evoked potential amplitudes during painful stimulation (reviewed in 15).

This work has led to the development of a model of abnormal pain perception in fibromyalgia that encompasses interactions among genetic, environmental, psychological, and physiologic factors. Only recently, however, have tests of this model been undertaken. Thus, while psychophysiological assessments are reliable and contribute to our understanding of pain, they generally are not appropriate at present for clinical purposes.

COMPREHENSIVE PAIN MANAGEMENT

Effective treatment of chronic pain usually requires professionals from multiple disciplines to provide appropriate interventions in a coordinated fashion. Goals are to reduce inflammation, pain, and physical or emotional impairments while maintaining function. Most patients with rheumatic disease will require pharmacologic and exercise therapies as well as education. Many patients also will require and benefit from psychological and behavioral therapies (see Chapter 10, Cognitive Behavioral Interventions). There are many unresolved issues regarding which combinations of treatment work best for specific individuals during the early and later stages of disease (5).

The psychological and behavioral therapies that have been developed for rheumatic disease pain tend to share similar treatment components. These components include education, training in relaxation and other coping skills, and rehearsal of these newly learned skills. The effects of nearly all of the interventions have been assessed relative to those produced by waiting-list or attention-placebo control conditions. The following discussion examines the interventions used for patients with RA, OA, and fibromyalgia that have been subjected to the most stringent testing procedures.

Rheumatoid Arthritis

One of the first psychological therapies was a biofeedback-assisted group therapy intervention that trained patients with RA and their family members in relaxation and behavioral problem-solving skills (16). Relative to attention–placebo and no adjunct treatment conditions, the intervention produced significant reductions in pain behavior and disease activity (i.e., joint counts). At one-year follow-up, patients who received the intervention reported significantly lower usage of health care resources and incurred lower medical service costs than patients in the other two study conditions (17). These patients also reported significantly lower levels of pain intensity and depression than patients who received no adjunct treatment. However, post-treatment reductions in pain behavior and disease activity produced by the group therapy intervention were not maintained at follow-up.

Several other investigators have reported that psychological and behavioral therapies produce significant symptom reductions in patients with RA. Until recently, however, few of these therapies produced outcomes that were maintained for extended time periods following treatment termination.

Keefe and Van Horn have proposed a model of relapse of treatment gains among patients with rheumatic disease (18). This model posits that relapse tends to occur when patients' symptoms increase in intensity and their perceptions of control are compromised. Patients are then likely to experience psychological distress, reduce their efforts to cope with symptoms, and subsequently experience a major relapse in pain, function, or emotional status. This suggests that psychological and behavioral interventions might produce better maintenance of treatment gains if they include components designed specifically to help patients cope with potential relapse. Specifically, all phases of treatment should include 1) identification of high-risk situations that are likely to tax patients' coping resources; 2) identification of the early signs of relapse, such as increases in pain or depression; 3) rehearsal of cognitive and behavioral skills for responding to these early relapse signs; and 4) training in self-reinforcement for effective performance of coping responses to possible relapse (18).

Stress management training and a post-treatment maintenance program, relative to attention–placebo and no adjunct treatment conditions, can produce significant improvements in pain ratings and reports of helplessness and coping strategy usage among patients with RA that have been shown to persist for 15 months following treatment (19).

Osteoarthritis

Two investigations have examined the effects of coping skills training on patients with OA of the knee (20,21). This training, relative to arthritis education and standard care, produced significant reductions in patients' ratings of pain and psychological disability that generally were maintained at 6 months. Patients who received coping skills training reported significant reductions in physical disability from post-treatment to follow-up.

The Arthritis Self-Management Program (ASMP) is a standardized intervention that has been evaluated primarily with OA and RA patients. It focuses particular attention on enhancing patients' beliefs that they can perform specific behaviors to achieve their health-related goals. These beliefs are known as perceptions of *self-efficacy* (see Chapter 9, Patient Education). It has been shown that the ASMP produces significant increases in self-efficacy for pain and other symptoms as well as significant reductions in pain ratings and arthritis-related physician visits among patients with OA and RA that persist for up to 4 years (22).

Telephone-based counseling interventions represent a new, inexpensive method for improving patients' health status. The first of these interventions, developed for patients with OA, reviewed educational information, medications, and clinical problems with patients. It also taught them strategies for increasing their involvement in encounters with physicians (23). This intervention produced significant improvements in patients' reports of pain and functional ability and did not substantially increase health care costs.

Use of telephone interventions in other rheumatic diseases has yielded mixed results (24). It remains to be determined whether more directive interventions, such as telephone-based coping skills training, may produce beneficial effects similar to those found with OA patients.

Fibromyalgia

Two studies have shown that cognitive behavioral therapy produces significant improvements in pain, psychological distress, and functional ability in patients with fibromyalgia (25,26). Although neither of the studies used attention–placebo control groups, it was found that the therapeutic effects of one intervention was maintained for one year following treatment (25). It is unlikely, then, that the positive effects of cognitive behavioral therapy were due solely to nonspecific or placebo factors. This type of intervention appears to be promising and deserves further study using rigorous experimental methodology.

Exercise therapies also have been used successfully with fibromyalgia patients. A cardiovascular fitness training program (27) and a combined program of education, motion exercise, pool therapy, and fitness training (28) can produce significant improvements in patients' ratings of disease activity and physical function. The improvements in function were maintained for 4 to 8 months after treatment (28). Thus, it appears that structured exercise programs that emphasize aerobic fitness training produce sustained improvements in patients with fibromyalgia.

PREVENTION OF CHRONIC PAIN

The recent development of behavioral interventions for the secondary prevention of chronic musculoskeletal pain among injured workers represents an important advance that may have a positive impact on the high health care costs of treating this condition (29). A controlled study of a secondary prevention program for injured nurses who had been sicklisted for back pain during the previous 2 years included intensive training in exercise and ergonomics as well as a cognitive behavioral intervention designed to help the nurses manage their pain and reduce their risk of reinjury (30). The program also included four post-treatment "booster sessions" to aid in relapse prevention.

It was found at a 6-month follow-up assessment that the program, relative to a waiting list control condition, produced significant improvements in nurses' displays of pain behavior, pain-related work absenteeism, and ratings of pain intensity, fatigue, anxiety, helplessness, and satisfaction with daily activities. At 18 months, the nurses maintained their improvements in ratings of pain intensity, fatigue, helplessness, and satisfaction with daily activities. Moreover, a cost-benefit analysis suggested that the program produced financial savings to the nurses' employers that were approximately twice as large as the costs of the program.

A small number of independent studies of secondary pre-

vention programs have produced positive effects similar to those noted above (reviewed in 29). Although the development of secondary prevention programs is a recent phenomenon, it currently appears that successful programs share three features. First, these programs emphasize increasing patient activity levels soon after injury (preferably 4–12 weeks after pain onset). Second, successful programs elicit patients' participation as active partners with the treatment providers. Finally, effective prevention programs emphasize relapse prevention and good adherence with newly learned strategies for managing pain.

SUMMARY

There is consistent evidence that psychological and behavioral therapies produce significant reductions in ratings of pain and psychological distress among patients with rheumatic disease. These therapies, however, do not consistently produce improvements in functional ability. Nevertheless, the small number of studies that have evaluated treatment-related changes in medical care costs have produced positive findings.

Several issues concerning psychological and behavioral therapies will receive greater attention from clinicians and investigators during the next 5 years. First, greater emphasis will be devoted to the prevention of patient relapse following treatment. The second issue involves the health care usage and related costs incurred by patients with rheumatic disease. It is expected that psychological and behavioral therapies will place increasing emphasis on documenting treatment-related reductions in health care utilization as well as in the direct and indirect costs of pain. Special attention will be devoted to the development and evaluation of "minimal" interventions, such as telephone-based counseling, that may contribute to substantial cost savings. Finally, it is expected that the secondary prevention of chronic musculoskeletal pain will continue to be of great interest to health care providers and investigators. As positive evidence accrues that secondary prevention may be achieved in persons with recent injuries, clinicians and investigators will begin to develop and evaluate early intervention therapies for managing pain among patients with newly diagnosed RA, OA, and fibromyalgia.

REFERENCES

1. Bradley LA: Introduction: the challenges of pain in arthritis. Arthritis Care Res 6:169–170, 1993
2. Kazis LE, Meenan RF, Anderson JJ: Pain in the rheumatic diseases: investigation of a key health status component. Arthritis Rheum 26:1017–1022, 1983
3. Bradley LA, Haile JM, Jaworski TM: Assessment of psychological status using interviews and self-report instruments. In, Handbook of Pain Assessment. Edited by DC Turk, R Melzack. New York, Guilford, 1992
4. Bradley LA: Pain measurement in arthritis. Arthritis Care Res 6:178–186, 1993
5. Bellamy N, Bradley LA: Workshop on chronic pain, pain control, and patient outcomes in rheumatoid arthritis and osteoarthritis. Arthritis Rheum 39:357–362, 1996
6. Varni JW, Thompson KL, Hanson V: The Varni/Thompson Pediatric Pain Questionnaire. I. Chronic musculoskeletal pain in juvenile rheumatoid arthritis. Pain 28:27–38, 1987
7. Melzack R: The McGill Pain Questionnaire: major properties and scoring methods. Pain 1:277–299, 1975
8. Melzack R: The short-form McGill Pain Questionnaire. Pain 30:191–197, 1987

9. Keefe FJ, Caldwell DS, Queen K, et al: Osteoarthritic knee pain: a behavioral analysis. Pain 28:309–321, 1987

10. McDaniel LK, Anderson KO, Bradley LA, et al: Development of an observation method for assessing pain behavior in rheumatoid arthritis patients. Pain 24:165–184, 1986

11. Jaworski TM, Bradley LA, Heck LW, et al: Development of an observation method for assessing pain behaviors in children with juvenile rheumatoid arthritis. Arthritis Rheum 38:1142–1151, 1995

12. Anderson KO, Bradley LA, Turner RA, et al: Observation of pain behavior in rheumatoid arthritis patients during physical examination: relationship to disease activity and psychological variables. Arthritis Care Res 5:49–56, 1992

13. Harrington L, Affleck G, Urrows S, et al: Temporal covariation of soluble interleukin-2 receptor levels, daily stress, and disease activity in rheumatoid arthritis. Arthritis Rheum 36:199–203, 1993

14. Moldofsky H: Sleep and the fibrositis syndrome. Rheum Dis Clin North Am 15:91–103, 1989

15. Bradley LA, Alarcón GS: Fibromyalgia. In, Arthritis and Allied Conditions. Thirteenth edition. Edited by WJ Koopman. New York, Lippincott, 1996

16. Bradley LA, Young LD, Anderson KO, et al: Effects of psychological therapy on pain behavior of rheumatoid arthritis patients: treatment outcome and six-month followup. Arthritis Rheum 30:1105–1114, 1987

17. Young LD, Bradley LA, Turner RA: Decreases in health care resource utilization in patients with rheumatoid arthritis following a cognitive-behavioral intervention. Biofeedback Self Regul 20:259–268, 1995

18. Keefe FJ, Van Horn Y: Cognitive-behavioral treatment of rheumatoid arthritis pain: maintaining treatment gains. Arthritis Care Res 6:213–222, 1993

19. Parker JC, Smarr KL, Buckelew SP, et al: Effects of stress management on clinical outcomes in rheumatoid arthritis. Arthritis Rheum 38:1807–1818, 1995

20. Keefe FJ, Caldwell DS, Williams DA, et al: Pain coping skills training in the management of osteoarthritic knee pain: a comparative study. Behav Ther 21:49–62, 1990

21. Keefe FJ, Caldwell DS, Williams DA, et al: Pain coping skills training in the management of osteoarthritic knee pain. II. Follow-up results. Behav Ther 21:435–447, 1990

22. Lorig KR, Mazonson PD, Holman HR: Evidence suggesting that health education for self-management in patients with chronic arthritis has sustained health benefits while reducing health care costs. Arthritis Rheum 36:439–446, 1993

23. Weinberger M, Tierney WM, Cowper PA, et al: Cost-effectiveness of increased telephone contact for patients with osteoarthritis: a randomized, controlled trial. Arthritis Rheum 36:243–246, 1993

24. Maisiak R, Austin JS, West SG, Heck L: The effect of person-centered counseling on the psychological status of persons with systemic lupus erythematosus or rheumatoid arthritis: a randomized, controlled trial. Arthritis Care Res 9:60–66, 1996

25. Nielson WR, Walker C, McCain GA: Cognitive behavioral treatment of fibromyalgia syndrome: preliminary findings. J Rheumatol 19:98–103, 1992

26. Goldenberg DL, Kaplan KH, Nadeau MG, et al: A controlled study of a stress-reduction, cognitive-behavioral treatment program in fibromyalgia. J Musculoskeletal Pain 2:53–66, 1994

27. McCain GA, Bell DA, Mai FM, Halliday PD: A controlled study of the effects of a supervised cardiovascular fitness training program on the manifestations of primary fibromyalgia. Arthritis Rheum 31:1135–1141, 1988

28. Burckhardt CS, Mannerkorpi K, Hendenberg L, Bjelle A: A randomized, controlled clinical trial of education and physical training for women with fibromyalgia. J Rheumatol 21:714–720, 1994

29. Linton SJ, Bradley LA: Strategies for the prevention of chronic pain. In, Psychological Treatments for Pain: A Practitioner's Handbook. Edited by RJ Gatchel, DC Turk. New York, Guilford, 1996

30. Linton SL, Bradley LA, Jensen I, et al: The secondary prevention of low back pain: a controlled study with follow-up. Pain 36:197–207, 1989

Additional Recommended Reading

1. Turk DC, Melzack R, editors: Handbook of Pain Assessment. New York, Guilford, 1992

2. Gatchel RJ, Turk DC, editors: Psychological Treatments for Pain: A Practitioner's Handbook. New York, Guilford, 1996

Fatigue

BASIA L. BELZA, PhD, RN

Fatigue is a frequent and bothersome problem for individuals with rheumatic disease. This chapter examines the impact and prevalence of fatigue, causes of fatigue, types of measurement, and management strategies for fatigue reduction in rheumatic diseases. Researchers in the rheumatic diseases have only recently begun to conduct studies in this area. Fatigue has important implications for overall disease management, because it may be a factor in discontinuing or not fully participating in rehabilitation programs, reducing quality of life, impairing functional status, and being sedentary.

Health professionals need to address the complaint of fatigue. Whereas physicians' expertise lies in management of the medical aspects of illness, symptom management is shared and is within the domain of allied health professionals. Symptoms such as pain, fatigue, disability, and depressed moods are the consequences of the illness. Health professionals are trained to help patients better understand and adjust to the consequences of disease. Collaborative efforts can lead to better utilization of the expertise of our colleagues. Disciplines such as nursing, physical therapy, occupational therapy, and mental health play pivotal roles. For example, nurses coordinate care, physical therapists prescribe activity programs, occupational therapists teach energy conservation behaviors, and mental health professionals treat mood changes and anxiety.

IMPACT

Fatigue is a perception arising from the complex interplay of somatic and psychological factors (1). To some, fatigue is the end result of excessive energy consumption, depleted hormones or neurotransmitters, or the diminished ability of muscles cells to contract (2). To others, fatigue is the subjective state of weariness related to reduced motivation, prolonged mental activity, or boredom. The functional impact of fatigue is significant. It is associated with moderate impairment in functional capacity and reduced productivity. One patient with rheumatoid arthritis (RA) describes the impact of fatigue as follows: "When I am fatigued everything is too great an effort. Ordinary tasks loom as overwhelming. Feelings of helplessness and hopelessness dominate." The presence of fatigue also makes the management of associated symptoms more challenging. Some patients would even prefer to do an activity and have pain rather than face the lack of control associated with fatigue. Fatigue may also be related to increased human error and associated with increased falls (3).

PREVALENCE

The prevalence and severity of fatigue in the rheumatic diseases varies by type of disease. Although the diagnostic criteria for RA do not include fatigue, one criterion for clinical remission is the absence of fatigue (4). The prevalence of fatigue in patients with RA has been found to range from 88% to 93% (4,5). The American College of Rheumatology 1990 multicenter study for fibromyalgia used a definition of fatigue as "usually or always being too tired to do what you want," and found that 81% of persons with fibromyalgia reported fatigue (6). Fatigue is also present in 80% to 100% of patients with systemic lupus erythematosus and is one of the most disabling symptoms for patients (7,8). Fatigue has been found in at least one-half of patients with ankylosing spondylitis (9). The occurrence of fatigue across diagnostic categories at all phases of life underscores the need for empirically based interventions.

ETIOLOGY

Fatigue is a complex phenomenon with multiple causes that include physiological, psychological, and environmental factors. Components of the inflammatory process may contribute to fatigue. Multiple contributors to fatigue have been examined; in one study of patients with RA, over 60% of the variance in fatigue could be explained by pain, sleep disturbance, inactivity, comorbidities, poorer functional status, and newly diagnosed disease (5). When in pain, people expend more energy to complete even the simplest of tasks. Disturbed night sleep leads to daytime fatigue. Inactivity leads to deconditioning and muscle atrophy.

As a result of reduced use or disuse, changes in the cardiorespiratory system reduce the body's energy producing capacity and mechanical efficiency, thus contributing to decreased endurance. Muscle function is impaired, probably due to an accumulation of metabolic products, which leads to impaired muscle contractility. Functional impairment is associated with less efficient use of the musculoskeletal system or use of less developed muscle groups to keep pain at a minimum. Potential psychological causes of fatigue, such as depression and anxiety, have been noted in patients with rheumatic disease. One of the diagnostic criteria for depression includes the presence of fatigue. Impairment in cognitive function, including decreased attention and impaired perception and thinking, has been associated with fatigue (10). Individuals with rheumatic disease may report cognitive impairment such as difficulty in thinking and inability to concentrate (8).

MEASUREMENT

The accurate measurement of fatigue is important for several reasons: 1) to understand the correlation of fatigue with other symptoms such as pain and depression, 2) to monitor its natural history over time, 3) to screen or classify, 4) to assess individual health status, 5) to distinguish between disease conditions, 6) to guide management decisions, and 7) to evaluate the magnitude of change in response to treatment. In addition to assessing degree, duration, and severity of fatigue, several related areas need to be determined (11). Key questions to ask patients presenting with fatigue are: What is the status of the rheumatic disease? Is there any associated disorder(s) such as hypothyroidism? Are there sleep disturbances? Is there a minor or major mood disturbance? Are there major psychosocial stressors? What is the exercise/activity level? Familiarity with the several different fatigue measures allows clinicians and researchers to select the scale that best meets provider and patient needs.

Traditionally, single items have been used to measure fatigue in rheumatology. One question frequently used to evaluate outcomes in clinical trials for rheumatic diseases is how many hours elapse from the time of arising to the time of fatigue onset. Various scales have been used to measure fatigue or energy, such as determining energy level on a 10-point scale from "not at all" to "a lot," or determining fatigue intensity on a four-point scale from none to severe. Although these approaches require minimal patient time and are simple to score, most of the measures have not been subject to stringent psychometric evaluation. Additionally, this type of questioning allows for the measurement of a single dimension of fatigue (such as severity) but fails to capture other dimensions (such as intensity or timing). More recently, there has been a move toward measuring fatigue within a multidimensional framework. A number of measures of fatigue are found in the literature; some have been tested in the rheumatic diseases.

The Multidimensional Assessment of Fatigue (MAF) scale measures five dimensions of fatigue as experienced during the past week: degree, severity, distress, impact on daily activities, and frequency. Fourteen questions use numerical rating scales with unipolar endpoints of 1 (not at all) to 10 (a great deal), and two have multiple choice responses. Possible scores range from 1 (no fatigue) to 50 (severe fatigue). The reliability and validity of MAF have been demonstrated in a sample of adults with RA (5).

The Activity Record (ACTRE) is a functional assessment tool that follows a daily log format designed to quantify how much physical activity a person is doing and how strenuous it is. Each activity is further characterized by whether it is associated with pain or fatigue, or perceived as enjoyable, meaningful, difficult to perform, or well done (12–14). The ACTRE is most useful when included as one of several evaluations for determining function. The benefit of the ACTRE is its ability to capture a sequence of activities comprising a day in the individual's life. The amount can be quantified, and specific abilities can be rated in terms of the presence and amount of associated symptoms. This index offers the health care professional and patient a more complete profile of function and defines problem areas based on the patient's perceived level of competence and satisfaction.

The Fatigue Severity Scale (FSS) is a nine-item scale measuring symptoms associated with fatigue and its impact on work, family, and social life (8,15). It is based on the characteristics of fatigue in systemic lupus erythematosus and multiple sclerosis. This scale can distinguish between patients with these two conditions and has internal consistency and stability over time. The FSS measures one dimension of fatigue as compared with the MAF, which measures five dimensions.

A brief unidimensional measure is the seven-item fatigue subscale of the Profile of Mood States (POMS) (16). The POMS, which has been tested in a variety of clinical populations and healthy subjects, contains subscales measuring tension, anger, vigor, fatigue, confusion, and depression. The internal consistency coefficients of these six subscales are excellent, and factor analytic studies have established the independence of the six states. Although the POMS is widely used, it measures only the severity of fatigue.

Another published measure is the Fatigue Scale, a 14-item instrument with physical and mental symptom subscales derived by principal components analysis (17). The scale focuses on the symptoms associated with the presentation of fatigue. This measure was tested initially in patients with chronic fatigue syndrome (CFS) and those attending a general medical clinic. The Fatigue Scale has good face validity and sensitivity to change.

The Profile of Fatigue-related Symptoms is a 96-item multidimensional illness-specific instrument incorporating the symptoms associated with CFS (18). The instrument was developed to assess the severity and pattern of illness, relate subjective symptoms to immunologic and clinical findings, evaluate the effects of treatment, and compare symptoms of CFS with other fatiguing illnesses. The four subscales of emotional distress, cognitive difficulty, fatigue, and somatic complaints have demonstrated good convergence with comparison measures, high reliability, and high internal consistency. Although extremely comprehensive, the length of the Profile of Fatigue-related Symptoms makes it impractical for use in clinical settings.

MANAGEMENT STRATEGIES

Treatment goals for the management of fatigue include resolving the underlying problem(s), helping the patient better understand fatigue, and reducing or alleviating the fatigue. If there is a single underlying problem causing fatigue, such as thyroid condition or anemia, it needs to be diagnosed and treated. If there is a component of depression, the patient should be advised to receive counseling and appropriate antidepressant therapy. The clinician and patient need to develop mutually agreed-upon treatment strategies to reduce or alleviate fatigue with the goal of maintaining or improving quality of life.

Self-appraisal of Fatigue. Monitoring changes in one's own body is a basic activity of self-care (19). Completing a fatigue care wheel may help a person understand the relationship between specific causes and solutions to fatigue. Using standardized measures to assess fatigue or maintaining a log may help note patterns, and variations and contributors to fatigue. Suggesting that patients read the story "My Bowl of Marbles" (Appendix A) may serve as a starting point for them to articulate how they perceive their own energy level.

Optimal Control of Inflammation. Although the mechanism is unknown, it is speculated that the release of interleukin-1, associated with the body's immune response, contributes to fatigue. Whatever the contributing factors, the resulting inflammation has been associated with fatigue. Appropriate type and amount of medications must be taken to control the inflammatory process.

Symptom Reinterpretation. Self-efficacy theory is the belief in one's capability to exercise control over motivation and environmental demands. One of the strategies to improve self efficacy is symptom reinterpretation, which allows an individual to reconceptualize what he or she thinks about fatigue. People with high self-efficacy approach difficult tasks as challenges, set challenging goals, increase effort in face of difficulties, and experience low stress and depression. Patients redefine physiological symptoms and signs. For example, fatigue may be a warning sign of an impending increase in disease activity that should stimulate a patient to seek earlier medical treatment.

Energy Conservation Behaviors. Energy conservation is the process of saving energy and improving the distribution of energy over the time it is needed (20). Proper body positioning conserves energy. Energy is used when the body is in poor posture, such as with the use of incorrect work height, poor posture, or hunched shoulders. Rest breaks may reduce pain and stress to damaged joints (see Chapter 12, Rest and Exercise). Activity analysis allows the examination of activities that might drain excessive time and energy. Strategies to alter work patterns include pacing, planning ahead, prioritizing, using adaptive equipment, and job simplification. Workbooks such as the *Rehabilitation Through Learning: Energy Conservation and Joint Protection* are valuable resources for clinicians and patients who want to learn more about the principles of energy conservation and joint protection, and the application of these principles to individual situations (20).

Modifying Sleep and Rest Behaviors. Resting and sleeping are intuitively logical approaches to managing fatigue. Examples of sleep hygiene are included in Chapter 21, Sleep Disturbance. For sleep apnea, myoclonus, or other suspected sleep disturbances, refer to a sleep clinic for evaluation and treatment.

Physical Activity. Evidence shows that individuals with rheumatic disease who are involved in aerobic exercise of moderate intensity note improvements in pain and fatigue (21). Additionally, improvements have been noted in muscle strength and functional status (22). Providers need to encourage patients with arthritis to safely increase their activity level. The level of aerobic conditioning also has a significant influence on performance capability. Individuals with limited aerobic capacity due to pathologic state or a sedentary life style can increase their endurance through training. Following an evaluation of the cardiorespiratory and musculoskeletal systems, and in consultation with an exercise specialist, patients can start a training program. Training produces improved heart rate, ventilation, and oxygen transport and utilization. Specific improvements in coordination and functional efficiency may also occur, depending on type of activity and muscle groups trained. Endurance training thus allows a lower energy expenditure for a given effort, resulting in reduced fatigue and enhanced performance.

SUMMARY

Effective management of fatigue is possible. Consideration should be given to the multiple causes of fatigue and varied management strategies. More research is need on factors that contribute to fatigue, as well as the testing of interventions to determine which are most effective in alleviating or reducing fatigue. Treating fatigue requires an understanding of the inflammatory process, the impact of the rheumatic disease on the psychological system, and the personal attributes and motivations of the individual with arthritis.

REFERENCES

1. Potempa K, Lopez M, Reid C, Lawson L: Chronic fatigue. Image J Nurs Sch 18:165–169, 1986
2. Poteliakhoff A: Adrenocortical activity and some clinical findings in acute and chronic fatigue. J Psychosom Res 25:91–95, 1981
3. Fessel KD: Fear of falling and activity limitation among persons with rheumatoid arthritis (abstract). Arthritis Rheum 38 (suppl 9):S305, 1995
4. Pinals RS, Masi AT, Larsen RA, The Subcommittee for Criteria of Remission in Rheumatoid Arthritis of the American Rheumatism Association Diagnostic Therapeutic Criteria Committee: Preliminary criteria for clinical remission in rheumatoid arthritis. Arthritis Rheum 24:1308–1315, 1981
5. Belza B, Henke C, Yelin E, Epstein W, Gilliss C: Correlates of fatigue in older adults with rheumatoid arthritis. Nurs Res 42:93–99, 1993
6. Wolfe F, Smythe HA, Yunus MB, et al: The American College of Rheumatology 1990 criteria for the classification of fibromyalgia: report of the Multicenter Criteria Committee. Arthritis Rheum 33:160–172, 1990
7. Shur P: Clinical features of systemic lupus erythematosus. In, Textbook of Rheumatology. Edited by W Kelly, E Harris, S Ruddy, C Sledge. Philadelphia, WB Saunders, 1993
8. Krupp LB, LaRocca NG, Muir J, Steinberg AD: A study of fatigue in systemic lupus erythematosus. J Rheumatol 17:1450–1452, 1990
9. Calin A, Edmonds L, Kennedy LG: Fatigue in ankylosing spondylitis—why is it ignored? J Rheumatol 20:991–995, 1993
10. Yoshitake H: Three characteristic patterns of subjective fatigue symptoms. Ergonomics 21:231–233, 1978
11. Goldenberg D: Fatigue in rheumatic disease. Bull Rheum Dis 44:4–8, 1995
12. Gerber L, Furst G, Shulman B, Smith C, Thornton B, Liang M, Cullen K, Stevens MB, Gilbert N: Patient education program to teach energy conversation behaviors to patients with rheumatoid arthritis. Arch Phys Med Rehabil 68:442–445, 1987
13. Gerber LH, Furst GP: Scoring methods and application of the activity record (ACTRE) for patients with musculoskeletal disorders. Arthritis Care Res 5:151–156, 1992
14. Gerber LH, Furst GP: Validation of the NIH Activity Record: a quantitative measure of life activities. Arthritis Care Res 5:81–86, 1992
15. Schwartz JE, Jandorf L, Krupp LB: The measurement of fatigue: a new instrument. J Psychosom Res 37:753–762, 1993
16. McNair D, Lorr R, Dropplemen L: Edits Manual for the Profile of Mood States. San Diego, Education and Industrial Testing Service, 1992
17. Chalder T, Berelowitz G, Pawlikowska T: Development of a fatigue scale. J Psychosom Res 37:147–153, 1993
18. Ray C, Weir W, Phillips S, Cullen S: Development of a measure of symptoms in chronic fatigue syndrome: the profile of fatigue related symptoms (PFRS). Psychol Health 7:27–43, 1992
19. Keller M, Ward S, Baumann L: Processes of self care: monitoring sensations and symptoms. Adv Nurs Sci 12:54–66, 1989
20. Furst GP, Gerber LH, Smith C: Rehabilitation Through Learning: Energy Conservation and Joint Protection. Washington DC, US Department of Health and Human Services, 1985
21. Robb-Nicholson LC, Daltroy L, Eaton LL, Gall E, Hartley LH, Schur PH, Liang MH: Effect of aerobic conditioning on lupus fatigue: a pilot study. Br J Rheumatol 28:500–505, 1989
22. Harkcom TM, Lampman RM, Banwell BF, Castor CW: Therapeutic value of graded aerobic exercise training in rheumatoid arthritis. Arthritis Rheum 28:32–39, 1985

APPENDIX A

My Bowl of Marbles
by Linda Jean Frame

I begin by thinking of energy as marbles. Each small, expendable amount of energy becomes a marble. I have a limited number of marbles to use each day and while the number of marbles may vary from day to day, I can pretty well judge each morning just how many marbles I will have to use that day. I then place my day's supply in an imaginary fish bowl and begin my day.

With each activity—washing my face, combing my hair, etc.—I use energy. When I expend one marble's worth of energy, I extract one marble from the bowl. (I value each marble at a certain amount and can judge when I use that amount of energy. You might give a different value to each of your marbles, but it will all work out the same way in the end.) Bigger projects require more marbles, however, on bad days you will find that even small activities will demand the use of more marbles than those same activities will require on your good days. There are times when it is very frustrating to have so little energy and to have to use so much of it to do even simple things, but that's the way it is!

Starting each day with an awareness of your energy supply will enable you to choose what is really important to you, and you can plan accordingly. Try to avoid frustration by accepting your limitations. Frustration is a form of stress and stress is a marble user! Comfort yourself with the thought that you won't always have so few marbles to use. Tomorrow may be a better day. *Remember* to remove marbles during the day for any type of stress. Remove marbles for anything that causes tension or fear. (I throw out a couple of marbles every time I have to drive in rush-hour traffic; not because the traffic bothers me, but because I know that I must be a little more alert and stressed than when I drive at other times of the day. If something really BIG happens, and I am *really* stressed or shocked, I may throw the whole bowl away and give myself the rest of the day off.)

If you should see me or phone me at one of those times when I have resigned from the human race, you might say, "Linda has lost her marbles!"—and you would be exactly right!

Sleep Disturbance

STEPHEN T. WEGENER, PhD

Sleep disturbances are prevalent in persons with painful chronic disease. Certain sleep disturbances are associated with specific rheumatic diseases. Clinicians working with rheumatic disease patients will encounter a range of sleep disturbances requiring a basic knowledge of sleep physiology, cycles, and disturbances as well as diagnostic and intervention techniques.

SLEEP PHYSIOLOGY

Sleep Architecture and Cycles

Human sleep is not a static or unidimensional experience. Healthy adults move through a series of stages during the sleep period. These sleep stages are characterized by distinct patterns of behavioral and physiological states measured by electroencephalography (EEG), electro-oculography (EOG), and electromyography (EMG). A usual night's sleep is divided into the two broad categories of rapid eye movement (REM) and non-REM sleep. Non-REM sleep is further subdivided into four stages. Stage 1 or alpha sleep is a transitory phase during which the individual moves from wakefulness to sleep. Stage 1 ranges from 30 seconds to 7 minutes in duration and is marked by decreased EEG and EMG activity. The individual may report being awake and is easily aroused by environmental stimuli. During stage 2 there is further decrease in EEG activity and both researchers and subjects report that true sleep begins. After 15 to 30 minutes, most adults enter stage 3 and 4 sleep. Stages 3 and 4 are grouped together and are called deep or delta sleep, due to the predominance of delta wave patterns (high amplitude, low frequency EEG activity). There is little movement and the person may be very difficult to arouse. Stage 3/4 sleep is thought to play an important role in physical restoration. Adults typically pass briefly through stages 1 and 2, followed by a period of 30 to 60 minutes in stage 3/4 sleep.

The typical sleeper returns briefly to stage 2 sleep and then enters the first REM period. The REM or dream sleep is characterized by mixed EEG patterns similar to stage 1; however, EMG measured muscle tension is at its lowest level. REM sleep is thought to be critical in the maintenance of mental health and memory consolidation. Individuals who are deprived of REM sleep tend to become overly aroused, anxious, and irritable, and they tend to have other psychological disturbances. The four sleep stages and REM occur in cycles each night. Early in the night stage 3/4 sleep is dominant. As sleep progresses, REM periods increase in length and frequency. The average adult has four to six cycles per night depending on age, previous sleep history, and medications. Typical adult sleep is allocated as follows: 5% stage 1, 50% stage 2, 20% deep sleep, and 25% REM.

Sleep Requirements

There is no fixed amount of sleep that is necessary for all individuals. In the U.S., adults average 7 to 8 hours of sleep per night; however, there are large variations in individual requirements. Our society has a significant sleep debt due to the lack of adequate sleep, particularly among school-age children and working adults. The typical sleep-wake cycle is approximately 24 hours and is related to the presence of sunlight. Sleeping during the dark hours of the day is most natural; peak alertness occurs during daylight hours.

Sleep Across the Life Span

As people age, there is a growing variability in their quality and quantity of sleep. Babies and young children have a higher percentage of stage 3/4 sleep, and there is less variation in sleep patterns. As the individual ages, there is an increasing tendency to spend less time in deep sleep and to sleep for shorter periods. The adolescent experiences a dramatic drop in the amount of time asleep to the adult range of 7 to 8 hours. Throughout middle age there is a decrease in *sleep efficiency*, which is the amount of sleep divided by the amount of time in bed. Older people have greater variability in their sleep patterns, but they often maintain their usual amount of sleep through daytime napping. The elderly are also subject to more frequent mid-sleep awakenings. It is not known whether older people need less sleep or are simply less able to achieve the same amount and quality of sleep as before. Factors contributing to changes in sleep quantity and quality include: degeneration of the nervous system, increasing prevalence of physical illness, alteration of sleep patterns, reduced level of physical activity, and continued expectation of previous sleep patterns (1).

SLEEP DISTURBANCES

Clinicians observe a wide variety of sleep disturbances within the population of persons with rheumatic disease that may, or may not be, related to the disease. The four main categories of sleep disturbances are listed in Table 1. The *International Classification of Sleep Disorders: Diagnostic and Coding Manual* suggests classifying the presenting sleep problem in terms of insomnia, excessive sleepiness, or abnormal event during the sleep period (2). Different types of sleep disorders are seen in various age groups. The most common problems in children are night terrors, enuresis, and fears related to separation at bedtime. Adolescents tend to suffer from sleep deprivation with the related problems of difficulty rising and daytime sleepiness. In adults, there is increasing prevalence of sleep apnea, restless leg sleep syndrome, and insomnia.

Table 1. The four main categories of sleep disturbances based on the International Classification of Sleep Disorders (2).

I. **Dyssomnias**—including disorders of initiating and maintaining sleep (DIMS) and disorders of excessive sleepiness (DOES)

II. **Parasomnias**—disorders that are not primarily associated with insomnia or excessive sleepiness such as sleepwalking, rhythmic movement disorder, nightmares, or sleep bruxism

III. **Sleep disorders associated with medical or psychiatric disorders**—such as alcoholism, mood disorders, Parkinsonism, sleep-related asthma, or gastroesophageal reflux

IV. **Proposed sleep disorders**—those disorders without sufficient data to include in the classification at this time

Epidemiology

Insomnia includes difficulty initiating sleep, frequent mid-sleep awakenings, and nonrestorative sleep. Due to the various definitions used in epidemiologic studies, the true incidence and prevalence of insomnia is not known. In sleep disorder centers, 15% of individuals presenting with sleep disturbance have true psychophysiological insomnia (3). Transient insomnia is common, as is the use of hypnotic medication. In the U.S., approximately 35% of the population indicate trouble sleeping during the past year; 50% of this group describe it as serious problem (4). Individuals with serious sleep problems have an approximately 50% comorbidity rate of psychological distress, anxiety, depression, and medical illness (4). Insomnia is best conceptualized as a symptom, and effective management of the sleep problem begins with accurate diagnosis of the underlying illness.

Sleep Disturbances and Rheumatic Disease

Individuals with rheumatic disease are at risk for sleep disturbance due to chronic pain and increased incidence of depression. Pain is the most commonly cited cause of sleep disturbance by patients (5). Certain sleep disturbances have been linked with specific rheumatic diseases.

Fibromyalgia has the most consistent and well documented association with sleep disturbances. There is a pattern of increased nocturnal vigilance, light nonrestorative sleep, and a high frequency of subjective sleep disturbances. Sleep apnea and periodic limb movements have also been associated with fibromyalgia (6). Several studies have documented the intrusion of alpha waves during non-REM sleep in persons with fibromyalgia (6,7). This alpha EEG non-REM sleep anomaly is not found in all patients with fibromyalgia, however (8,9). While sleep disturbances are quite common in this population, a sleep disorder alone does not produce fibromyalgia (10). These sleep anomalies may reflect a hyper arousability during sleep and may result in the daytime experience of unrefreshing sleep and pain. Whether this hyper arousability is due to the underlying disease or some related process remains unclear. Recently, disruption of the growth hormone somatomedin C neuroendocrine axis has been identified and may serve as a potential link between disturbed sleep and muscle pain (11).

Sleep fragmentation—light, easily disrupted sleep with multiple mid-sleep awakenings—has been observed by EEG and by self-report in samples of persons with rheumatoid arthritis (12–14). This sleep disruption has been associated with increased rheumatic disease activity (12), night time movements (15), fatigue (16), morning stiffness (17), and other sleep disturbances; however, these specific findings remain to be replicated. Two studies have observed sleep disturbances in persons with osteoarthritis (18,19). There is one report of mid-sleep awakenings and less efficient sleep in persons with primary Sjögren's syndrome (20). The incidence and prevalence of sleep disturbances in other forms of rheumatic disease remain to be determined.

ASSESSMENT

A review of sleep parameters should be included in the initial patient history. Critical information for the diagnosis of sleep problems is provided by the individual's medical, psychiatric, and family history; medication usage; and psychosocial assessment. A complete history should also include an interview with the patient's bed partner. Short-term complaints and difficulties should be distinguished from chronic problems. Inquiry regarding what steps the patient has taken to address the sleep disturbance will indicate the chronicity and severity of the problem. Sleep patterns may be affected by pain, respiratory problems, psychiatric or neurological conditions, medications, or environmental stimuli. Careful review of medications is necessary to identify pharmacologic agents that may be disrupting sleep patterns. Some medications disrupt sleep during active use; others affect sleep during the withdrawal period.

Sleep diaries are useful in assessing sleep disturbance. A daily record of the individual's sleep patterns including bedtime, rising time, mid-sleep awakenings, pain, mood, and medication use are essential. It is also useful to keep track of daytime fatigue, drowsiness, and functioning. As part of the history, assess the patient's behavior in terms of eating, substance and exercise habits, sleep schedule, and pre-sleep activities. An assessment of the individual's sleep environment in light of good sleep hygiene should also be undertaken.

A full physical and neurological examination with emphasis on detecting disorders of the nervous system is indicated for those with severe sleep problems. Evaluation of anxiety and depression are critical, because psychiatric illness is common in persons with sleep disturbances (4). If a severe mood disturbance is identified, referral for psychiatric evaluation and medication is indicated.

The need for sleep laboratory evaluation depends on factors such as the individual's presenting complaint, response to initial sleep hygiene, and behavioral and pharmacologic interventions. Due to the close association between excessive daytime sleepiness and potentially serious organic pathology, individuals with this presenting problem should be referred to a sleep medicine specialist. Primary complaints of delayed sleep onset and mid-sleep awakenings may be initially treated with sleep hygiene education or behavioral therapy if sleep apnea, movement disorders, or disorders of excessive sleepiness such as narcolepsy can be ruled out. The clinician should develop a list of potential causes for the sleep disturbance and seek to understand and treat them in turn.

Table 2. Sleep hygiene principles.

Regular Sleep Patterns
  Go to bed and arise the same time each day
  Avoid naps except for brief 10–15 minute period 8 hours after rising
  Take a hot bath to raise temperature 2°C within 2 hours of bedtime
  A hot drink may help
  Establish a bedtime ritual

Environmental Factors
  Avoid large meals 2–3 hours before bedtime
  Avoid bright light if you have to arise during the sleep period
  Keep clock face turned away
  Make sure sleeping environment is dark, quiet, and comfortable

Exercise
  Exercise regularly each day
  Avoid vigorous exercise 2 hours prior to bedtime

Drug Effects
  Give up smoking entirely or avoid smoking several hours before bedtime
  Do not smoke if you have a mid-sleep awakening
  Limit use of alcoholic beverages
  Discontinue caffeine use
  Avoid use of over-the-counter sleep medications
  Use prescribed sleep medication only occasionally

Aging
  Educate patients regarding changes in sleep parameters that occur with age to reduce unrealistic expectations and anxiety

TREATMENT

Treatment is dictated by the underlying cause or causes of the sleep disturbance. Treatment of medical, psychiatric, or environmental problems should be the initial step in improving sleep parameters. It may be necessary to add sleep hygiene education or behavioral treatment for residual sleep disturbances due to learned maladaptive sleep patterns or anxiety arising from the expectation of sleep problems. A hierarchical approach to the management of residual sleep problems builds on good sleep hygiene, adds behavioral therapy, and progresses to pharmacologic intervention. Treatment recommendations are based on studies in non-rheumatic disease populations. There have been no replicated, controlled clinical trials of interventions for sleep problems in persons with rheumatic disease.

Sleep Hygiene Education

Poor sleep hygiene may be viewed as a primary cause of sleep disturbances or as a risk factor for developing these disturbances. Education regarding principles of good sleep hygiene is the foundation for treating sleep disturbance. Recommendations provided in brief oral or written form are unlikely to change behavior or have any impact on the sleep problem. Effective sleep hygiene intervention requires ongoing counseling and contact with the patient to translate the advice into behavior change. Sleep hygiene principles are listed in Table 2.

Behavioral Interventions

In adult populations, behavioral treatments may be effective in reducing sleep latency and improving subjective sleep parameters (21). Behavioral therapy generally employs sleep habit reconditioning known as stimulus control and relaxation training. Specialized training is required to teach patients these techniques, and referral to a specialist in behavioral medicine is necessary. The use of self-management techniques may have the additional benefit of promoting self-efficacy, thus leading to positive effects in other aspects of the rheumatic disease.

Pharmacologic Interventions

Optimal medical management of the rheumatic disease is the initial intervention for patients whose sleep disturbance is related to their primary disease process. Adequate doses and optimal timing of nonsteroidal anti-inflammatory drugs or analgesic medications to reduce pain and inflammation may facilitate restful sleep.

The most appropriate use of hypnotic medication is in individuals with sleep disturbance of recent origin. The role of hypnotics in chronic insomnia is less clear and should only be used as part of a coordinated clinical management strategy to address the underlying problem. Duration of activity is the primary consideration in choosing a hypnotic agent. This duration is determined by rates of absorption, distribution, and elimination. Special care must taken in the elderly due to slowing of metabolism, which may result in higher plasma levels and greater sensitivity of the central nervous system (22). The choice of medication is based on whether the intended effect is to reduce time to sleep onset, reduce mid-sleep awakenings, or decrease anxiety related to sleep disturbance. It is important to use the smallest dose possible and to avoid chronic use of hypnotic agents. If sleep disturbance persists, further diagnostic evaluation and treatment of underlying causes is indicated.

If chronic use is anticipated and the sleep disturbance is related to pain or fibromyalgia, consider the use of a tricyclic antidepressant. Sedating tricyclic antidepressants such as amitriptyline, doxepin, or nortriptyline in small doses (10–50 mg at bedtime) can be effective in reducing pain and sleep disturbance (23). The effect of tricyclic antidepressants on alpha EEG non-REM sleep anomaly is unclear (9). Tricyclic antidepressants also depress REM sleep. The positive effects of these agents must be weighed against the side effects related to their anticholinergic activity, particularly in the elderly. Cyclobenzaprine (10–40 mg/day) has also demonstrated improvement in total sleep time in persons with fibromyalgia; however, it did not affect pain, mood, or alpha intrusion (24). Serotonin reuptake inhibiting compounds have not yet been demonstrated effective in reducing pain and improving sleep parameters in individuals with chronic pain conditions. These compounds increase wakefulness and may interfere with sleep in some individuals (25).

REFERENCES

1. Regestein QR: Sleep and insomnia. J Geriatr Psychiatry 13:153–171, 1980
2. American Sleep Disorders Association, Diagnostic Classification Steering Committee, Thorpy MJ, Chairman: International Classification of Sleep Disorders: Diagnostic and Coding Manual. Rochester, MN, American Sleep Disorders Association, 1990
3. Partinen M: Sleep disorders and stress. J Psychosom Res 38 (suppl 1):89–91, 1994
4. National Institute of Mental Health, Consensus Development Conference: Drugs and insomnia: the use of medications to promote sleep. JAMA 251:2410–2414, 1984
5. Leigh TJ, Bird HA, Hindmarch I, Wright V: A comparison of sleep in rheumatic and non-rheumatic patients. Clin Exp Rheumatol 5:363–365, 1987

6. Moldofsky H: Sleep and fibrositis syndrome. Rheum Dis Clin North Am 15:91–103, 1989

7. Branco J, Atalaia A, Paiva T: Sleep cycles and alpha-delta sleep in fibromyalgia syndrome. J Rheumatol 21:1113–1117, 1994

8. Jennum P, Drewes AM, Andreasen A, Nielsen KD: Sleep and other symptoms in primary fibromyalgia and in healthy controls. J Rheumatol 20:1756–1759, 1993

9. Carette S, Oakson G, Guimont C, Steriade M: Sleep electroencephalography and the clinical response to amitriptyline in patients with fibromyalgia. Arthritis Rheum 38:1211–1217, 1995

10. Alvarez LB, Teran J, Alonso JL, Alegre J, Arroya I, Viejo JL: Lack of association between fibromyalgia and sleep apnea syndrome. Ann Rheum Dis 51:108–111, 1992

11. Bennett RM, Clark SR, Campbell SM, Burkhardt CS: Low levels of somatomedin C in patients with the fibromyalgia syndrome: a possible link between sleep and muscle pain. Arthritis Rheum 35:1113–1116, 1992

12. Crosby LJ: Factors which contribute to fatigue associated with rheumatoid arthritis. J Adv Nurs 16:974–981, 1991

13. Mahowald MW, Mahowald ML, Bundlie SR, Ytterberg SR: Sleep fragmentation in rheumatoid arthritis. Arthritis Rheum 32:974–983, 1989

14. Hirsch M, Carlander B, Vergé M, Tafti M, Anaya J-M, Billiard M, Sany J: Objective and subjective sleep disturbance in patients with rheumatoid arthritis: a reappraisal. Arthritis Rheum 37:41–49, 1994

15. Lavie P, Epstein R, Tzischinsky O, Gilad D, Nahir M, Lorber M, Scharf Y: Actigraphic measurements of sleep in rheumatoid arthritis: comparison of patients with low back pain and healthy controls. J Rheumatol 19:362–365, 1992

16. Belza BL: Comparison of self-reported fatigue in rheumatoid arthritis and controls. J Rheumatol 22:639–643, 1995

17. Moldofsky H, Lue FA, Smythe HA: Alpha EEG sleep and morning symptoms in rheumatoid arthritis. J Rheumatol 10:373–379, 1983

18. Moldofsky H, Lue FA, Saskin P: Sleep and morning pain in primary osteoarthritis. J Rheumatol 14:124–128, 1987

19. Leigh TJ, Hindmarch I, Bird HA, et al: Comparison of sleep in osteoarthritic patients and age and sex matched healthy controls. Ann Rheum Dis 47:40–42, 1988

20. Gudbjornsson B, Broman JE, Hetta J, Hallgren R: Sleep disturbances in patients with primary Sjögren's syndrome. Br J Rheumatol 32:1072–1076, 1993

21. Lacks P: Behavioral Treatment for Persistent Insomnia. New York, Pergamon Press, 1987

22. Nicholson AN: Hypnotics: clinical pharmacology and therapeutics. In, Principles and Practice of Sleep Medicine. Second edition. Edited by MH Kryger, T Roth, WC Dement. Philadelphia, WB Saunders, 1994, pp. 355–363

23. Carette S, McCain GA, Bell DA, Fam AG: Evaluation of amitriptyline in primary fibrositis: a double-blind, placebo-controlled study. Arthritis Rheum 29:655–659, 1986

24. Reynolds WJ, Moldofsky H, Saskin P, Lue FA: The effects of cyclobenzaprine on sleep physiology and symptoms in patients with fibromyalgia. J Rheumatol 18:452–454, 1991

25. Nicholson AN, Pascoe PA: 5 hydroxytryptamine and noradrenaline uptake inhibition: studies on sleep in man. Neuropharmacology 25:1079–1083, 1986

Additional Recommended Reading

1. Kryger MH, Roth T, Dement WC, editors: Principles and Practice of Sleep Medicine. Second edition. Philadelphia, WB Saunders, 1994

Mood Disorders

ROBERT G. FRANK, PhD; and KRISTOFER J. HAGGLUND, PhD

Mood disorders are commonly experienced by persons with chronic illness, including those with rheumatic disease. Depression is, arguably, the mood disorder with the most personal and societal impact. In fact, depression is a major health problem associated with excessive mortality and morbidity. Impairment and disability associated with depression are equal to that associated with cardiovascular disease and are greater than that due to other chronic disorders such as hypertension or diabetes mellitus (1). Depressed and anxious individuals utilize higher levels of health care services (2). Despite the high personal and fiscal costs associated with depression, it may go undetected and untreated in as many as 50% of depressed individuals seen in medical settings.

Research indicates that patients with undetected depression tend to be only slightly less depressed than those treated for this disorder (3). Furthermore, individuals who are treated for their depression by general medical providers are less likely to receive appropriate, high-quality care (4). Recent emphasis on cost-effective care for both primary care and chronic illness demands careful examination of co-morbid conditions and aggressive, high-quality treatment of conditions like depression that can be detected and treated effectively.

Depression is common in individuals with all types of rheumatic disease, but it is most clearly documented among individuals with rheumatoid arthritis (RA) (5,6). Research indicates that regardless of the type of rheumatic disease, mood disturbance is associated with increased pain, functional impairment, and poorer outcomes (7,8).

CHARACTERISTICS

The common usage of the term *depression* has necessitated the establishment of clear criteria for depressive illness. The frequently utilized appellate "clinical depression" has no true descriptive value. In general usage, depression describes transient mood changes in response to life's vagaries. The clinical syndrome of depression with persistent impairment of mood and the presentation of associated symptoms is markedly different from normal mood variations and grief. As shown in Table 1, clinical features include impairment in mood, cognition behavior, and somatic functioning (9).

Epidemiology of Depression

The incidence of depressive disorders is increasing. Research data suggest there are increasing rates of depressive disorders among successive birth cohorts throughout this century. These data also indicate an earlier age of onset for the most recent birth cohorts and a persistence of higher prevalence among women, although a less pronounced gender difference is apparent in recent cohorts (10). In family studies, cohorts under

Table 1. Four clinical features of depression.

Feature	Description
Mood (affect)	Sad, blue, depressed, unhappy, down in the dumps, empty, worried, irritable
Cognition	Loss of interest, difficulty concentrating, low self-esteem, negative thoughts, suicide ideation and, less commonly, hallucinations and delusions
Behavior	Psychomotor retardation or agitation, crying, social withdrawal, dependency, suicide
Somatic (physical)	Sleep disturbance, fatigue, appetite disturbance, weight change, pain, gastrointestinal upset, decreased libido

40 years of age have been found to have rates three times as high as the oldest cohort (10). In addition, it appears that the lifetime rate of any disorder declines with age, with the lowest rates being found among elderly people. This pattern of decreased lifetime rate with age is particularly pronounced for affective disorders. For men and women, the lifetime rates for affective disorders are 6% and 11%, respectively. In the 18 to 19 age group, 7% and 15% had affective disorders; in the 45 to 64 age group, only 4% and 9%; and in the 65 and older age group, 2% and 3% had affective disorders (11).

Depression is a disabling syndrome. Depressed individuals are less able to perform the activities of daily living than patients with medical conditions such as diabetes and rheumatic disorders alone (1). In one study, patients with dysthymia were significantly more limited in physical and social role functioning 2 years after diagnosis than patients with hypertension, despite significant deterioration of function for those with hypertension. Individuals who recover from depressive disorders tend to be employed, have a lower intake of alcohol, use active coping strategies, and have a higher level of physical activity and social support in comparison with individuals who do not recover over time (1).

Depression is a potentially lethal disorder; about 15% of individuals with primary affective disorder eventually kill themselves. Approximately 50% of persons who commit suicide have a primary diagnosis of depression (9). Long-term risk factors for suicide include hopelessness, suicidal ideation, and prior suicide attempts.

Anxiety has received less empirical attention than depression in persons with rheumatic diseases, despite evidence that anxiety disorders can be significantly disabling. Clinically noteworthy levels of anxiety have been reported among large samples of people with rheumatic diseases (12). A longitudinal investigation involving 400 persons with RA found that initial anxiety scores were related to pain and predicted subsequent physician utilization (13). Other investigations in persons with RA (7) and osteoarthritis (OA) (14) found that anxiety and depression were the strongest predictors of pain and impairment, even when considering objective measures of disease.

More research is needed to address the prevalence of anxiety, its co-morbidity and mood disorders, and its relationships to disease status.

Major Depressive Episode

Major depressive episode (MDE) is the most common mood disorder. Diagnosis of MDE is based on operational criteria including the presence of either a depressed mood or the loss of pleasure/interest and at least four other major symptoms of depression over a 2-week period. The symptoms also must cause significant impairment in social, occupational, or other roles, and they must not be due to a "general" medical condition such as hypothyroidism, to bereavement, or to the physical effects of a mood-altering substance (15).

Based on a survey of over 18,000 adults in five U.S. communities, epidemiologic studies found a 1-month prevalence of 1.6% and a lifetime prevalence of 4.4% for MDE (11). The mean age at onset for MDE was 27 years with little difference between men and women. The prevalence of depression in women was found to be uniformly higher than in men, with twice as many women having major depression. An average untreated episode lasts 6 or more months, although 21% of patients studied were still experiencing depression 2 years later.

Major depressive episode is a recurrent disorder; the likelihood of experiencing a single episode is less than 50%, but the risk of further episodes increases with each subsequent episode. Frequently, MDE occurs with other conditions. For example, patients with dysthymic disorder may have MDE superimposed (double depression). Anxiety disorders also coexist with MDE. A person with a major depressive episode is estimated to have between 9 to 19 times increased risk of an anxiety disorder (16).

Dysthymic Disorder

Dysthymic disorder is characterized by a chronic disturbance involving depressed mood for most of the day, more days than not, for at least 2 years. In addition to depression, two or more of the following symptoms are necessary: decreased appetite or overeating, hypersomnia or insomnia, fatigue, poor self-esteem, impaired concentration or difficulty with decision making, and feelings of hopelessness. Dysthymic disorder differs from MDE in the number and intensity of the symptoms.

A distinction is made between early onset (before age 21) and late onset (age 21 or older) dysthymia (15), although the value of this distinction is unclear. A 3% lifetime prevalence of dysthymia was found in the adult population, with women affected 1.5 to 3 times more often than men. Dysthymia was more common in women under 65, unmarried persons, and young persons with low income. Dysthymia also was associated with greater use of general health and psychiatric services, and with psychotropic drug use. Dysthymic disorders are often accompanied by other psychiatric disorders. Up to 75% of persons with dysthymia may have other conditions, including MDE, panic and other anxiety disorders, and substance abuse (11).

Adjustment Disorder with Depressed Mood

Adjustment disorder with depressed mood refers to a maladaptive reaction to an identified psychosocial stressor or stressors, which occurs within 3 months after the onset of the stressor and has persisted no longer than 6 months. The depressive reaction must either impair the person's occupational or social function or be overreactive in light of the nature of the stressor. Symptoms include depressed mood, tearfulness, and feelings of hopelessness. The distinction between adjustment disorder with depressed mood and MDE is often not clear; stressors play an important role in the onset of both conditions. If the full criteria for MDE are met, that diagnosis takes precedence (15).

Uncomplicated Bereavement

Uncomplicated bereavement is considered a normal reaction to a major loss, such as the death of a family member. It is not classified as a mental disorder, although some symptoms may be identical to those of MDE. In general, uncomplicated bereavement is not associated with the pervasive sense of guilt and worthlessness, marked functional impairment, and suicidality (9). Guilt is sometimes associated with things done or not done at the time of death of a loved one (6). Marked or prolonged functional impairment is uncommon. Bereavement usually begins shortly after the loss and improves over several months.

Organic and Psychoactive Substance Induced Mood Disorders

Organic mood syndromes are characterized by mood disturbance created by medical conditions. The clinical presentation mimics functional depression and may range from mild to severe. A common example of organic mood syndrome in rheumatic disease is a depressive effect associated with high doses of corticosteroids in individuals with RA (6). A variety of nonpsychiatric medical conditions are thought to be accompanied by depression, for example, endocrine disorders (including those of the pituitary, adrenal, and thyroid) and collagen-type disorders such as systemic lupus erythematosus.

PREVALENCE

Assessment

Estimates of depression among persons with rheumatic disease vary widely, depending on the assessment methodology. Most studies have relied on self-report questionnaires, which tend to produce higher estimates of the prevalence of depression compared to structural interviews. Self-report approaches to the assessment of depression are flawed in several ways (17). First, the administration of a single questionnaire, even at multiple times, is insufficient to measure depression validly and reliably even as a syndrome (i.e., signs and symptoms that cluster together). Structured and semi-structured interviews like the Diagnostic Interview Schedule (DIS) are more sensitive and specific (5). The DIS can be used by lay interviewers, provides a lifetime as well as a current diagnosis, and helps investigators differentiate mood changes associated with alcohol and other substance abuse.

Another problem with the use of depression questionnaires is the lack of valid cut-off scores. Most questionnaires have a range of cut-off scores for the designation of depression, depending on the population studied. In addition, designations such as non-depressed, mildly depressed, moderately depressed, severely depressed, or dysphoric are used to describe test results. Comparison between self-report questionnaires and structured interviews becomes almost impossible given the lack of research examining the validity of these diagnostic designations. Moreover, scores in the mild or moderately depressed ranges can be obtained without endorsement of key symptoms, including depressed mood, hopelessness, or feelings of worthlessness. Research has indicated that common self-report measures of depression and anxiety may be measuring global emotional distress, rather than specific emotional states. Among patients with RA, common measures of depression demonstrated good convergent validity, but poor discriminant validity.

The symptoms of depression and other mood disorders overlap with symptoms from rheumatic diseases such as RA, fibromyalgia, ankylosing spondylitis, and systemic lupus erythematosus. Most self-report questionnaires of mood disturbance were initially developed and validated among individuals without chronic illness, resulting in possible criterion contamination (18).

Rheumatoid Arthritis

Most examinations of depression among individuals with rheumatic disease have focused on RA. In one of the larger studies involving 137 patients with RA, 42% met criteria for some form of depression, using a structured interview (DIS) (5). Forty-one percent met criteria for dysthymic disorder, and 17% met criteria for MDE. These findings support previous work (19), although another study in which the DIS interview system was administered to a small group of outpatients with RA found no current cases of major depression (20). Limitations in this study include a small sample recruited from the practices of participating rheumatologists that may not have been representative of the population of individuals with RA. The rate of depression in clinical samples varies substantially from community samples that have been found to have prevalence of about 5.6%, but it approximates the rate found in other types of serious chronic illness.

Using the Arthritis Impact Measurement Scales (AIMS) depression scale in a sample of 6,153 consecutive patients with rheumatic disease (including 1,152 with RA), 25% of the RA patients self-reported depressive symptoms at a level analogous to possible depression, and 20.4% reported depressive symptoms analogous to probable depression (21). Patients with RA do not appear to be more depressed than patients with other rheumatic diseases.

Osteoarthritis

Depression scores for individuals with OA vary according to the area of the body affected, although all exceed the percentage reported in community samples. Only 14% of individuals with OA reported levels of depression on the AIMS analogous to probable depression, while 17% and 23%, respectively, of individuals with OA of the knee/hip and neck indicated depression analogous to probable depression. In a community sample, with OA (22), most individuals reported few depressive symptoms. A small minority (less than 20%) reported many symptoms of depression.

Fibromyalgia

Almost one of every three patients with fibromyalgia reports symptoms of depression analogous to probable depression (21). Similar studies have demonstrated a wide range in prevalence rates of depression among individuals with fibromyalgia. In one study, a lifetime prevalence of depression was found to be approximately 43% (23), whereas another reported 78% of the sample had scores suggestive of MDE when a "community" norm was applied (24). Differences in methodology are likely to account for these discrepancies. When contamination by rheumatic disease items is controlled, the MDE rate was 22% and 29% on the Beck Depression Inventory (25). An unadjusted Beck Depression Inventory indicated a prevalence of 55% of depression among this sample. In fibromyalgia, scores on common self-reported measures of depression are likely to be contaminated by disease-related symptoms. Caution should be used when generalizing results from studies susceptible to this methodologic problem.

Ankylosing Spondylitis

In a sample of 177 individuals with ankylosing spondylitis, rates of depression comparable to other types of rheumatic disease and chronic illness were observed, despite the possibly widespread belief that individuals with ankylosing spondylitis are better adjusted than others with chronic illness (26). Using the Center for Epidemiological Studies-Depression Scale, 31% of the subjects exceeded criteria for depression, with women reporting higher levels of depressive symptoms.

Systemic Lupus Erythematosus

Psychiatric symptoms in systemic lupus erythematosus may result from generalized or localized involvement of the central nervous system, secondary phenomena caused by other manifestations of the disease, therapy, or emotional reactions to the chronicity, uncertainty, and severity of the disease. A recent review noted that depression was the most common symptom reported in nearly half of the 19 studies reviewed (27). Depression rates ranged from 20% to 55% of the patients with systemic lupus erythematosus.

PSYCHOLOGICAL FACTORS

Function and Depression

It is widely speculated that the more disabling the disease, the higher the prevalence of depression. Among individuals with RA, those with depressive symptoms have poorer function and are more likely to have a major physical limitation, spend more days in bed, and report joints with pain as well as higher levels of pain (28). Depression and anxiety predict pain and functional impairment in RA, even after disease activity is considered (7). Conversely, disability has been found to the single most important predictor of depression (29).

The component of functional impairment most associated with risk for depressive symptoms is loss of valued activities (8). Patients with higher levels of depressive symptoms perform 12% fewer valued activities than those with lower levels of depressive symptoms (30). A decline in basic activities of daily living appears to be a risk factor for the development of depressive symptoms in women with RA; the most critical risk factor is the loss of the ability to perform valued activities (8). Similar patterns may exist among populations with other forms of rheumatic disease, but further research is needed.

Sleep

There is a widely recognized link between sleep pathology and depression, but the causal direction of the relationship is poorly understood. A recently proposed model of fatigue in systemic lupus erythematosus suggests that depression and sleep problems, precipitated or exacerbated by disease activity, act as mediators that worsen fatigue (31). Sleep problems, including sleep disruption and anxiety about sleep, are the proximal link to fatigue. An affective component, characterized by depression and anxiety, can become linked to sleep disruption in a cyclic process. In systemic lupus erythematosus, disease manifestations appear to have a more proximal effect on depression, sleep disruption, and/or sleep anxiety, which then act on more proximal causes of fatigue. This model may have applications to other types of rheumatic disorders. (See also Chapter 21, Sleep Disturbance.)

Depression, Cognition, and Pain

Disease-related factors such as pain or disability often are associated with the manifestation of mood disorders. Numerous investigations suggest that depression makes an independent contribution to predicting pain when both are assessed concurrently among individuals with RA (5,7), fibromyalgia, and osteoarthritis (14). Pain makes an independent contribution to predicting depression when both are assessed concurrently, but its effects on subsequent depression are mediated by passive coping strategies (32,33).

Cognitive theory suggests that individuals in pain displaying high levels of cognitive distortion are more likely to develop depressed mood. Individuals with RA who have high levels of depressed mood may exhibit increased concurrent levels of cognitive distortion. Similarly, perceptions of helplessness are associated with higher levels of depression. Patients with a tendency toward cognitive distortion such as inaccurate overgeneralization, selective abstraction, personalization, and catastrophizing are more prone to symptoms of depression (34). The tendency toward cognitive distortion increasing the likelihood of depressive symptoms appears to be independent of illness-related disability.

PSYCHOBIOLOGY OF DEPRESSION

Advances in the pharmacotherapy of affective disorders over the last four decades have illuminated the psychobiology of depressive disorders. Evidence indicates that depression involves dysregulation of two major neurobiologic systems: the hypothalamic–pituitary–adrenal axis and the sympathetic–adrenal–medullary axis (6).

Beginning in the 1950s, tricyclic antidepressants replaced monamine oxidase inhibitors as the treatment of choice for unipolar depression. The tricyclic antidepressants have relatively high affinity for muscarinic, histaminergic, and adrenergic receptors, causing the side effects and toxicity associated with this class of drug. More recently, the selective serotonin reuptake inhibitors and the dual action serotonin–norepinephrine reuptake inhibitors were introduced. These drugs are widely accepted by patients because they lack the side effects that are common with tricyclic antidepressants, and they are simpler to administer. Despite these advantages, as many as 30% to 40% of patients fail to respond satisfactorily to pharmacologic therapy, and a significant number of patients fail to achieve long-term remission.

The development of antidepressant medications has underscored the role of neurotransmitters in the pathophysiology of depression. It now is accepted that serotonin neuronal systems are involved in many episodes of depression. It is unlikely that only this single neurotransmitter underlies the neurochemical basis of all depressions; other neurotransmitters thought to be involved in depression include norepinephrine, dopamine, and a variety of neuropeptides, most prominently corticotropin releasing factor.

Although most current research on the psychobiology of depression focuses on the role of serotonin and norepinephrine, there is substantial interdependence among neurotransmitter systems. Currently, no theory adequately describes the role of neurotransmitters in depression. Abnormalities in the hypothalamic–pituitary–adrenal axis have been commonly observed in depression, but possible links with rheumatic disease remain unknown (6).

TREATMENT

Despite a plethora of studies assessing depression in rheumatic disease, few studies address the treatment of depression associated with rheumatic disease (6). Several studies have examined analgesic effects of antidepressant medication in patients with RA who may also meet criteria for depression. These studies of analgesia have used low doses of antidepressants, less than effective for the treatment of depression. Fifty-seven percent of depressed patients with RA who were treated with a combination of chlorimipramine and supportive psychotherapy significantly improved (35). In contrast, another study found no significant difference in depression between RA patients receiving psychotherapy and age-matched controls (36). Six weeks of treatment with low doses of imipramine (75 mg) resulted in lower levels of depression (37). Unfortunately, the treatment group had higher initial depression scores (6). A randomized, double-blind trial to examine the effects of low-dose trimipramine (25–75 mg) in 36 depressed patients with RA found that joint pain and tenderness were reduced, but depression did not improve (38).

A double-blind, cross-over study compared response to low doses of trazodone, desipramine, and amitriptyline in 47 RA patients. All conditions produced improvement on pain measures, but only amitriptyline exceeded placebo. Post-hoc analyses revealed that depressed subjects responded best to amitriptyline in contrast to non-depressed patients. Because depressed subjects did not improve more than non-depressed subjects on measures of depression, it was concluded that amitriptyline produced analgesic effects independent of its effect on mood.

Life stressors and psychological adjustment are thought to play important roles in illness resistance and disease course. Younger adults are more likely than older adults to become depressed when challenged with chronic medical illness. Chronic illness can lead to demoralization, feelings of hopelessness, self-blame, and sensitivity to interpersonal conflict. Sensitivity to conflict can be heightened in those dependent on others for help with daily life activities. Depression has been viewed as an outcome of chronic illness, while depressive symptoms have been used as a measure of the severity of stressors or the ability of the individual to cope with the stressors.

Over the last decade a number of studies have investigated psychotherapeutic interventions in patients with rheumatic disease, most often RA. These studies have focused on improving rheumatic disease, not depression. Most often, depressive symptoms have been assessed using self-report instruments. While this approach lacks sensitivity, it provides some insight regarding the value of the interventions in reducing depressive symptoms (33). In general, these interventions have utilized cognitive and behavioral interventions in groups of patients with RA, although several studies have utilized similar interventions in patients with OA. There has been remarkable consistency in reports indicating reduction of pain. Cognitive variables appear to serve as mediators that result in low and decreased arthritis helplessness and improved self-efficacy.

The relatively meager outcome literature examining interventions for depression associated with arthritis leaves most treatment issues unanswered. There is limited evidence that tricyclic antidepressants (notably amitriptyline) are effective in reducing pain. Higher doses of these antidepressants are likely to be required to adequately treat depression. Similarly, there is evidence that cognitive-behavioral interventions administered in groups may be effective in reducing depressive symptoms. However, there is no evidence to indicate that treatments found to ameliorate or treat depression in other populations are not effective in depressed individuals with rheumatic diseases.

Psychological Therapy

Two forms of psychotherapy, interpersonal psychotherapy and cognitive therapy, have been found to be effective in the treatment of mild to moderate major depressive episodes. Interpersonal psychotherapy is derived from the interpersonal approach of Harry Stack Sullivan (9). The goal of treatment is to relieve depression by reducing interpersonal conflicts. Treatment length is relatively brief, typically lasting several months. The focus is on current relationships, although historic relationships may be addressed. Interpersonal psychotherapy has been found to be effective in the treatment of major depression and similar to tricyclic antidepressants in overall effectiveness. The combination of interpersonal therapy and antidepressants has proven most effective in the treatment of depression. Cognitive therapy also has been shown to be effective in treating depression in ambulatory settings and, more recently, in inpatient settings (9). This model of therapy emphasizes

identification and reduction of negative thoughts and beliefs. In several studies, cognitive therapy and pharmacotherapy have been found to be equally effective in the treatment of depressed outpatients.

Antidepressant Therapy

All antidepressants marketed in the U.S. have established efficacy for major depression in placebo-controlled studies. When compared to each other, none has proven superior. Outcome studies typically report that 60% to 80% of subjects improve, while 30% to 40% of placebo subjects improve (9). As the severity of depression increases, active drug/placebo differences become more apparent. As yet there is no method to identify those who will respond to specific regimens. Little guidance is available to help clinicians determine appropriate antidepressant medication for individuals with rheumatic disorders.

Because there is no evidence to suggest relative advantage of any antidepressant, choice of drug should be determined by factors such as: 1) previous positive response; 2) similar pharmacogenetics to a drug that has been helpful; 3) depressive subtype; 4) side effects and toxicity of the drug; and 5) cost. Selective serotonin reuptake inhibitors (fluoxetine, paroxetine, sertraline) tend to have fewer side effects and can be started at what is usually an effective dose, but maintenance on the medication for at least 4 months after full remission is important.

For older individuals with rheumatic disorders, medications must be used with caution and adjusted appropriately. Side effects are more common due to increased age and the complicated medical regimen common to the treatment of rheumatic disorders. Moreover, 42% of the subjects screened to participate in one study (39) were excluded because of medical regimens likely to interact with tricyclic antidepressants (including heart disease, renal failure, and glaucoma).

CONCLUSION

Alone or in combination, mood disorders and rheumatic disorders are costly to individuals and to society. Our understanding of both of these disorders grows rapidly, but further research is needed, especially for mood disorders other than depression and for rheumatic diseases other than RA. Fortunately, effective treatment for depression and other mood disorders is available. However, mood disorders often are undetected, especially in settings not focused on mental health (4). Changes in the delivery of health care and behavioral health care may further exacerbate accurate detection and treatment of depression. Patients, health care providers, health care payors and vendors, and policy makers would benefit from further research examining the common neurobiological, behavioral, and socioecological substrates of mood disorders and rheumatic disorders. Finally, outcome research comparing various treatments and health care delivery systems is needed.

REFERENCES

1. Hays RD, Wells KB, Sherbourne CD, Rogers W, Spritzer K: Functioning and well-being outcomes of patients with depression compared with chronic general medical illnesses. Arch Gen Psychiatry 52:11–19, 1995

2. Simon G, Ormel J, VonKorff M, Barlow W: Health care costs associated with depressive and anxiety disorders in primary care. Am J Psychiatry 152:352–357, 1995

3. Wells KB, Burnam AM, Camp P: Severity of depression in prepaid and fee-for-service general medical and mental specialty practices. Med Care 33:350–364, 1995

4. Wells KB, Sturm R: Care for depression in a changing environment. Health Aff 14:78–89, 1995

5. Frank RG, Beck NC, Parker JC, Kashani JH, Elliott TR, Haut AE, Smith E, Atwood C, Brownlee-Duffeck M, Kay DR: Depression in rheumatoid arthritis. J Rheumatol 15:920–925, 1988

6. Morrow KA, Parker JC, Russell JL: Clinical implications of depression in rheumatoid arthritis. Arthritis Care Res 7:58–63, 1994

7. Hagglund KJ, Haley WE, Reveille JD, Alarcón GS: Predicting individual differences in pain and functional impairment among patients with rheumatoid arthritis. Arthritis Rheum 32:851–858, 1989

8. Katz PP, Yelin EH: The development of depressive symptoms among women with rheumatoid arthritis: the role of function. Arthritis Rheum 38:49–56, 1995

9. Jefferson JW, Greist JH: Mood disorders. In, The American Psychiatric Press Textbook of Psychiatry. Second edition. Edited by RE Hales, SC Yudofsky, JA Talbott. Washington, DC, American Psychiatric Press, 1994, pp. 465–495

10. Fombonne E: Increased rates of depression: update of epidemiological findings and analytical problems. Acta Psychiatr Scand 90:145–156, 1994

11. Weissman MM, Livingston BM, Leaf PJ, Florio LP, Holzer C III: Affective disorders. In, Psychiatric Disorders in America: The Epidemiologic Catchment Area Study. Edited by LN Robins, DA Regier. New York, Free Press, 1991, pp. 328–366

12. Wells KB, Golding JM, Burnam MA: Affective, substance use, and anxiety disorders in persons with arthritis, diabetes, heart disease, high blood pressure, or chronic lung conditions. Gen Hosp Psychiatry 11:320–327, 1989

13. Hawley DJ, Wolfe F: Anxiety and depression in patients with rheumatoid arthritis: a prospective study of 400 patients. J Rheumatol 15:932–941, 1988

14. Summers MN, Haley WE, Reveille JD, Alarcón GS: Radiographic assessment and psychologic variables as predictors of pain and functional impairment in osteoarthritis of the knee or hip. Arthritis Rheum 31:204–209, 1988

15. American Psychiatric Association: Diagnostic and Statistical Manual of Mental Disorders. Fourth edition. Washington, DC, American Psychiatric Association, 1994

16. Reiger DA, Burke JD Jr, Burke KC: Comorbidity of affective and anxiety disorders in the NIMH Epidemiologic Catchment Area Program. In, Comorbidity of Mood and Anxiety Disorders. Edited by JD Maser, CR Cloninger. Washington, DC, American Psychiatric Press, 1990, pp. 113–122

17. Tennen H, Hall JA, Affleck G: Depression research methodologies in the Journal of Personality and Social Psychology: a review and critique. J Pers Soc Psychol 68:870–884, 1995

18. Callahan LF, Kaplan MR, Pincus T: The Beck Depression Inventory, Center for Epidemiological Studies Depression scale (CES-D), and General Well-Being Schedule depression subscale in rheumatoid arthritis. Arthritis Care Res 4:3–11, 1991

19. Rimon R, Laakso RL: Overt psychopathology in rheumatoid arthritis: a fifteen year follow-up study. Scand J Rheumatol 13:324–328, 1984

20. Hudson JI, Hudson MS, Pliner LF, Goldenberg DL, Pope HG: Fibromyalgia and major affective disorder: a controlled phenomenology and family history study. Am J Psychiatry 142:441–446, 1985

21. Hawley DJ, Wolfe F: Depression is not more common in rheumatoid arthritis: a 10-year longitudinal study of 6,153 patients with rheumatic disease. J Rheumatol 20:2025–2031, 1993

22. Dexter P, Brandt K: Distribution and predictors of depressive symptoms in osteoarthritis. J Rheumatol 21:279–286, 1994

23. Ahles TA, Khan SA, Yunus MB, Spiegel DA, Masi AT: Psychiatric status of patients with primary fibromyalgia, patients with rheumatoid arthritis, and subjects without pain: a blind comparison of DSM-III diagnoses. Am J Psychiatry 148:1721–1726, 1991

24. Ercolani M, Trombini G, Chattat R, Cervini C, Piergiacomi G, Salaffi F, Zeni S, Marcolongo R: Fibromyalgic syndrome: depression and abnormal illness behavior. Psychother Psychosom 61:178–186, 1994

25. Burckhardt CS, O'Reilly CA, Wiens AN, Clark SR, Campbell SM, Bennett RM: Assessing depression in fibromyalgia patients. Arthritis Care Res 7:35–39, 1994

26. Barlow JH, Macey SJ, Struthers GR: Gender, depression, and ankylosing spondylitis. Arthritis Care Res 6:45–51, 1993

27. Wekking EM: Psychiatric symptoms in systemic erythematosus: an update. Psychosom Med 55:219–228, 1993

28. Katz PP, Yelin EH: Prevalence and correlates of depressive symptoms among persons with rheumatoid arthritis. J Rheumatol 20:790–796, 1993

29. Newman SP, Fitzpatrick R, Lamb R, Shipley M: The origins of depressed mood in rheumatoid arthritis. J Rheumatol 16:740–744, 1989

30. Katz PP, Yelin EH: Life activities of persons with rheumatoid arthritis with and without depressive symptoms. Arthritis Care Res 7:69–77, 1994

31. McKinley PS, Ouellette SC, Winkel GH: The contributions of disease activity, sleep patterns, and depression to fatigue in systemic lupus erythematosus: a proposed model. Arthritis Rheum 38:826–834, 1995

32. Brown GK, Nicassio PM, Wallston KA: Pain coping strategies and depression in rheumatoid arthritis. J Consult Clin Psychol 57:652–657, 1988

33. Young LD: Psychological factors in rheumatoid arthritis. J Consult Clin Psychol 60:619–627, 1992

34. Smith TW, Christensen AJ, Peck JR, Ward JR: Cognitive distortion, helplessness, and depressed mood in rheumatoid arthritis: a four-year longitudinal analysis. Health Psychol 13:2113–2117, 1994

35. Rimon R: Depression in rheumatoid arthritis. Ann Clin Res 6:171–175, 1974

36. Kaplan S, Kozin F: A controlled study of group counseling in rheumatoid arthritis. J Rheumatol 8:91–99, 1981

37. Fowler PD, MacNeill A, Spencer D, Robinson ET, Dick WC: Imipramine, rheumatoid arthritis and rheumatoid fact. Curr Med Res Opin 5:241–246, 1977

38. Macfarlane JG, Jalai S, Grace EM: Trimipramine in rheumatoid arthritis: a randomized double-blind trial in relieving pain and joint tenderness. Curr Med Res Opin 10:89–93, 1986

39. Frank RG, Kashani JH, Parker JC, Beck NC, Brownlee-Duffeck M, Elliott TR, Haut AE, Atwood C, Smith E, Kay DR: Antidepressant analgesia in rheumatoid arthritis. J Rheumatol 15:1632–1638, 1988

Deconditioning

JUDITH A. FALCONER, PhD, MPH, OTR

Deconditioning is a generalized physical debilitation that occurs in response to disease and/or to diminishing or habitually low levels of physical (muscular) activity. In healthy young adults (1) and patients with acute or chronic illness (2), prolonged immobilization significantly impairs all physiologic and selected psychologic functions. Hallmarks of physical deconditioning include diminished cardiorespiratory efficiency (increased resting heart rate, decreased VO_2 max), decreased muscle and connective tissue function, bone loss, increased percent body fat, and low endurance.

Stimuli from muscular activity and postural (gravitational) stress with daily activities regulate musculoskeletal and cardiorespiratory function. When muscular activity is reduced or is below threshold levels for prolonged periods of time, Type II (fast twitch, force production) muscle fibers atrophy, especially in the weight-bearing muscles, with a corresponding loss of muscle mass and function. Loss of aerobic enzymes, mitochondrial density (cellular energy), and capillary density render the muscles less able to use oxygen efficiently. When the muscular demand for oxygen and blood flow is diminished by immobilization or disuse, cardiac stroke volume, cardiac output, and plasma volume decrease with a proportionate increase in resting and submaximal heart rate. These changes interfere with the capacity of the cardiorespiratory system to deliver oxygen and nutrition to working muscle.

In addition to regulating cardiorespiratory and musculoskeletal function, physical activity (muscular contraction) regulates bone and joint integrity. Physical activity provides the mechanical loading that is essential to bone formation and maintenance of joint flexibility. Inadequate bone loading decreases bone mass and the supporting matrix, thus increasing the risk for injury and fracture. Immobility of joints causes contracture of the joint capsule and periarticular muscles (stiffness) and interferes with cartilage nutrition.

Deconditioning or poor physical fitness contributes to excess fatigue, low functional status, injury risk (impairments in neuromuscular protective responses), incoordination, low pain threshold, sleep disturbances, and selected diseases such as obesity, coronary heart disease, osteoporosis, and depression. Deconditioning may also impair immune system functioning, including the response to illness and injury.

Deconditioning and rheumatic disease activity are related, but the nature of this relationship is unclear. Deconditioning may increase the products of inflammation (such as cytokines and tumor necrosis factor), or deconditioning may be a product of the inflammation. Deconditioning is generally worse in inflammatory than non-inflammatory diseases, suggesting a role for inflammation in the deconditioning process. The role of physical activity in deconditioning has also been shown. Increased physical fitness in persons with inflammatory and non-inflammatory rheumatic disease is associated with improved physical performance, elevated mood, and possibly a slower rate of joint destruction (3,4).

Deconditioning in the chronic inflammatory diseases may be confounded by associated comorbidities such as cardio-pulmonary involvement and gastrointestinal complications that alter nutritional state. Medications used to manage inflammatory disease and associated comorbidities, such as corticosteroids (steroid myopathy), beta blockers, or chemotherapy, may also be factors in the deconditioning process.

Although research findings on deconditioning in the rheumatic diseases are limited, available evidence and clinical observations suggest that it is more prevalent and serious than commonly acknowledged. Low levels of physical fitness have been reported in all of the rheumatic disease groups studied including rheumatoid arthritis (5), osteoarthritis (OA) (5), juvenile rheumatoid arthritis (6), fibromyalgia (7), and systemic lupus erythematosus (8).

Prevention and management of deconditioning is deceptively simple: daily physical activity of sufficient intensity, duration, frequency, and mode to improve or maintain physical fitness. Patient directives "to be more active" or "get more exercise" are necessary, but they provide limited guidance in terms of therapeutic intervention. Key issues to examine include the patient's reasons for inactivity and possible methods to become more active.

FACTORS LIMITING PHYSICAL ACTIVITY

Disease-specific factors; psychological, social, and environmental factors; and aging influence the level of habitual physical activity. The relative importance of each factor in a particular individual suggests the course of action.

Rheumatic disease alters the energy supply and demand balance required to support muscular (physical) activity and prevent fatigue. Lean body mass, a primary energy supply source, is often diminished with rheumatic disease. Loss of muscle mass and muscle strength may be caused by primary inflammation (elevated cytokine production, reduced growth hormone production, increased resting energy expenditure, or increased whole-body protein breakdown rates), reflex inhibition due to pain, changes in muscle metabolism (e.g., polymyositis), neuropathic complications of disease such as entrapment neuropathies, medications (e.g., steroid myopathy), or muscle wasting due to disuse atrophy. Smaller muscles have a lower cross-sectional area to generate force as well as fewer mitochondria for muscle respiration, which contributes to muscle weakness and fatigue. Strength loss explained by disuse is significant and rapid—perhaps as much as 1.5% to 5% strength loss per day of immobilization (9).

Caloric intake, especially for proteins, is another important source of energy that may be diminished with rheumatic disease due to appetite loss or protein malnutrition. Recent evidence suggests that *cachexia*, a general lack of nutrition and wasting associated with excess disability and increased mortality risk, may be more common and severe with chronic inflammatory disease than has been previously known (10). In the presence of adequate caloric and protein intake, rheumatoid cachexia may be related to the inflammatory process and not to physical activity level.

Excess body weight may lower physical activity, increase risk for many diseases (such as OA of the knee), worsen joint symptoms, and increase energy expenditure per unit of force; it is probably both a contributing factor and a consequence of deconditioning. Rheumatic disease and physical inactivity may increase the percentage of storage fat with or without a change in body weight (deconditioning). Recommended body fat content is about 27% for young women and 15% for young men; these percentages increase with age (11).

In addition to low energy supply, energy demand with physical activity is increased by rheumatic disease. Rheumatic disease symptoms such as pain, stiffness, and weakness alter joint biomechanics, particularly in the spine and lower extremities, and significantly add to the energy costs of movement. For example, limping or other abnormal gaits may double the energy needed to ambulate.

Chronic inflammation may also cause a *hypermetabolism*, a primary metabolic abnormality that increases energy expenditure in the resting state (elevated resting heart rate) (10). The elevated resting energy expenditure rate plus the increased energy demand with activity result in an energy deficit, early onset or excess fatigue, and diminished physical activity. Physical training decreases resting and submaximal heart rate. Recent evidence also suggests that exercise or physical training may help to re-set the basal metabolic thermostat in chronic inflammation (12).

Psychological, social, and environmental factors propel the deconditioning process by their influence on physical activity. The pain and fatigue accompanying rheumatic disease limit the drive for physical activity. The natural response to pain and fatigue is to rest or limit physical activity. Ironically, physical inactivity contributes to the pain and low endurance, yet the deconditioned individual often feels too bad or too tired to exercise.

Few individuals know intuitively the appropriate level of physical activity for their disease state. Anxiety or fear of damaging the joints or increasing pain often restricts physical activity in an otherwise motivated person. Painful or exhausting experiences following activity, such as delayed onset exercise-induced pain, further discourages this behavior.

Attitudes and beliefs about physical activity influence habitual activity behaviors and the willingness to change activity behaviors. Persons who believe that their activity level can be improved and that increasing physical activity improves their health are likely to initiate a fitness program. Continued involvement in physical activities depends on many factors including the level of enjoyment, convenience, social support, and symptom relief or feeling of well-being that accompanies the activity (see also Chapter 24, Adherence).

Social and environmental factors act as stimuli or constraints to physical activity. For example, physical activity level correlates with occupational requirements, amount and type of leisure pursuits, and social characteristics such as gender, education, and cultural expectations. Environmental factors such as physical barriers and seasonal trends encourage or discourage physical activities in daily life and help to explain overall physical activity level.

Aging may compound the deconditioning effects of rheu-

Table 1. Clinical indications of deconditioning.

Fatigue, daytime tiredness, lack of energy for usual activities
Prolonged bed rest or joint immobilization
Less than 30 minutes per day of moderate physical activity
Decreased daily physical activity
Decreased physical fitness

matic disease and physical inactivity. Age-correlated losses in cardiorespiratory and musculoskeletal functions may include decline in aerobic capacity, muscle weakness, joint stiffness, and bone demineralization. These losses are similar to physiologic deconditioning and are, at least in part, also thought to be caused by diminishing physical activity with age (13). Age-related decline in physical activity is partially explained by attitude toward physical activity; perceptions of health, fitness, and activity needs; anxiety and emotional health; and level of encouragement and social support (14).

ASSESSMENT

Prolonged immobilization, self-reports of fatigue or low or diminishing physical activity, and physical fitness and physical activity assessments are used clinically to determine the presence and severity of deconditioning (Table 1).

Some level of deconditioning occurs after any prolonged bed rest or joint immobilization that is volitional or enforced by acute inflammation, comorbid illness, splinting, or surgery. Although the illness or condition dictating the immobilization contributes to the deconditioning effects (and at one time was thought to explain deconditioning), we now know that prolonged immobility is an independent cause of deconditioning. Bed rest experiments conducted by the National Aeronautics and Space Administration to study the effects of immobilization and weightlessness during space travel demonstrated the severe physiologic deconditioning inherent in inactivity even in young healthy adult volunteers (1). Largely because of the risk of deconditioning, prolonged bed rest in the management of rheumatic disease is rare.

In the ambulatory adult or child, initial indications of deconditioning may not be readily apparent by physical appearance or from a clinical examination. General self-reports of daytime tiredness, lack of energy for usual daytime activities, prolonged exercise recovery, or excessive fatigue with physical exertion may signal deconditioning in the otherwise healthy person. Self-reports of habitually low physical activity or of a recent loss or dwindling of physical activity in usual daily living also implicate deconditioning.

The recommended public health guidelines for physical activity provide a benchmark for interpreting low physical activity in individuals with rheumatic disease. All adults should accumulate 30 minutes or more of moderate intensity physical activity (3.0 to 6.0 metabolic equivalents of task [METs]) on most, preferably all, days of the week (15). Examples of moderate physical intensity activities include walking briskly (3–4 mph), bicycling (≤10 mph), golf (pulling cart), swimming, and home care or repair. Guidelines for healthy children (16) and adolescents (17) are higher and include moderate to vigorous and continuous physical activities.

Physical fitness testing is necessary to quantify deconditioning and to determine appropriate and safe exercise recommendations. Comprehensive physical fitness testing consists of tests of cardiorespiratory function (resting heart rate, submaximal heart rate, VO_2 max), muscle strength, endurance, joint flexibility, and body composition (weight and percent body fat). The assessed physical fitness level is compared either with the individual's previous physical fitness level or with age- and gender-specific physical fitness normative data to evaluate the relative degree of deconditioning. Laboratory-based physical fitness assessment is the most reliable and valid method, but requires specialized equipment, expertise, and conditions that are seldom available for the routine management of deconditioning in rheumatic disease. Standardized field-based or clinical physical fitness tests require minimal equipment, tester training, and time to administer. With minor modifications, these tests appear to be safe and reliable for use with adults (18) and children (6). Due to the importance of physical activity and physical fitness to normal growth and development, regular school-based physical fitness testing is recommended for children with rheumatic disease. (See Chapter 12, Rest and Exercise, for discussion of specific tests of physical fitness.)

Because deconditioning is common and preventable, routine monitoring for physical activity is recommended as part of all health care for individuals with rheumatic disease. Simple screening questions about the level of habitual physical activity and regular exercise behaviors help determine the need for assessment or intervention and alert the patient to the importance of physical activity.

Physical activity may be assessed by many methods (19), but diary or activity logs, activity questionnaires, behavioral observations, and mechanical monitoring are among the more common methods used in clinical practice. Diaries and activity logs involve prospective self-recording of daily behaviors. One diary method specifically used in rheumatic disease is the Activity Record (ACTRE) (20), which requires the participant to record activity level and type, amount of pain and fatigue, perception of performance, level of difficulty, meaningfulness and enjoyment, and number of rest periods for each half-hour increment of waking time. From these data, frequency and duration of activity and rest, frequency of pain and fatigue with specific activities, and difficulty and motivation levels are computed for daily routines.

Activity questionnaires can be used to quantify participation in physical activities and to estimate average daily energy expenditure. For example, the Human Activity Profile for adults is a survey of 94 activities common in daily life (21). The items are ranked according to the required METs. Respondents rank each item as "still doing the activity," "have stopped doing the activity," or "never did the activity." Average daily energy expenditure can be determined and compared with age and sex percentile data. These METs provide an estimate of activity intensity and energy demands, but probably underestimate energy expenditure for an individual with rheumatic disease because of the metabolic and mechanical abnormalities described earlier.

Mechanical monitoring is less common than diary or questionnaire methods in rheumatic disease practice, but is a potentially informative assessment method. Mechanical monitoring involves the use of lightweight motion sensor systems that quantify in real time physical movement. For example, an accelerometer, a small mechanical device attached to the trunk or limbs, enables direct quantification of the frequency and intensity of physical movement in various planes of motion during daily activity.

Physical activity assessments in children usually involve parent or self-report activity measures, heart rate or motion monitors, or direct observation (22). Direct observation methods typically include recording and coding the physical activity type and intensity that is observed at home, school, or the recreational setting during a time-sampling interval. Energy expenditure is then derived by associating the specific activity with an estimated rate of energy expenditure.

Perception of physical exertion provides additional clues about the experience of physical activity that underlies voluntary effort. Borg's RPE scale (Rating of Perceived Exertion), a 15-grade categorical scale with ratings from "no exertion at all" to "maximal exertion," is one simple method to assess perceived exertion (23).

MANAGEMENT STRATEGIES

In the absence of evidence to the contrary, it is reasonable to assume clinically that individuals with rheumatic disease are either at risk for deconditioning or that they would benefit from improved physical activity level. Some individuals unavoidably lose physical performance capacities and the ability to run or participate in strenuous physical activities. Although the disease process itself imposes a physical fitness ceiling, few individuals with rheumatic disease accumulate sufficient levels of physical activity to maintain maximal physical fitness capacity.

Newly diagnosed patients are usually anxious to retain or regain their previous physical activity capacity. Early intervention prevents excess deconditioning and safely rebuilds exercise tolerance and confidence. Patients with established disease tend to adapt to low levels of physical activity, unnecessarily relinquishing valued activities and functional ability. In this group, the goal of intervention is to restore activity initiative and habit as a prerequisite to improving physical fitness, health, and function.

Deconditioning interventions are targeted to the factors contributing to physical inactivity. A combination of methods is used to alleviate obstacles to physical activity, such as disease factors and psychological, social, or environmental issues, and to motivate and counsel patients towards healthful overall physical activity levels. The healthful activity level for a specific individual is one that controls or diminishes the disease symptoms, maximizes physical fitness potential, and is adequate for personal and social needs and preferences.

Physical fitness and physical activity assessments are used to set the goals of intervention, to mark progress toward goals, and to guide the choice of interventions. An understanding of current fitness and activity (baseline performance) and activity interests and needs (performance goals) promotes awareness and insight into daily routines and suggests ideas and directions for specific changes.

Therapies that relieve disease symptoms and restore joint function address some of the disease-specific factors inhibiting physical activity. For example, pain management, joint replacement surgery, or functional activity and gait training are expected to indirectly increase overall activity level by reducing pain and energy expenditure and improving joint mechanics.

Structured exercise is indicated to overcome one or more of

the physical performance deficits (i.e., cardiorespiratory efficiency, strength, and flexibility) underlying deconditioning. All individuals, regardless of disability status, can participate in some form of exercise. The type, frequency, duration, and intensity of exercise, however, should be guided by a health professional who is knowledgeable in exercise prescription with rheumatic disease. Individuals may also need "permission" to exercise or reassurance that exercise will not worsen symptoms. Learning to regulate exercise builds confidence and is essential to a safe and effective exercise program.

Physical activity and exercise, combined with dietary regulation, are used to alter the percentage of body fat/lean and to safely eliminate excess body fat. In addition to the physical and psychologic health benefits of weight control, regulation of body weight and percent body fat may improve physical activity levels.

Improving the economy of movement increases overall physical activity by maximizing the efficiency of energy use and preventing fatigue (24). Energy conservation training refers to programs designed to teach movement economy (ratio of energy expended per unit of force generated). Principles of movement economy include pacing, delegating, prioritizing, and balancing physical activity and rest. These principles should be integrated into home and workplace organization and design.

Understanding the social and environmental context for physical activity sets the stage for meaningful and realistic therapeutic recommendations. For example, walking is a safe and excellent method to build physical fitness. However, even something as simple as walking may be unrealistic or undesirable in winter climates or high-crime neighborhoods. The challenge is to help the individual find and participate in some activity—preferably many activities—that are enjoyable, accessible, safe, appropriate, and sufficiently active and varied to increase physical fitness within the limits imposed by the rheumatic disease.

The social and environmental context for physical activity can also be modified. For instance, the camaraderie provided by group exercise promotes exercise adherence in some individuals. In children, parental and school support reinforces appropriate physical activities in an able child.

Becoming more physically active involves overcoming habit by learning and practicing new behaviors that create new physical activity patterns. Learning begins when the problem is personally experienced and meaningful to the patient. Experiential or problem-based learning promotes the development and mastery of the attitudes, skills, and behaviors required to incorporate new physical activity patterns. Physical activities that can be integrated into daily routines are likely to be rewarding and sustained. Sometimes one small change in a daily routine, such as climbing a flight of stairs or taking a walk around the block, provides the initial impetus and motivation for meaningful change.

GUIDELINES FOR REFERRAL

Routine office-based management of deconditioning by a physician or nurse-clinician who is trained in exercise prescription may be sufficient to prevent deconditioning or to treat mild to moderate deconditioning. Referral to other health care specialists or programs may be warranted under the following general conditions: resource expertise or intensity is not available in the office setting; deconditioning is moderate to severe and requires immediate and intensive training and supervision; patient appears overwhelmed by disease management and requires intensive or specialized assessment and management; or the patient's fitness status declines or fails to improve with office-level intervention after a trial of 3 months.

Although there is overlapping expertise among arthritis health care professionals, physical therapists generally focus on disorders of movement and possess expertise in physical fitness assessment, exercise prescription, and physiologic issues underlying deconditioning. Occupational therapists focus on disorders of human performance and offer expertise in physical activity analyses, energy conservation training, and behavioral issues underlying deconditioning. Community-based or group activity programs are recommended because they are cost-efficient, socially supportive, and they are safe and effective when properly instructed and supervised. Because these programs may be conducted by many different disciplines, specific programs should be evaluated for their appeal to patients and competence in exercise and physical activity prescription in rheumatic disease.

REFERENCES

1. Sandler H, Vernikos J: Inactivity: Physiological Effects. Orlando, FL, Academic Press, Inc., 1986
2. Steinberg FU: The Immobilized Patient: Functional Pathology and Management. New York, Plenum Publishing Corporation, 1980
3. Minor MA, Hewett JE, Webel RR, Anderson SK, Kay DR: Efficacy of physical conditioning exercise in patients with rheumatoid arthritis and osteoarthritis. Arthritis Rheum 32:1396–1405, 1989
4. Kovar PA, Allegrante JP, MacKenzie CR, Peterson MGE, Gutin B, Charlson ME: Supervised fitness walking in patients with osteoarthritis of the knee. Ann Intern Med 116:529–533, 1992
5. Minor MA, Hewett JE, Webel RR, Dreisinger TE, Kay DR: Exercise tolerance and disease related measures in patients with rheumatoid arthritis and osteoarthritis. J Rheumatol 15:905–911, 1988
6. Klepper SE, Giannini MJ: Physical conditioning in children with arthritis: assessment and guidelines for exercise prescription. Arthritis Care Res 7:226–236, 1994
7. Bennett RM, Clark SR, Goldberg L, Nelson D, Bonafede RP, Porter J, Specht D: Aerobic fitness in patients with fibrositis: a controlled study of respiratory gas exchange and ^{133}xenon clearance from exercising muscle. Arthritis Rheum 32:454–460, 1989
8. Robb-Nicholson LC, Daltroy L, Eaton H, Gall V, Wright E, Hartley LH, Schur PH, Liang MH: Effects of aerobic conditioning on fatigue: a pilot study. Br J Rheumatol 28:500–505, 1989
9. Muller EA: Influence of training and of inactivity on muscle strength. Arch Phys Med Rehabil 51:449–462, 1970
10. Rall LC, Roubenoff R: Body composition, metabolism, and resistance exercise in patients with rheumatoid arthritis. Arthritis Care Res 9:151–156, 1996
11. McArdle WD, Katch FI, Katch VL: Exercise Physiology. Fourth edition. Baltimore, William & Wilkins, 1996
12. Rall LC, Lundgren N, Joseph L, Dolnikowski G, Kehayias JJ, Roubenoff R: The metabolic cost of rheumatoid arthritis: reversal with progressive resistance exercise (abstract). Arthritis Rheum 37 (suppl 9):S222, 1994
13. Wagner EH, LaCroix AZ: Effects of physical activity on health status in older adults. Annu Rev Public Health 13:451–468, 1992
14. Shephard RJ: Physical Activity and Aging. Second edition. Rockville, MD, Aspen, 1987
15. Pate RR, Pratt M, Blair SN, Haskell WL, Macera CA, Bouchard C, Buchner D, Ettinger W, Heath GW, King AC, Kriska A, Leon AS, Marcus BH, Morris J, Paffenbarger RS, Patrick K, Pollock ML, Rippe JM, Sallis J, Wilmore JH: Physical activity and public health. JAMA 273:402–407, 1995
16. Corbin CB, Pangrazi RP, Welk GJ: Toward an understanding of appropriate physical activity levels for youth. Phys Act Fit Res Dig 8:1–6, 1994
17. Sallis JF, Patrick K: Physical activity guidelines for adolescents: consensus statement. Pediatr Exerc Sci 6:302–314, 1994

18. Burckhardt CS, Clark SR, Nelson DL: Assessing physical fitness of women with rheumatic disease. Arthritis Care Res 1:38–44, 1988

19. LaPorte RE, Montoye HJ, Caspersen CJ: Assessment of physical activity in epidemiologic research: problems and prospects. Public Health Rep 100:131–146, 1985

20. Gerber LH, Furst GP: Scoring methods and application of the activity record (ACTRE) for patients with musculoskeletal disorders. Arthritis Care Res 5:151–156, 1992

21. Fix AJ, Daughton DM: Human Activity Profile. Odessa, FL, Psychological Assessment Resources, Inc., 1988

22. Pate RR: Physical activity assessment in children and adolescents. Crit Rev Food Sci Nutr 33:321–326, 1993

23. Borg G: Psychophysical scaling with application in physical work and the perception of exertion. Scand J Work Environ Health 16 (suppl):55–58, 1990

24. Gerber L, Furst G, Shulman B, Smith C, Thornton B, Liang M, Cullen K, Stevens MB, Gilbert N: Patient education program to teach energy conservation behaviors to patients with rheumatoid arthritis: a pilot study. Arch Phys Med Rehabil 68:442–445, 1987

Additional Recommended Reading

1. Sandler H, Vernikos J: Inactivity: Physiological Effects. Orlando FL, Academic Press, Inc., 1986

2. Steinberg FU: The Immobilized Patient: Functional Pathology and Management. New York, Plenum Publishing Corporation, 1980

3. Exercise and Arthritis. Arthritis Care Res Vol. 7, No. 4, 1994

CHAPTER 24

Adherence

MICHAEL A. RAPOFF, PhD

Treatment regimens for adult and pediatric rheumatic diseases are complex, demanding, costly, and the benefits are often delayed (1–3). These factors characterize regimens that are likely to foster nonadherence (4–6).

Adherence has been defined as "…the extent to which a person's behavior (in terms of taking medications, following diets, or executing lifestyle changes) coincides with medical or health advice" (7). This definition has heuristic value because it: 1) specifies the range of adherence behaviors required for various regimens (such as medications, therapeutic exercises, and splinting in rheumatic diseases); 2) requires an evaluation of the "extent" of adherence, emphasizing that adherence is relative and can vary within persons over time, between persons, and across different regimen requirements; and 3) implies there is a standard (that which coincides with medical advice) for determining acceptable adherence.

MEASURES OF ADHERENCE

A variety of methods have been used to measure adherence, including drug assays, behavioral observations, automated devices, pill counts, treatment outcome, provider estimates, and patient report (2,6,8,9). As shown in Table 1, each of these methods have assets and liabilities.

Drug Assays. Serum drug levels or inert substances added to drugs as tracers are used to assess adherence (6,10,11). They are quantifiable, useful for dosing adjustments, and do not rely on provider or patient estimates. However, assays can be expensive, invasive (particularly for children), and intermittently obtained, thereby reflecting more recent ingestion. In addition, drug levels may be affected by factors other than patient adherence, such as inadequate dosing, non-steady state concentrations, pharmacokinetic variations due to the medication preparations (e.g., enteric coating), gastric pH levels, interactions with other medications, patient age, or patient behaviors such as smoking (12).

Behavioral Observations. Direct observations are preferable for non-pharmacologic regimens (such as therapeutic exercises), because the provider can evaluate how patients are carrying out treatments and provide corrective feedback as needed (2). A major drawback of observations is the limited access providers have to observe patients. Family members can provide reliable observations of patient adherence if they are provided with a specific and relatively simple observational strategy and are adequately trained (13).

Automated Devices. Technological advances in microprocessors has led to the development of automated adherence measures. Microelectronic monitors are now available for recording, storing, and downloading information on medication removal (8). These devices allow for continuous (real-time) and long-term assessments of adherence.

One such system is the Medication Monitoring System

Table 1. Assets and liabilities of adherence measures (adapted from 14).

Measure	Assets	Liabilities
Assays	1. Can adjust drug dosage 2. Gold standard in adherence measurement	1. Pharmacokinetics may affect absorption and excretion rates 2. Short-term, invasive, and expensive
Observation	1. Direct measure of non-medication regimen adherence 2. Can measure adherence on repeated occasions	1. Obtrusive and reactive 2. Clinically impractical
Automated Measures	1. Precise dosing and interdose interval data obtained 2. Continuous and long-term measurement is possible	1. Medication removal does not guarantee consumption 2. Reactive and mechanical failures
Pill Counts	1. Easily obtained 2. Inexpensive	1. Pill removal does not guarantee ingestion 2. Overestimates adherence
Treatment Outcomes	1. Evaluate regimen efficacy 2. Clinically feasible	1. Inexact or unknown relationship to adherence 2. Factors other than patient adherence can affect outcome
Physician Estimates	1. Clinically feasible 2. Generally more accurate than global patient estimates	1. Overestimates adherence 2. Physician experience or familiarity with patient unrelated to accuracy
Patient Report	1. Clinically feasible 2. Generally accurate for nonadherence	1. Overestimates adherence 2. Subject to reporting bias—"faking good"

(MEMS). The MEMS contains two components: a monitor and communicator. The monitor consists of standard vial caps with a microelectric circuit recessed in the cap that records the date and time of each vial opening. The current monitor has a life of 18 months and can store 1,800 dosing events. The communicator is an electronic reader that transfers data from the monitor to a personal computer where software programs can read, display, and print dosing records.

These automated devices present an exciting new avenue for adherence assessment, but opening vials does not guarantee ingestion and the cost is prohibitively expensive for routine clinical use. When supplemented by periodic assays, these measures are likely to become the "gold standard" in adherence research (6).

Pill Counts. Pill counts or volume measurements have been used extensively in adherence research (6,9). They are simple and can be routinely done during clinic visits or by phone (2). As with automated measures, the major liability is that medications removed are not necessarily ingested (14).

Treatment Outcome. Outcomes such as active joint counts, duration of morning stiffness, and functional status measures have been viewed as indirect measures of adherence (14). These measures are well integrated into clinical practice and research. However, there is not necessarily a close correspondence between patient adherence and treatment outcome. Poorly adherent patients may have acceptable outcomes, and fully adherent patients may have bad ones (5,6). Adherence and treatment outcome are two separate phenomena and need to be assessed separately to determine the optimal level of adherence necessary to achieve desired therapeutic effects (14).

Provider Estimates. Provider estimates generally involve a global rating of the degree to which patients are adherent to a regimen (6,15). Busy providers may find this the most feasible way to assess adherence (14). However, provider estimates consistently underestimate levels of nonadherence (6). This may be due to reliance on treatment outcomes for estimating adherence and to positive bias or expectancies, such as wanting to believe patients are adhering to recommendations.

Patient Report. Consistent with the emphasis on history-taking in clinical practice, it is not surprising that patient and family reports are often used to assess adherence (6,16). Such estimates are inadequate in that they tend to overestimate the degree of adherence (2,17). This may be due to social desirability effects whereby patients and families want to preserve their relationships with providers by reporting socially approved behaviors.

However, patient reports have received a "bad rap" in the adherence literature, in part due to how patients are questioned. Questions that are nonjudgmental, specific, and time limited may yield more accurate information about adherence and lead to a discussion of obstacles to adherence that can be addressed. For example, questions about adherence can be prefaced by stating that "Most people—including the interviewer—miss doses of their medication for one reason or another" (18). In contrast, a judgmental and/or global approach without time referents can be useless or actually induce deception.

An alternative is to have patients or their families monitor and record specific adherence behaviors. These can even be done using computerized diaries (8). The accuracy of such records can be improved by clearly specifying target behaviors, using simple monitoring strategies, emphasizing the importance of accuracy and honesty, demonstrating and having patients practice the monitoring strategy, and periodic and independent checks on accuracy (19).

ADHERENCE RATES

Adherence rates range from 16% to 84% for medications; from 39% to 65% for therapeutic exercises; and from 25% to 65% for splint usage in the treatment of adults with rheumatoid arthritis (RA) (1,20). Adherence rates for medications in the treatment of juvenile rheumatoid arthritis (JRA) range from 38% to 59% (2,21,22). No comparable adherence data have been reported for therapeutic exercises or splint usage in JRA, but parents report lower adherence to exercises relative to medications (23,24).

CONSEQUENCES OF NONADHERENCE

The consequences of nonadherence include compromised efficacy of regimens, increased health care costs and utilization,

Table 2. Patient/family, disease, and regimen factors associated with nonadherence to medical regimens (adapted from 6).

Patient/Family Factors
Dissatisfaction with medical care
Limited financial and social resources
Lack of knowledge
Low self-esteem
Learned helplessness and pessimism
Negative overall adjustment
Poor coping strategies
Family dysfunction

Disease Factors
Decrements in compliance over time
Patient asymptomatic or in remission
Increased number of symptoms
Younger age at disease onset
Disease not perceived as severe by patient and/or family

Regimen Factors
Complex and demanding regimens
Costly regimens
Questionable efficacy of regimen
Lack of continuity of care
Limited provider supervision of regimen
Shorter duration of subspecialty care
Negative regimen side effects

and compromised clinical trials (6). Increased morbidity and possibly mortality (such as with abrupt discontinuation of corticosteroids) can be attributed to nonadherence (25). The cost-effectiveness of health care can also be adversely affected. Money may be wasted on treatments that are not followed, or families may incur the costs of unnecessary diagnostic and treatment procedures (26). These unnecessary costs may further burden society in the form of increased insurance premiums and taxes. Treatment nonadherence can also interfere with clinical trials of therapeutic regimens by complicating judgements of efficacy and adding to the sample sizes needed to detect clinical effects (27,28).

FACTORS RELATED TO ADHERENCE

Much of the adherence literature has focused on identifying factors that promote or impede adherence (2,4,5). Typically this is done by correlating various factors with adherence or contrasting adherent and nonadherent patients along factorial dimensions (2). As seen in Table 2, patient/family, disease, and regimen factors have been most frequently studied as correlates of adherence. Studies of this type can be useful for several reasons: 1) they can help determine risk profiles for adherence problems; 2) they can help formulate or augment theoretical models; and 3) they can suggest potentially modifiable variables for adherence intervention trials (2).

Patient/Family Factors. Adherence is likely to be compromised when patients and their families are not well informed, are dissatisfied with care, lack financial and social resources, and experience adjustment problems such as low self-esteem, decreased self-efficacy, and family disharmony. The search for a "typical" nonadherent patient has not been particularly fruitful (5); therefore, providers are cautioned to examine these patient/family factors in terms of their relevance for specific patients.

Disease Factors. Persons with rheumatic diseases are prime candidates for adherence problems due to the chronicity and fluctuations of disease activity. This is particularly troublesome when adherence is found to be inconsistently related to disease activity (20). Patients may have little natural incentive to adhere to prescribed regimens.

Regimen Factors. The list of these factors in Table 2 suggests that regimens for rheumatic diseases are prototypical nonadherence inducers because they are complex, costly, of significant duration, and provide delayed beneficial effects. Delayed benefits may particularly undermine patient adherence, as in the case of nonsteroidal anti-inflammatory drugs in the treatment of JRA requiring at least an 8-week trial (29). How providers manage regimens is also critical; limited supervision, feedback, and comprehensive subspecialty care has been associated with nonadherence (2).

ADHERENCE IMPROVEMENT STRATEGIES

Adherence intervention studies are rare in the rheumatology literature (see references 1,2, and 20 for reviews). However, extrapolating from this meager database and a wider database in clinical medicine, some suggestions for improving adherence can be made.

Adherence improvement strategies can be broadly classified as educational, organizational, and behavioral (30). *Educational strategies* rely on verbal and written instructions designed to inform patients and their families about the illness, regimen requirements, and the importance of consistent adherence. These strategies are necessary but not sufficient to improve adherence.

Organizational strategies address the way health care is delivered, including increasing accessibility to health care services, simplifying and reducing the negative side-effects of regimens, and countering sources of dissatisfaction for patients and their families. Organizational strategies are promising, particularly those that emphasize greater supervision and feedback to patients and their families.

Behavioral strategies refer to procedures designed to alter specific adherence behaviors by monitoring, prompting or cueing, shaping, and reinforcing adherence. These behavioral strategies, such as teaching patients and their families to monitor, prompt, and positively reinforce adherence, seem to be the most effective (2,5,6). Behavioral strategies are often combined with educational strategies and can be effectively merged with organizational strategies.

Table 3 provides specific recommendations for improving adherence by type of strategy. Clearly, providers can have a substantial impact on patient adherence. However, adherence does not occur in a clinical or social vacuum. Patients may experience personal and family adjustment problems that may need to be addressed in addition to or prior to addressing adherence problems (6).

CONCLUSIONS

Rheumatology providers have an important role to play in assessing and managing adherence problems. Potentially the most important benefit is that patient care and outcomes will be enhanced. Providers will also be able to more accurately evaluate the efficacy and cost-effectiveness of their therapeutic endeavors.

Table 3. Adherence improvement strategies for rheumatic disease regimens (adapted from 2).

Educational Strategies
  Provide clear verbal and written information
  Make sure patients have the skills to carry out regimens
  Re-educate about treatments and adherence as needed
  Emphasize the importance of adherence, especially when patients are asymptomatic or in remission
  Increase education about rheumatic diseases in the community to foster early diagnosis and referral for subspecialty care

Organizational Strategies
  Minimize costs of treatments (e.g., use generic medications)
  Reduce the complexity of regimens (e.g., reduce number of exercises)
  Reduce negative side-effects of regimens (e.g., use coated medications)
  Address barriers to adherence and sources of patient/family dissatisfaction on a continuing basis
  Link families to resources that can reduce financial and service accessibility barriers to adherence

Behavioral Strategies
  Self-management training to encourage autonomy and self-esteem
  Demonstrate and have patients behaviorally rehearse complex regimens such as exercises
  Increase provider and family member supervision of regimens
  Have patients monitor adherence
  Provide social and other reinforcers (such as token systems) to increase adherence, especially when treatment benefits are delayed

Health care providers must only ask patients to adhere to regimens that have demonstrable efficacy. At the minimum, they should be congruent with the Hippocratic Oath: "I will follow that system of regimen which, according to my ability and judgment, I consider for the benefit of my patients, and abstain from whatever is deleterious and mischievous" (31).

To further treatment of rheumatic diseases, providers need to be technically informed and competent as well as sensitive and caring. Patients and their families now demand and deserve a more active role in their health care. The term *compliance* lost favor in the literature because it implied an authoritative approach to health care that required unquestioned obedience by patients to providers' recommendations (33). It was replaced by the term *adherence*, which implies a cooperative partnership between patients and providers as reflected in the following perspective by Cassell: "Doctors do not treat chronic illnesses. The chronically ill treat themselves with the help of their physicians; the physician is part of the treatment. Patients are in charge of themselves. They determine their food, activity, medications, visits to their doctor—most of the details of their own treatment" (32).

Finally, as rheumatology providers, we may need to entertain the possibility that failing to adhere to prescribed regimens may be strategic, rational, and adaptive in selected cases (34). As noted by Cousins, "The history of medicine is replete with accounts of drugs and modes of treatment that were in use for many years before it was recognized that they did more harm than good" (35). Perhaps, when our patients are nonadherent, we need to closely examine what we are recommending and why. This examination may lead us to evaluate the goals and methods for reaching treatment objectives that more appropriately address improvements in the day-to-day quality of life of our patients.

Acknowledgment. Preparation of this manuscript was supported in part by grant MCJ-200617 from the Maternal and Child Health Bureau (Title V, Social Security Act), Health Resources and Services Administration, Department of Health and Human Services.

REFERENCES

1. Bradley LA: Adherence with treatment regimens among adult rheumatoid arthritis patients: current status and future directions. Arthritis Care Res 2:S33-S39, 1989
2. Rapoff MA: Compliance with treatment regimens for pediatric rheumatic diseases. Arthritis Care Res 2:S40-S47, 1989
3. Thompson SM, Dahlquist LM, Koenning GM, Bartholomew LK: Brief report: adherence-facilitating behaviors of a multidisciplinary pediatrics rheumatology staff. J Pediatr Psychol 20:291-297, 1995
4. Haynes RB, Taylor DW, Sackett DL, editors: Compliance in Health Care. Baltimore, The Johns Hopkins University Press, 1979
5. Meichenbaum D, Turk DC: Facilitating Treatment Adherence: A Practitioner's Guidebook. New York, Plenum Press, 1987
6. Rapoff MA, Barnard MU: Compliance with pediatric medical regimens. In, Patient Compliance in Medical Practice and Clinical Trials. Edited by JA Cramer, B Spilker. New York, Raven Press, 1991
7. Haynes RB: Introduction. In, Compliance in Health Care. Edited by RB Haynes, DW Taylor, DL Sackett. Baltimore, The Johns Hopkins University Press, 1979
8. Cramer JA: Overview of methods to measure and enhance patient compliance. In, Patient Compliance in Medical Practice and Clinical Trials. Edited by JA Cramer, B Spilker. New York, Raven Press, 1991
9. Dunbar J, Dunning EJ, Dwyer K: Compliance measurement with arthritis regimen. Arthritis Care Res 2:S8-S16, 1989
10. Dubbert PM, King A, Rapop SR, Brief D, Martin JE, Lake M: Riboflavin as a tracer of medication compliance. J Behav Med 8:287-299, 1985
11. Pullar T, Peaker S, Martin MF, Bird HA, Feely MP: The use of a pharmacological indicator to investigate compliance in patients with a poor response to antirheumatic therapy. Br J Rheumatol 27:381-384, 1988
12. Backes JM, Schentag JJ: Partial compliance as a source of variance in pharmacokinetics and therapeutic drug monitoring. In, Patient Compliance in Medical Practice and Clinical Trials. Edited by JA Cramer, B Spilker. New York, Raven Press, 1991
13. Rapoff MA, Lindsley CB, Christophersen ER: Improving compliance with medical regimens: case study with juvenile rheumatoid arthritis. Arch Phys Med Rehabil 65:267-269, 1984
14. Rapoff MA, Christophersen ER: Compliance of pediatric patients with medical regimens: a review and evaluation. In, Adherence, Compliance and Generalization in Behavioral Medicine. Edited by RB Stuart. New York, Brunner/Mazel, 1982
15. Feinberg J: Effect of the arthritis health professional on compliance with use of resting hand splints by patients with rheumatoid arthritis. Arthritis Care Res 5:17-23, 1992
16. Feinstein AR: Clinical Judgment. New York, Robert E. Krieger Publishing Co., 1967
17. Caron HS: Compliance: the case for objective measurement. J Hypertens 3:11-17, 1985
18. Lorish CD, Richards B, Brown S: Missed medication doses in rheumatic arthritis patients: intentional and unintentional reasons. Arthritis Care Res 2:3-9, 1989
19. Mahoney MF, Arnkoff DB: Self-management. In, Behavioral Medicine: Theory and Practice. Edited by OF Pomerleau, JP Brady. Baltimore, Williams and Wilkins, 1986
20. Belcon MC, Haynes RB, Tugwell P: A critical review of compliance studies in rheumatoid arthritis. Arthritis Rheum 27:1227-1233, 1984
21. Litt IF, Cuskey WR: Compliance with salicylate therapy in adolescents with juvenile rheumatoid arthritis. Am J Dis Child 135:434-436, 1981
22. Litt IF, Cuskey WR, Rosenberg BA: Role of self-esteem and autonomy in determining medication compliance among adolescents with juvenile rheumatoid arthritis. Pediatrics 69:15-17, 1982
23. Hayford JR, Ross CK: Medical compliance in juvenile rheumatoid arthritis: problems and perspectives. Arthritis Care Res 1:190-197, 1988
24. Rapoff MA, Lindsley CB, Christophersen ER: Parent perceptions of problems experienced by their children in complying with treatments for juvenile rheumatoid arthritis. Arch Phys Med Rehabil 66:427-429, 1985
25. Ruley EJ: Compliance in young hypertensive patients. Pediatr Clin North Am 25:175-182, 1978
26. Smith M: The cost of noncompliance and the capacity of improved compliance to reduce health care expenditures. In, Improving Medication Compliance: Proceedings of a Symposium. Washington, DC, National Pharmaceutical Council, 1985
27. Haynes RB, Dantes R: Patient compliance and the conduct and interpretation of therapeutic trials. Control Clin Trials 8:12-19, 1987
28. Probstfield JL: Adherence and its management in clinical trials: implications for arthritis treatment trials. Arthritis Care Res 2:S48-S57, 1989
29. Lovell DJ, Giannini EH, Brewer EJ Jr: Time course of response to nonsteroidal antiinflammatory drugs in juvenile rheumatoid arthritis. Arthritis Rheum 27:1433-1437, 1984
30. Dunbar JM, Marshall GD, Hovell MF: Behavioral strategies for improving compliance. In, Compliance in Health Care. Edited by RB Haynes, DW Taylor, DL Sackett. Baltimore, The Johns Hopkins University Press, 1979
31. The oath. In, The Genuine Works of Hippocrates. Vol. II. Translated by F Adams. New York, William Wood, 1886
32. Cassell EJ: The nature of suffering and the goals of medicine. New York, Oxford University Press, 1991
33. DiMatteo MR, DiNicola DD: Achieving Patient Compliance: The Psychology of the Medical Practitioner's Role. New York, Pergamon Press, 1982
34. Deaton AV: Adaptive noncompliance in pediatric asthma: the parent as expert. J Pediatr Psychol 10:1-14, 1985
35. Cousins N: Anatomy of an Illness as Perceived by the Patient. New York, Bantam, 1979

Work Disability

SARALYNN H. ALLAIRE, ScD, RN, CRC

Work disability is commonly defined as unemployment due to the effects of health conditions such as rheumatic diseases. Other indicators of work disability include reduced work hours, diminished opportunity for promotion, increased sick leave use, and frequent job change.

WORK DISABILITY RATES

Work disability is a major problem for persons with rheumatic diseases and a challenge in terms of social and health policy. Arthritis is the leading cause of work loss and the second leading cause of work disability payments (1,2). In a national, community-based sample of persons self-reporting health problems, labor force participation was 20% lower among men and 25% lower among women with arthritis (1). Furthermore, the rate of arthritis-related work disability has been rising, especially among middle-aged and older men (1).

In clinical samples of individuals with rheumatoid arthritis (RA), work disability prevalence rates varied between 25% and 50% after one decade of disease (3–5), increasing to 90% with longer disease duration (3). The rate of work disability associated with osteoarthritis approaches that of RA (6). In a French sample, most persons with ankylosing spondylitis were employed, although work capacity was reduced (7). In a Finnish sample, 64% of individuals with RA were work disabled 8 years after disease onset, compared to 31% of those with psoriatic arthritis and 10% to 15% of those with ankylosing spondylitis, seronegative oligoarthritis, or reactive arthritis (8). Among Canadians with systemic lupus erythematosus, 37% were work disabled after a mean disease duration of 5.5 years (9).

Adults with a history of juvenile rheumatoid arthritis (JRA) and other childhood rheumatic diseases appear to be employed at rates close to peers without illness (10,11). Many employed individuals reported having difficulty doing their jobs, and 21% had resigned from a job due to JRA (12).

Other musculoskeletal conditions, notably back injuries and cumulative trauma disorders, are also important causes of work disability. Back injuries are the leading industrial injury, and 2.6 million persons are permanently disabled by back pain (13). Rates for both back injuries and cumulative trauma disorders continue to increase. Work performance studies of persons with fibromyalgia show reduced capacity to do repetitive activities (14), but a low work disability rate (11%) has been reported (15).

RISK FACTORS

Risk factors that affect work disability can be useful in determining whether and how rate reductions can be achieved. Risk factors exist at both the level of the individual and at a societal level.

Among adults with RA, the most substantial individual risk factors for work disability are poor disease status as measured by functional status or number of involved joints, greater job physical demand, and older age (3,16,17). Other risk factors include greater commuting difficulty, low job autonomy (lack of control over work pace and other work activities), less education, less support from family members or co-workers, depression, and desire to be at home. For adults with JRA, continued disease activity, polyarticular JRA, and female gender were predictors of unemployment and lower salaries (10,11), while poor psychological status and pain predicted productivity loss in those with systemic lupus erythematosus (18). Physically demanding jobs and a greater number of involved joints were predictors of work disability in individuals with ankylosing spondylitis (7). Investigation of the work attitudes and job satisfaction of people with arthritis revealed that these aspects of work commitment were similar to those without arthritis (19).

Societal risk factors include economic conditions, attitudinal and architectural barriers, types of jobs available, employer practices, and the characteristics of disability pension plans. When the economy is poor, applications to disability pension plans increase, a reflection of the effect of the unemployment rate on work disability. Discrimination, as well as inaccessible work places, transportation systems, and homes, make it difficult for persons with chronic health conditions to continue to work. A study of employers' attitudes about different impairments suggested they view arthritis less negatively than many other conditions (20). However, because arthritis is common among older persons, age discrimination may produce a combined discriminatory effect. Gender may be an additional basis for discrimination among women (16). The physical demand and autonomy characteristics of the jobs available in a national economy influence the number of employment opportunities available to those with health impairments.

The disability management practices used by an employer determine in part the job retention rate among employees with health conditions. Early return to work, temporary light duty, and job accommodation programs promote retention, while early retirement through use of disability pension plans promotes work disability. Many employers do offer help to employees with arthritis, but the types of help given to those with RA—reduction in work hours for example—did not preserve employment, possibly because it lowered productivity (17). Other types of help, such as providing adaptive equipment, may be more beneficial.

Work disability rates are higher in countries where disability pension compensation levels are high relative to wages (up to 100%). In the U.S., the Social Security Disability Insurance (SSDI) program compensates at an average of 45% of salary.

Only 25% of U.S. employees are covered by additional employer disability pension plans.

EMPLOYMENT OUTLOOK

Although the employment rate of persons with arthritis and musculoskeletal conditions has been declining, opportunities for employment may increase in the future. U.S. demographics predict that shortages of skilled, experienced workers and increased use of technologies such as robots and computers should expand job opportunities for those with limited function. Furthermore, the Americans with Disabilities Act (ADA), which prohibits discrimination and requires that reasonable accommodation be provided, now covers the majority of employers. The fact that job physical demand and autonomy are important predictors of work disability suggests job loss could be prevented or delayed through accommodation in some cases.

ASSESSMENT

The usual goal is to preserve or facilitate employment, which provides important financial, psychological, and other benefits. Goal setting needs to be individualized, however, because employment is not possible or desirable for all.

Prevention and early intervention are the best approaches to managing work disability related to rheumatic diseases (21). Unfortunately, the potential for work disability often is not addressed until job loss is imminent and intervention is more difficult, if not too late. Chances for return to work diminish as time away from work lengthens.

Evaluation of employment problems should begin prior to job loss. Initial assessment focuses on the presence of immediate problems, and priority should be given to persons who are currently on sick leave or who cannot do their job. Adults without immediate employment problems (especially those who are younger) and adolescents need guidance to help them factor in the long-term impact of their disease on employment and to consider jobs or careers that are appropriate.

The person's health status should be evaluated, including frequency of acute illness episodes; degree of symptom control, notably pain, stiffness and fatigue; functional status; and scheduling of surgery, if any. The short- and long-term suitability of the individual's current job can then be examined. Assessment topics include the following: 1) difficulty getting to and from work, beginning within the patient's home; 2) physical barriers encountered at work; 3) job physical demand and autonomy, including number of work hours; 4) relationship with the employer, including employer's attitude toward disability; 5) relationships with co-workers; and 6) employer and co-worker awareness of the patient's condition. If employment problems are likely, opportunity for change with the current employer should be examined, such as the employee's length of tenure, availability of other jobs, and any job training or educational benefits. Previous work history, educational background, specialized job training, and interests should also be assessed.

Family support and financial need should be included in the evaluation. The beliefs of family members about the ability of the patient to be employed can be explored. Especially among women, assessment should include the accomplishment of household work, including the proportion done by the patient, the willingness and availability of family members to do tasks, and role perceptions.

Even if they are currently unemployed, patients may have a need or desire for employment. In such cases, evaluation should cover stability of the rheumatic condition, work history pertaining to earning potential, types of benefits received, and possible alternative sources of health insurance.

Areas of assessment for children and adolescents include histories of helping at home and inclusion in educational, social, and recreational activities. Other factors to assess are summer and after-school work, volunteer experiences, parental beliefs about the child's ability to work, and the child's interests and academic achievement.

INTERVENTION

The goal of intervention is to facilitate patient decision making. This may be accomplished by initiating discussion about actual or potential interactions between the person's rheumatic disease and employment, as well as by active listening, examination of alternatives, and referral for vocational services. To avoid misunderstandings, any communication with employers can be conducted through the patient.

Primary Prevention for Future Job Loss

Because individuals without current employment difficulties may encounter problems in the future, actions taken to reduce risk of job loss may be preventive. The first step is to promote awareness of this potential. Persons with energy limitations can be counseled about reducing demand in various life spheres, such as at work, during commuting, in household responsibilities, in social activities, and in health self-care. To some extent this means managing the demands more efficiently, although reduction of activities in at least some spheres may also be required.

If the individual's job is demanding, exploration of future job change options should be initiated. Available resources, including the person's employer, should be exploited early in the disease course when patients are more likely to be employable. Career counseling and vocational testing services of the state–federal vocational rehabilitation program, which exists in all states, should be available at no cost to many persons with rheumatic diseases (Table 1). Private vocational counseling is another alternative. Administrative and professional jobs often are characterized by low physical demand and high autonomy and therefore meet the needs of those with rheumatic diseases. These positions may also be more stressful, but, as circumstances dictate, additional training or education needed to obtain such positions is advisable.

Pre-vocational interventions are extremely important for children and adolescents with rheumatic diseases (22). Parents can be instructed to assign appropriate household chores to the child and can be helped to obtain any assistive technology needed to carry out these and other activities. Parents should also observe the activities the child enjoys doing as a preliminary guide to future vocational interests. The child's inclusion in academic, social, and recreational activities should be facilitated to build vocational experience and social skills.

Assistance can be given to adolescents in obtaining summer

Table 1. Primary resources.

Government-sponsored Vocational Rehabilitation Services

Although differences in administration of the state-federal vocational rehabilitation program exist among the states, most persons with rheumatic diseases should be eligible for the following services:

Vocational counseling and testing

Job placement

Assistance with resume construction, interview preparation, and job seeking support

Payment for job accommodations, training, education, and travel when financial eligibility criteria are met

Independent Living Centers

These centers provide advocacy services and services that strive to enable persons with disabilities to live on their own.

Information

The Arthritis Foundation can provide excellent pamphlets about employment challenges for adults and teenagers, and about Social Security benefits; 1-800-283-7800.

The President's Committee on Employment of People with Disabilities operates the Job Accommodation Network (JAN), a free consulting service about the Americans with Disabilities Act and types of job accommodations; 1-800-526-7234 (V/TDD).

Disability and Business Technical Assistance Centers are available in each region of the country to advise businesses and individuals about accommodations; 1-800-949-4232.

The U.S. Equal Employment Opportunity Commission has information available about employment aspects of the Americans with Disabilities Act; 1801 L Street, NW, Washington, DC 20507.

and after school work or volunteer experiences. At age 15 (one year prior to eligibility), the teen can be referred to the state–federal vocational rehabilitation program for vocational counseling, transitional services, and, depending on financial criteria, funding of vocational education or training. Early referral is crucial, as eligibility can take time to establish and there may be waiting lists. Parents may need education regarding their child's abilities, the value of employment, and possible problems or difficulties that may exist. Career choices that seem unrealistic can be managed by exploring the appeal of the chosen field, encouraging volunteer experience, and by helping the teen interview people currently working in the field. Positive attitudes on the part of professionals and parents and attempts to facilitate the child's choice are more successful than ready dismissal.

Secondary Prevention for Immediate Job Loss

Employed persons who are experiencing problems at work need immediate attention to prevent or delay job loss. The individual's employer is the first resource, but if the employer is unaware of the person's condition, the pros and cons of providing such information must be weighed. Employees are often pleasantly surprised at the positive reaction of their employers, but the possibility of discrimination exists. Repercussions, such as not being considered for promotions, can occur. More positive reactions are ensured if the employee can present ways of managing disease effects that will maintain productivity.

Retaining the individual's current job is often the best option. In some cases, changes in non-employment life spheres are sufficient. Ways of reducing energy used in commuting to and from work can be sought, such as obtaining a handicapped license plate or special transportation. For some jobs, working

at home may be an option. Family meetings can result in better management of household work responsibilities. Continuation of the household role can be facilitated by encouraging a "manager" rather than a "doer" role.

Job accommodations (modifications) may also be required. Categories of job accommodations include job restructuring, assistive devices, training for new job duties, provision of a personal assistant, modification of the work environment, and job reassignment. Occupational therapists can provide individual work evaluations and prescribe specific accommodations. Vocational rehabilitation counselors can intercede with the employer on behalf of an employee to obtain needed accommodations. Employers may not know that the overwhelming majority of accommodations are inexpensive and that the ADA requires only that an accommodation be adequate to accomplish the job. If an expensive accommodation is needed, cost sharing with the employer is possible. In some cases, funding can be obtained from the state–federal vocational rehabilitation program.

Good management of paid vacation time, accumulated sick time, and short-term sick leave benefits (when available) can help the individual with disease flares continue working; a few days of rest when a flare is beginning or during periods of stress can sometimes avert longer periods of disability. The Family Medical Leave Act legislation can be utilized by covered employees to obtain medical leave. For persons currently on sick leave, inquiry should be made about early return-to-work, transitional work, and/or job accommodation programs.

When keeping a current job is no longer possible, the next best option is often a job change with the same employer. A good work history is an asset, and persons with RA who were able to change their jobs within the same employer had a higher job retention rate than those who changed employers (3). In addition to low physical demand and high autonomy, other desirable job characteristics are avoidance of repetitive physical tasks and jobs in which position changes are possible. Jobs involving communication skills and/or thought processes are good choices. Job changes may be accompanied by salary reduction; although this seems difficult to accept or financially unfeasible, the resulting amount is often higher than other jobs or disability pension plans offer. Some employers provide job training opportunities that can lead to better future jobs. The ADA requires that employees with disabilities be considered for vacant positions for which they are prepared, but it does not mandate that they be given those positions.

When continuing employment with the individual's current employer is not possible or desirable, the remaining employment option is change of employers, possibly including change of job type or career. Referral for government-sponsored or private vocational rehabilitation services should be considered, because physical restoration and vocational training services have been linked to employment gain among clients with arthritis (23). Working at home avoids the energy expenditure of commuting; however, it can be socially isolating. Starting a business is appealing to many people, but while this would meet job autonomy needs, the time requirements are often great and failure rates are high.

Tertiary Prevention for Return to Work

It can be difficult for persons who have not been employed for an extended period to return to work, but it is possible. Among persons with RA, 10% of those who left the work force returned to work at a later time (3). Persons receiving Supplemental Security Income (SSI) benefits can work and continue to receive health insurance and partial income payments depending on the amount earned. Part-time work is thus supported, a valuable option for persons with energy limitations. Trial work programs are available to SSDI program recipients; permanent continuation of benefits after return to work is not allowed, but Medicare health insurance can be purchased for $3,400 per year (as of 1994). Individuals can contact local Social Security offices for information about return-to-work programs, the state–federal vocational rehabilitation program for employability evaluation, an independent living center for advocacy services, and state employment offices for job listings.

Stopping Work

Employment cessation may be the best, or only, option for some. Persons with severe RA may find that joint symptoms and functional status improve somewhat following withdrawal from work (17). Individuals with health problems that necessitate frequent hospitalization may find their productivity is lowered by job interruptions. The family and financial circumstances of some patients require and permit a family care rather than employment role. Finally, older workers with disease of long duration may find it especially difficult to work, both because of their physical condition and discrimination against older, disabled workers.

For persons who are considering leaving the work force, discussion can focus initially on the benefits of working versus not working. Employment almost always provides greater financial return and, for younger persons, greater future financial security. Other advantages include personal achievement, group health insurance coverage and other employee benefits, and opportunities for socialization. On the other hand, stopping work provides health advantages for some people, including additional time for self care. Volunteer activities can provide fulfillment.

Individuals under the age of 65 who are unable to engage in substantial gainful activity (a monetary amount that changes annually) because of an impairment expected to last at least 12 months or result in death, and who have contributed sufficiently to Social Security, are eligible to apply for SSDI. Those who have not contributed (including children) but who meet financial need criteria are eligible to apply for SSI. Approval is based primarily on medical disease criteria, such as a positive rheumatoid factor test and x-rays showing joint damage. When such criteria do not exist, approval is based on residual functional capacity and the person's age, education, and prior work experience. For children, approval is based on an individualized functional assessment.

Persons with RA are more likely to obtain initial approval than those with systemic lupus erythematosus, in which test results are often nonspecific. Although pain with positive examination findings, such as in fibromyalgia, can now be an acceptable criterion, only 7% of the 19.7% of persons with fibromyalgia applying for disability pensions obtained them (14). Several levels of appeal are available, and pursuit of appeal is often fruitful. Persons receiving SSDI or SSI are subject to continuing disability reviews; the timing of reviews (every 6 months to 7 years) depends on the recipient's age and the nature and severity of impairment. Those receiving SSDI are eligible for Medicare benefits after 2 years, while those receiving SSI are immediately eligible for Medicaid. Recipients of SSDI can earn a very limited amount of income from employment without losing benefits.

REFERENCES

1. Yelin E: Arthritis: the cumulative impact of a common chronic condition. Arthritis Rheum 35:489–497, 1992
2. US Department of Health and Human Services: Social Security Annual Statistics Supplement. Washington, DC, Social Security Administration, 1991
3. Yelin E, Henke C, Epstein W: The work dynamics of the person with rheumatoid arthritis. Arthritis Rheum 30:507–512, 1987
4. Reisine ST, Grady KE, Goodenow C, Fifield J: Work disability among women with rheumatoid arthritis: the relative importance of disease, social, work, and family factors. Arthritis Rheum 32:538–543, 1989
5. Wolfe F, Anderson J, Hawley DJ: Rates and predictors of work disability in rheumatoid arthritis: importance of disease, psycho-social and workplace factors (abstract). Arthritis Rheum 37 (suppl 9):S231, 1994
6. Pincus T, Mitchell J, Burkhauser RV: Substantial work disability and earnings losses in individuals less than age 65 with osteoarthritis: comparisons with rheumatoid arthritis. J Clin Epidemiol 42:449–457, 1989
7. Guillemin F, Briançon S, Pourel J, Gaucher A: Long-term disability and prolonged sick leaves as outcome measurements in ankylosing spondylitis: possible predictive factors. Arthritis Rheum 33:1001–1006, 1990
8. Kaarela K, Lehtinen K, Luukkainen R: Work capacity of patients with inflammatory joint diseases: an eight-year followup study. Scand J Rheumatol 16:403–406, 1987
9. Clarke AE, Esdaile JM, Bloch DA, Lacaille D, Danoff DS, Fries JF: A Canadian study of the total medical costs for patients with systemic lupus erythematosus and the predictors of costs. Arthritis Rheum 36:1548–1559, 1993
10. Hill RH, Herstein A, Walters K: Juvenile rheumatoid arthritis: follow-up into adulthood—medical, sexual, and social status. Can Med Assoc J 114:790–794, 1976
11. Miller JJ, Spitz PW, Simpson U, Williams GF: The social function of young adults who had arthritis in childhood. J Pediatr 100:378–382, 1982
12. Muney K, Hanson V, Mukamel M, Boone D: Health status and achievement in adult life of patients diagnosed with juvenile rheumatoid arthritis (abstract). Arthritis Rheum 30 (suppl 4):S200, 1987
13. National Institute on Disability and Rehabilitation Research: Chronic back pain. Rehab Brief 15(7), 1993
14. Wolfe F, Ross K, Anderson J, Russell IJ, Hebert L: The prevalence and characteristics of fibromyalgia in the general population. Arthritis Rheum 38:19–28, 1995
15. Kennedy MJ, Goldenberg DL, Felson DT: A prospective long-term study of fibromyalgia syndrome (abstract). Arthritis Rheum 37 (suppl 9):S213, 1994
16. Reisine A, McQuillan J, Fifield J: Predictors of work disability in rheumatoid arthritis patients: a five-year followup. Arthritis Rheum 38:1630–1637, 1995
17. Allaire SH, Anderson JJ, Meenan RF: Reducing work disability associated with rheumatoid arthritis: identification of additional risk factors and persons likely to benefit from intervention. Arthritis Care Res 9:349–357, 1996
18. Clarke AE, Bloch DA, Danoff DS, Esdaile JM: Decreasing costs and improving outcomes in systemic lupus erythematosus: using regression trees to develop health policy. J Rheumatol 21:2246–2253, 1994
19. Yelin E, Epstein W: Do people with arthritis lack commitment to work? (abstract) Arthritis Rheum 28 (suppl 4):S79, 1985
20. Yuker HE: The disability hierarchies: comparative reactions to various types of physical and mental disabilities. Hempstead, NY, Hofstra University, 1987
21. Boschen KA: Early intervention in vocational rehabilitation. Rehabil Couns Bull 32:254–265, 1989
22. White PH, Shear ES: Transition/job readiness for adolescents with juvenile arthritis and other chronic illness. J Rheumatol 19 (Suppl 33):23–27, 1992
23. Straaton KV, Harvey M, Maisiak R: Factors associated with successful vocational rehabilitation in persons with arthritis. Arthritis Rheum 35:503–510, 1992

Additional Recommended Reading

1. Allaire SH, Partridge AJ, Andrews HF, Liang MH: Management of work disability: resources for vocational rehabilitation. Arthritis Rheum 36: 1663–1670, 1993
2. Cooper C: Occupational activity and the risk of osteoarthritis. J Rheumatol 22 (Suppl 43):10–12, 1995
3. Greenwald S, Gerber L: The Americans with Disabilities Act. Bull Rheum Dis 41:5–7, 1992
4. Reisine S, Fifield J: Expanding the definition of disability: implications for planning, policy, and research. Milbank Q 70:491–508, 1992
5. Social Security Administration: Disability evaluation under Social Security. Office of Public Affairs, Room 4-J-10 West High Rise Building, 6401 Security Boulevard, Baltimore, MD 21235
6. Straaton KV, Maisiak R, Wrigley JM, Fine PR: Musculoskeletal disability, employment, and rehabilitation. J Rheumatol 22:505–513, 1995

SECTION E: COMMON RHEUMATIC DISEASES

CHAPTER

26

Rheumatoid Arthritis

THEODORE PINCUS, MD

Rheumatoid arthritis (RA) is a systemic chronic disease, characterized by an acute inflammatory response, with symmetric polyarticular joint pain and swelling, morning stiffness, malaise, and fatigue. The inflammatory activity may be reversible over months, and patients may experience spontaneous remission. However, most patients whose disease has persisted for longer than 90 days experience a progressive disease, in which the reversible inflammatory activity leads to irreversible joint damage. While the disease course is highly variable in individual patients, many patients may experience joint damage within the first 2 years of disease. Joint damage in RA ultimately has resulted in work disability in more 50% of patients within 10 years, and subsequent premature death. Until recent years, the severity of RA has been underrated, while results of treatment have been overrated. However, considerable progress has been made over the last decade in characterization of the course, outcomes, and treatment of RA (1,2).

INCIDENCE, ETIOLOGY, AND PATHOGENESIS

Rheumatoid arthritis is found in approximately 0.5% to 1% of the population in many cultures. The disease can affect individuals at any age, including infants and aged individuals; however, the most common onset is in women aged 40 to 50 years.

The etiology of RA remains unknown. Historically, RA was called *chronic infectious arthritis*, because the clinical and pathologic features of disease resemble those seen in chronic infectious diseases such as tuberculosis. However, extensive efforts to identify an exogenous infectious agent, such as a bacterium, mycobacterium, mycoplasma, fungus, or virus, have been unsuccessful.

Even if an exogenous infectious agent or footprints of such an agent were identified consistently in tissues of people with RA, endogenous host variables would be of considerable importance in the pathogenesis. One important host variable is the major histocompatibility locus (HLA). The HLA genetic locus controls immune responses, and the association of HLA–DR1 and HLA–DR4 with RA may indicate an effect on T cell function in the immune response. However, the mechanism remains unknown, and the HLA type may simply provide a marker for people who are susceptible to dysregulations associated with inflammation.

A second host variable in pathogenesis is gender; about 70%

of people with RA are females in most cultures, and an improvement in clinical status is often seen during pregnancy. Recent data suggest that an incompatibility at the HLA–DR4 locus is associated with this improvement during pregnancy (3).

The pathogenesis of RA is based on a hypercellular pannus resulting from proliferative and inflammatory responses in the synovial tissue lining the joint (2). The synovial lining develops from a one-cell layer to an extensive cellular tissue, which contains many growth factors, as well as inflammatory cytokines. If spontaneous remission does not occur within a few months, a persistent inflammatory process results from apparently inappropriate signals and continues production of cytokines and other mediators, leading to destruction of cartilage and other structural components of the joint.

Further evidence that RA cannot be regarded simply as a result of exposure to an infectious or toxic agent, is seen in dysregulations of normal host constituents, such as growth factors and cytokines, without a requirement for any abnormal protein or cell. One possible explanation may involve dysregulation in the hypothalamic-pituitary-adrenal axis. Normally, endogenous corticosteroids are secreted by the adrenal glands in response to adrenocorticotropic hormone, which in turn is secreted by the pituitary gland in response to corticotropin releasing factor (CRF) produced by the hypothalamus. A stressful stimulus results in increased corticosteroid production. However, people with RA appear to have a blunted response to CRF, leading to insufficient corticosteroid production, which may explain why people with RA often respond to very low, sub-physiologic doses of corticosteroids. This observation also suggests that the pathogenesis of RA could be based on endogenous dysregulations, without any exogenous etiologic stimulus.

DIAGNOSIS AND MONITORING

There is no single diagnostic test available to establish the definitive diagnosis of RA, analogous to a blood glucose test in diabetes or a biopsy in cancer. As discussed below, rheumatoid factor is found in only 80% of patients with RA and is not a diagnostic test for the disease. Therefore, RA is best defined as a clinical entity in which a patient has symmetric polyarthritis (Figure 1), and morning stiffness that has persisted for more than 60 days. Various sets of criteria for RA (Table 1), described as "classification" criteria rather than "diagnostic" cri-

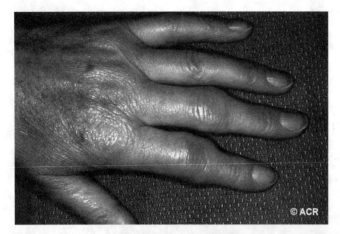

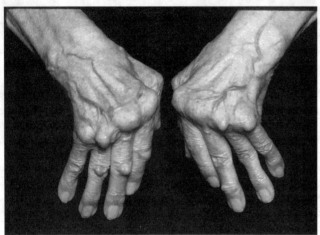

Figure 1. Hand of patient with early rheumatoid arthritis (RA) **(top)** and late RA **(bottom)**. Soft-tissue swelling is an early finding in RA and and usually appears as fusiform or spindle-shaped enlargement of the proximal interphalangeal joints. At bottom, ulnar deviation, metacarpophalangeal joint subluxation, and intrinsic muscle atrophy can be seen in longstanding RA. Rheumatoid nodules are seen over the right proximal interphalangeal joints, the metacarpophalangeal joints, and the left third distal interphalangeal joint (reprinted from the Clinical Slide Collection on the Rheumatic Diseases, copyright 1995).

teria, have been developed to promote uniformity in research studies.

Classification Criteria

The classification criteria for RA identify individuals with very heterogenous courses of disease. It has been suggested that there are at least three types of individuals who meet criteria for RA (Table 2) (4). Type I individuals have a self-limited inflammatory polyarthritis, which meets criteria at time of presentation. *Type I RA* is often a post-viral syndrome that resolves without a visit to a health professional. Nonetheless, it has been documented in population-based studies that at least one-half of people who met definite criteria for RA did not have evidence of disease 3 to 5 years later, suggesting that this disease type is quite common (5). *Type II RA* describes patients who have persistent disease that does not lead to significant long-term consequences and is manageable by traditional therapies. *Type III RA* is a progressive disease even with traditional therapies. The natural history of this type is characterized by radiographic damage, decline in functional status, work disability, and premature mortality in most patients. Type III RA is seen in more than 50% (up to 90%) of patients managed in clinical settings. Because it was recognized that some, if not many, people who meet criteria for RA had a self-limited or relatively mild disease, there has been considerable reluctance to initiate aggressive treatment for people with RA until recent years.

Clinical History

The clinical history of a patient with RA generally includes pain and symmetric swelling involving multiple joints. Any joint may be affected, but those most commonly involved are the second and third metacarpophalangeal (MCP) joints of the hand, second and third proximal interphalangeal joints (PIP) of the hand, foot metatarsophalangeal (MTP) joints, wrists, knees, elbows, and, less commonly, shoulder, hip, and distal interphalangeal joints (6). A characteristic finding is morning stiffness, which may last for several hours after arising.

Although RA is manifested primarily by joint involvement, it is a systemic inflammatory disease. Most patients note systemic symptoms such as fatigue, pain, and malaise, which may be as prominent as, or more prominent than joint pain in certain patients. Extra-articular involvement may be seen, including

Table 1. 1988 Revised ACR Criteria for Classification of Rheumatoid Arthritis* (RA).

Criteria	Definition
Morning stiffness	Morning stiffness in and around the joints lasting at least 1 hour before maximal improvement
Arthritis of three or more joint areas	At least three joint areas have simultaneously had soft tissue swelling or fluid (not bony overgrowth alone) observed by a physician. The 14 possible joint areas are (right or left): PIP, MCP, wrist, elbow, knee, ankle, and MTP joints
Arthritis of hand joints	At least one joint area swollen as above in wrist, MCP, or PIP joint
Symmetric arthritis	Simultaneous involvement of the same joint areas (as in 2) on both sides of the body (bilateral involvement of PIP, MCP, or MTP joints is acceptable without absolute symmetry)
Rheumatoid nodules	Subcutaneous nodules, over bony prominences, or extensor surfaces, or in juxta-articular regions, observed by a physician
Serum rheumatoid factor	Demonstration of abnormal amounts of serum "rheumatoid factor" by any method that has been positive in less than 5% of normal control subjects
	Radiographic changes typical of RA on postero-anterior hand and wrist x-rays, which must include erosions or unequivocal bony decalcification localized to or most marked adjacent to the involved joints (osteoarthritis changes alone do not qualify)

* For classification purposes, a patient is said to have RA if he or she satisfies at least four of the above seven criteria. Criteria 1 through 4 must be present for at least 6 weeks. Patients with two clinical diagnoses are not excluded. Designation as classic, definite, or probable RA is not to be made. PIP = proximal interphalangeal; MCP = metacarpophalangeal; MTP = metatarsophalangeal.

Table 2. Subtypes of clinical courses of patients who may meet classification criteria for rheumatoid arthritis (4).

	Type I	Type II	Type III
Type of polyarthritis	Self-limited process	Minimally progressive disease	Progressive disease
Predominant site of identification	Population studies; (occasionally in clinic)	Clinical settings (unusual)	Clinical settings (usual)
Estimated proportion of next 100 patients with Ra to be seen by a rheumatologist	5% to 20%	5% to 20%	60% to 90%
Rheumatoid factor positive (%)	<5%	60% to 90%	60% to 90%
Odds of HLA–DR4	1:1	3–5:1	3–5:1
Meet RA Criteria 3–10 years later (%)	0% (by definition)	90% to 100% (a few may have a different diagnosis)	90% to 100% (a few may have a different diagnosis)
Response to traditional treatment approach	Long-term treatment not needed	Good, although some progression usually seen	Disease progression continues, despite treatment
Markers to distinguish from other types	Rheumatoid factor; HLA–DR4	Course over 30–180 days; ?Baseline clinical markers	Course over 30–180 days; ?Baseline clinical markers

Sjogren's syndrome with dry eyes and dry mouth, and more rarely, Felty's syndrome with splenomegaly and leukopenia.

Physical Examination

Swelling and tenderness are generally noted in at least three joint areas, including at least one hand joint in most patients. A glossary committee of the American Rheumatism Association (now the American College of Rheumatology [ACR]) identified five types of joint abnormalities for recording on physical examination: tenderness, swelling, pain on motion, limited motion, and deformity. Studies of joint abnormalities indicate that pain on motion is correlated with joint tenderness and limited motion is correlated with deformity; thus, the observer may enumerate three types of abnormalities, i.e., tenderness or pain on motion, swelling, and limited motion or deformity (6).

The primary changes associated with inflammation are tenderness and swelling for all joints except the shoulder and hip joints, in which pain on motion is a primary indicator of inflammation. In clinical trials, it has been suggested that a core data set (7) should include counts of joint tenderness and swelling, which are responsive to change over relatively short periods. Joint limited motion or deformity are not necessarily included, as they are often unresponsive over short periods. Over long periods, however, joint tenderness and swelling may improve, while progressive deformity and disability may develop (8). Therefore, in order to assess long-term effects of disease, it is necessary to have a baseline measure of deformity or limited motion.

A general physical examination is indicated in all patients with RA, because of the systemic nature of the disease. Other associated comorbid diseases, such as cardiovascular and gastrointestinal disease, are more likely to be seen in people with RA than in the general population (1). The physical examination should include a search for rheumatoid nodules on the extensor surfaces of the arms and legs, dry eyes or dry mouth associated with Sjogren's syndrome, splenomegaly associated with Felty's syndrome, and evidence of vasculitis including abdominal tenderness and palpable purpura, which are quite unusual. Assessment of possible muscle weakness and neurologic abnormalities is also indicated.

Radiographic Abnormalities

Early radiographs in RA indicate juxta-articular osteopenia and soft tissue swelling, which should be evident from physical examination. Further disease progression results in cartilage destruction, manifested radiographically as joint space narrowing and erosion. Over time, radiographic evidence of malalignment, which is correlated with physical joint deformity, may be noted.

More than one-half of patients with RA develop radiographic abnormalities within the first 2 years of disease. However, there generally is no evidence of malalignment on the radiograph, or of joint deformity on physical examination; hence, potential damage from disease is underestimated. A normal radiograph does not exclude a diagnosis of RA, and indeed may indicate the optimal circumstances in which to initiate aggressive treatment.

Laboratory Tests

The diagnosis of RA can be made in the absence of any laboratory tests, and all laboratory tests may be normal in certain patients. Nonetheless, four types of laboratory data may contribute to the diagnosis and assessment of the severity of RA in an individual patient.

General Hematologic Data. Patients with RA often have a mild to severe anemia known as the *anemia of chronic disease*, which may occasionally be severe. In addition, patients with severe RA often have thrombocytosis, a high platelet count that accompanies inflammation. The white blood cell count generally is not elevated, as in an acute infection; a significant elevation may suggest an infected joint.

Acute Phase Reactants. Acute phase reactants such as the erythrocyte sedimentation rate (ESR) and C reactive protein (CRP) are elevated in the presence of active inflammation, which is characteristic of many patients with RA. However, as many as 40% of patients with RA have normal values for these tests, despite significant clinical evidence of inflammation. It is important to recognize that a normal ESR or CRP does not exclude a diagnosis of RA.

Rheumatoid Factor. Rheumatoid factor was identified in 1948 as immunoglobulin M (IgM) that binds to the Fc portion of Immunoglobulin G (IgG) as an "antiglobulin." Rheumatoid factor is found in approximately 70% to 90% of people with RA. Nonetheless, rheumatoid factor does not provide a specific diagnostic test for RA. In every clinical series (except those in which patients are excluded because they do not have rheumatoid factor), at least 10% to 20% of patients who are not distinct clinically have no evidence of rheumatoid factor. In population studies, only about 25% of people who meet criteria for RA have rheumatoid factor, and the absence of rheumatoid factor in no way excludes RA. Conversely, a positive rheumatoid factor test may be seen in many conditions associated with chronic immunologic stimulation, including chronic infections such as leprosy, tuberculosis, and chronic hepatitis, as well as pulmonary fibrosis and other diseases. Occasionally rheumatoid factor is found in a normal individual. Therefore, a positive rheumatoid factor does not establish a diagnosis of RA, although when seen in association with a typical clinical picture, it does help to confirm the clinical impression.

HLA–DR4. People with a specific haplotype at the HLA–DR4 locus (*0401 or *0101) have a five-fold higher likelihood of developing RA than an individual in the general population. However, HLA–DR4 also is not a diagnostic test for RA for several reasons. First, most people who have the *0401 or *0101 haplotype do not have RA. Second, only about 70% of people who have a diagnosis of RA have these haplotypes. Finally, although the *0401 and *0101 haplotypes are associated with a somewhat higher likelihood of radiographic damage and the presence of rheumatoid factor (9), they are not associated with greater severity of disease other than as a predictor of Type II or Type III (rather than Type I) RA. Therefore, a HLA typing test is not useful clinically in the diagnosis or management of patients with RA.

Functional Status Questionnaires

Over the last 15 years, an important development in rheumatology has been the development and use of functional status questionnaires completed by the patient to monitor clinical status. The most widely used questionnaires include the Health Assessment Questionnaire (HAQ), its modified version (MHAQ), and the Arthritis Impact Measurement Scales (AIMS). These questionnaires have been found to be effective in clinical trials to monitor disease status (see Chapter 5, Health Status Assessment). The HAQ and MHAQ have been found to be representative of other clinical measures to assess patient status (10). In a two-page format, the MHAQ provides a permanent record of functional status, pain, fatigue, global status, learned helplessness and other psychological distress, as well as medications, and is as effective as any clinical measure to predict mortality over 5 to 15 years in RA (1,11).

Functional status questionnaires have been used primarily as research tools, but some clinicians have incorporated them into routine clinical care (11). A self-report questionnaire can be given to the patient at each visit by the receptionist, and completed in 10 to 15 minutes (sometimes with help from a family member or the office staff) prior to being seen by the physician. A patient questionnaire is the only effective method to document such important clinical constructs as functional disability, pain, fatigue, and psychological distress, which are the primary concerns of patients and health professionals, and cannot be assessed by radiographs, laboratory tests, or physical examination. Therefore, a self-report questionnaire may be the optimal method to document effectiveness of care for people with RA.

Physical Measures of Functional Status

Physical measures of functional status have been available for many years and include grip strength, walk time, and button test. These measures, which have been termed *rheumatology function tests* (12), are effective in assessing clinical status and monitoring response to therapies. Poor results, as recorded by these measures, are associated with significantly decreased survival over the subsequent 5 to 15 years.

Differential Diagnosis

The primary considerations in differential diagnosis of RA include other types of inflammatory arthritis, as well as fibromyalgia and osteoarthritis (OA). The term *inflammatory polyarthritis* (ICD9 Code 714.9 versus 714.0 for RA) may be applied to patients who may have Type I RA with evidence of a self-limited inflammatory polyarticular disease, which may also be termed *reactive arthritis* or *post-infectious arthritis*.

Fibromyalgia can usually be distinguished from RA by the presence of generalized tenderness not limited to joints, a history of various forms of somatization disorders such as irritable bowel syndrome or migraine headaches, and a history of sleep difficulty (see Chapter 33, Common Soft Tissue Rheumatic Diseases). However, all these findings may be seen in patients with RA, and the differential diagnosis of fibromyalgia and RA may be quite difficult. Both types of patients present with generalized musculoskeletal pain, morning stiffness, and a suggestion of tender joints. There also appears to be a higher prevalence of fibromyalgia in RA, and many patients with RA have symptoms that are secondary to a noninflammatory fibromyalgia rather than RA. In most cases, the distinction between fibromyalgia and RA may become clear over several months, but some patients may have mild fibromyalgia and RA concomitantly.

Osteoarthritis is usually not generalized, and affects the DIP joints of the hands and other joints in a pauciarticular pattern (i.e., a few joints are affected). In general, OA is not associated with constitutional symptoms, and usually does not lead to as severe functional disability as RA, particularly in the hands. Severe OA of the hips or knees may lead to disability comparable to RA, however.

Other inflammatory rheumatic diseases to be considered in the differential diagnosis include ankylosing spondylitis, systemic lupus erythematosus (SLE), systemic sclerosis, polymyositis, and vasculitis. One source of confusion is the finding of a positive antinuclear antibody (ANA) test, a test that is positive in almost all patients with SLE (see Chapter 28, Connective Tissue Diseases). The ANA test may also be positive in many patients with RA, and does not indicate that the patient has SLE. Uncommon conditions that may simulate RA include hypothyroidism, subacute bacterial endocarditis, calcific periarthritis, familial Mediterranean fever, hemochromatosis, sickle cell disease, hypertrophic osteoarthropathy, and rheumatic fever. Polymyalgia rheumatica and giant cell arteritis may appear similar to RA, and some observers have suggested it is a form of seronegative (rheumatoid factor negative) RA. Gout, known as "the great masquerader", must always be considered in the differential diagnosis, particularly as tophaceous deposits may simulate rheumatoid nodules (see Chapter 31, Acute Inflammatory Arthritis).

COURSE AND PROGNOSIS

The course of RA tends to be uncertain for at least two reasons. First, the natural history of groups of patients includes at least three types, as noted above (4), which cannot be distinguished definitively by laboratory tests or other studies, although patients with Types II and III RA are more likely to have rheumatoid factor and be HLA–DR4 positive. Second, the courses of individual patients with Types II and III RA may vary considerably, from a rapidly severe course to a relatively undulating course, both from patient to patient and within the same patient at different periods.

Careful monitoring over 1 to 3 months is often the most helpful method to predict the course of disease, if evidence of progressive disease is not apparent at presentation. Clearly, a patient who has 10 swollen joints at presentation but had 30 swollen joints 2 weeks earlier differs in prognosis from a patient who has 10 swollen joints and had 3 swollen joints 2 weeks earlier. However, the rate of change in patient measures at the time of the first visit generally has been neglected in development of criteria.

For the most part, RA was regarded in the 1970s and 1980s as "a disease with a good prognosis," which "the majority of patients can control satisfactorily with well-accepted, conservative regimens" (1). This belief was based in part on the assumption that data from population-based studies—in which the majority of patients had Type I RA with a self-limited process—applied to most patients seen in clinical settings. However, the great majority of patients with clinical RA have a Type III progressive course.

It is important to distinguish between inflammatory activity and end organ long-term damage in assessment of outcomes (13). Measures of inflammatory activity, including ESR, number of tender joints, and patient global status, may improve even in the face of progressive radiographic structural joint damage and functional disability (8). Assessment of improvement in RA without a measure of functional disability and radiographic progression may lead to inappropriate optimism concerning the outcomes of therapy. Most patients with Type III RA show radiographic damage (14), severe functional declines (15–17), work disability (15,18), and premature mortality (19,20), in long-term clinical studies.

Radiographic damage in RA is often seen within the first 2 years (14). Increases in radiographic scores according to various quantitative methods appear more rapid in early disease than late in the disease course (21). Radiographic progression has been found in all longitudinal studies of patients with RA.

Over time, most patients with RA show severe declines in functional status that are not explained by age. For example, in analyses over 9 years in 75 patients (15), most declined in capacities to perform physical tests of function, grip strength, and the button test, as well as in functional status according to questions concerning activities of daily living (Figure 2). Many patients showed improvement in morning stiffness over 9 years, suggesting that the disease process may "burn-out" over time, but it may leave an individual with significant losses in functional capacity.

Work disability has been reported after 5 years in 60% to 70%

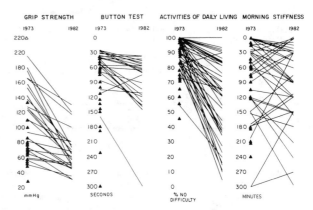

Figure 2. Changes over 9 years in patients with rheumatoid arthritis for grip strength, button test, activities of daily living, and morning stiffness. Patients who died over the 9 years are represented by triangles. Most patients show significant functional declines (reprinted from 10, with permission).

of patients with RA younger than 65 years who had been working at onset of disease (15,18). A high rate of work disability has been recognized not only in patients seen by rheumatologists who may have more severe RA, but also in individuals in the general population (22). More than 2 million individuals under age 65 in the U.S. population are unable to work because of RA.

Patients with RA appear to die from causes substantially similar to those in the general population, although with a higher likelihood of death attributed to infection, pulmonary, gastrointestinal or renal disease, as well as RA (19) (Table 3). However, patients with RA die at an earlier age than would be expected for persons of similar age and sex in the general population (1). Ten studies from diverse locations (Figure 3) all indicate premature mortality in patients with RA (one study incorporates comparisons with OA patients rather than with the general population, see Figure 3C).

Mortality, whether attributed to RA or other causes, is associated with more severe disease, rather than simply a random event in people with RA (23,24). In analyses over 15 years, significant high subsequent mortality was seen according to the baseline number of involved joints. Similar results were noted in counts that included 50, 36, 28, 12 or even 6 joints. Mortality was also predicted by poorer functional status, documented according to four measures: questionnaire responses regarding activities of daily living, grip strength, walking time, and

Table 3. Attributed causes of death (%) in 2,262 patients with rheumatoid arthritis in 13 series.*

Attributed Cause of Death	Patients with Rheumatoid Arthritis	1977 U.S. Population
Cardiovascular disease	42.1	41.0
Cancer	14.1	20.4
Infection	9.4	1.0
Renal disease	7.8	1.1
Respiratory disease	7.2	3.9
Rheumatoid arthritis	5.3	Not listed
Gastrointestinal disease	4.2	2.4
Central nervous system disease	4.2	9.6
Accidents	1.0	5.4
Miscellaneous	6.4	15.2
Unknown	0.6	Not listed

* Source: Pincus, T, Callahan LF: Early mortality in RA predicted by poor clinical status. Bull Rheum Dis 41:1–4, 1992

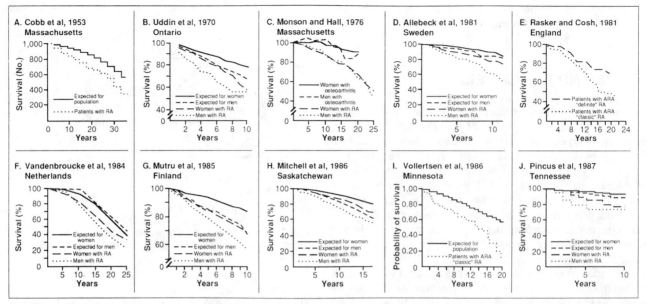

Figure 3. Analyses of survival in patients with rheumatoid arthritis compared to the general population (in C, patients are compared to patients with osteoarthritis; in E, two different groups of rheumatoid arthritis patients are compared). Note increased mortality rates in patients with RA over more than 35 years of studies from 10 diverse locales (reprinted from Br J Rheumatol 32:28–37, 1993, with permission).

button test. Earlier mortality was also predicted by high age, low socioeconomic status, and comorbid cardiovascular disease (24). Five-year survivals were in the range of 85% to 95% in individuals with favorable values, versus 45% to 55% in patients with unfavorable baseline values for these measures. The findings are not explained by age, disease duration, race, or clinical setting, although age, educational level, and cardiovascular comorbidity were also significant predictive markers for mortality in RA (24). Patients with poor clinical status according to measures of functional status or the number of involved joints, cardiovascular comorbidities, older age, and low socioeconomic status are 4.4 to 7.5 times more likely to die over the next 5 years than patients with more favorable status (24).

Long-term mortality rates in certain patients with severe RA may be similar to rates seen in cardiovascular and neoplastic diseases (Figure 4). Patients with more than 20 involved joints, or those who could perform fewer than 80% of activities of daily living without difficulty according to a questionnaire, had subsequent 5-year survival of about 50%, in the range of patients with 3-vessel coronary artery disease or Stage IV Hodgkin's disease (1). A smaller proportion of patients with RA appear in the poorest prognostic categories as compared to patients with cardiovascular or neoplastic diseases, and many patients with coronary artery disease and Hodgkin's disease were studied earlier in disease course than the patients with RA. Nonetheless, certain patients with RA have a poor prognosis for survival over 5 years, comparable to some patients with cardiovascular and neoplastic diseases.

TREATMENT

Non-drug Therapy

The foundation of therapy for RA does not involve drugs, but rather a therapeutic relationship with a caring and knowledge-

able health professional. It is important to overcome serious traditional misconceptions, such as beliefs that "there is nothing one can do about arthritis," or that "crippling is an inevi-

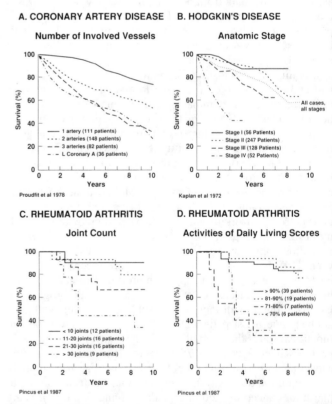

Figure 4. Examples of survival analyses in cardiovascular, neoplastic, and rheumatic disease based on specific disease markers at baseline, including **A)** number of coronary arteries involved, **B)** anatomic stage in Hodgkin's disease, **C)** number of involved joints, and **D)** functional status in rheumatoid arthritis (reprinted from Scand J Rheumatol 18 [Suppl 79]:67–95, 1989, with permission).

table consequence of arthritis and/or aging." It is also important to educate the patient regarding issues such as joint preservation through occupational therapy, exercise programs through physical therapists, impact of arthritis on work and family through a social worker, and education regarding disease course, drugs, and other matters through a nurse. Occasional intervention regarding vocational matters may involve a rehabilitation counselor.

These matters traditionally have been approached through a "team" of health professionals who interact with the patient. However, current health care reform in the U.S. has made it difficult to establish a team for each patient. Furthermore, it has not been definitively documented that a team is more helpful than one therapist who establishes a comprehensive therapeutic relationship. Therefore, it seems appropriate to recommend that any health professional who routinely interacts with RA patients should become familiar with the principles of various disciplines. Although an optimal situation might involve specialists from many fields to care for an individual patient, a health professional who interacts with a person with RA or other rheumatic disease may assume the role of an "arthritis therapist" in providing knowledge and information from many disciplines to the patient.

Drug Therapy

Drugs are an important component of the management of RA. Four types of drugs are important in patient management: analgesic drugs, nonsteroidal anti-inflammatory drugs, corticosteroids, and second-line agents for treatment of RA (see also Chapter 11, Pharmacologic Interventions).

Analgesic Drugs. Analgesic drugs are often ignored in treatment of patients; it is certainly desired that control of inflammation should result in control of pain. Nonetheless, patients with long-term disease may have joint damage which is unresponsive to anti-inflammatory therapy. It is often appropriate that patients be treated directly to control pain with such drugs as acetaminophen, propoxyphene (Darvon), and small amounts of narcotics when necessary. There is very little value in having a patient experience chronic pain, and there is considerable evidence that the capacity to control pain is important in enhancing self-efficacy and developing positive reinforcement for other therapeutic interventions.

Nonsteroidal Anti-inflammatory Drugs. The prototype nonsteroidal anti-inflammatory drug (NSAID) is aspirin, which was regarded traditionally as the mainstay of RA management. However, use of aspirin (particularly plain aspirin) is limited, because doses in the anti-inflammatory range required for disease control frequently result in gastrointestinal distress and bleeding. Newer forms of aspirin have been developed, including coated aspirin, aspirin with antacid or buffer, and long-acting preparations such as enteric coated Easprin® or zero-order release aspirin such as Zorprin®. These modified aspirin preparations are likely to have lower clinical toxicity than plain aspirin and thus are likely to be continued by patients longer.

Other NSAIDs show reduced gastrointestinal toxicity versus plain aspirin, but may not be as efficaceous as acetylated salicylates. Available NSAIDs include propionic acids such as ibuprofen, naproxen, and ketoprofen; a group of non-acetylated salicylates such as salsalate and trisilicate; indomethacin; diclofenac; meclofenamate; nabumetone; piroxicam; and sulindac. All NSAIDs have activity against prostaglandin syn-

thetase (cyclooxygenase), so that other adverse effects—including gastrointestinal irritation, interference with kidney function, and headaches and other unpleasant central nervous system effects—may emerge in some patients.

In an analysis of 1775 courses of various NSAIDs taken by 532 patients with RA in 7 practices, only 50% of the courses were continued 12 months, and only about 10% to 20% of courses were continued over 5 years (25). Acetylated salicylates were continued longest of all available NSAIDs. The most frequent combination of NSAID and second-line drug involved acetylated salicylates and methotrexate. Curiously, many computer-generated pharmacy lists suggest that these drugs are mutually incompatible due to protein binding interactions in the test tube; however, these protein binding interactions do not appear to be of clinical importance.

Corticosteroids. Corticosteroids have a long history in the treatment of RA. They were initially a "wonder drug" used in doses of 20–60 mg/day. Use of these doses longer than 6 months led to considerable toxicity and it was taught that corticosteroids should not be used at all in RA. In recent years the use of low-dose corticosteroid such as prednisone or prednisolone in doses of 7.5 mg or less has become widespread. Patients who take these low doses over periods of 10 years or longer have no higher prevalence of diabetes, hypertension, osteopenia, obesity, or other recognized complications of long-term corticosteroid therapy. Parenteral corticosteroids may be given periodically as an intramuscular injection of 40 to 80 mg of a long-acting preparation or as an intra-articular injection into a joint that shows disproportionate involvement compared to most other joints.

Second-line Drugs. A number of second line drugs are used to treat patients with RA. Second-line drugs are sometimes referred to as "disease modifying antirheumatic drugs" (DMARDs) and as "remission inducing" drugs. However, remission occurs in only a very small percentage of patients, and sustained remission is seen in fewer than 2% of patients over 3 years or more (26), and the term *remission inducing* should not be used.

Methotrexate is the most widely used second-line drug in the U.S., primarily because it is continued longer than other second-line drugs (27,28). The toxicity of methotrexate is low, in the range of many NSAIDs. The rationale for use of methotrexate initially was to destroy activated lymphocytes on the basis of its cytotoxic activity as an antifolic acid agent. Further research has documented that it also has anti-inflammatory properties, which probably represents the primary mode of action in RA. Initial dosage is 7.5 mg/week in three divided doses; this may be increased to 25 mg/week. The injectable form is considerably less expensive than pills, and may be taken orally. It is recommended that all patients who take methotrexate also take folic acid at a dose of 1 mg/day, which appears to reduce the likelihood of toxicity (29).

Potential toxicities include gastrointestinal distress and hair loss, which usually can be minimized through dosage reduction. Methotrexate is a liver toxin, but hepatotoxicity is uncommon unless the patient consumes more than one alcoholic drink per day; therefore, a liver biopsy is rarely indicated. Pulmonary toxicity (i.e., "methotrexate lung") may mimic a pulmonary infection and is the most serious clinical toxicity associated with the use of methotrexate in RA. Bone marrow suppression may occur rarely. Hematologic monitoring is indicated every 6 to 12 weeks. Methotrexate has the hypothetical potential to promote malignancy, although this has been found to be minimal in careful long-term studies.

The antimalarial drugs, chloroquine and hydroxychloroquine (Plaquenil), were discovered to be effective for patients with RA who where taking them for malaria prophylaxis. Chloroquine appears more powerful than hydroxychloroquine, but is more likely to be associated with ocular toxicity, including potential loss of visual fields and retinopathy. Hydroxychloroquine is rarely associated with ocular toxicity, although some gastrointestinal toxicity is seen. The dosage is 200 mg twice daily. Patients should see an ophthalmologist annually to monitor ocular status.

Injectable gold salts became a mainstay in the treatment of RA in the 1970s and early 1980s. Gold injections are given weekly at dosages of 10, 25, or 50 mg/week. After a response occurs they may be given less frequently, and traditionally were discontinued. However, many observers suggest that weekly, biweekly, or monthly maintenance may be appropriate to maintain a clinical response. Toxicities resulting from gold salts include an immediate flushing "nitritoid" reaction seen primarily with water-soluble rather than oil-soluble formulations. Other toxicities include hematologic cytopenia, glomerulitis, pulmonary toxicity, and rash. Blood counts and urinalysis should be monitored at least monthly.

Auranofin, an oral form of gold therapy, was introduced during the 1980s. Although auranofin has been shown to have efficacy in clinical trials, in practice it is generally effective only in patients with relatively mild or early disease. The primary toxicity involves diarrhea, although there may also be potential hematologic toxicity and nephritis, as seen with injectable gold. Auranofin is rarely continued over 5 years.

Sulfasalazine was developed to combat RA on the basis of containing an active salicylate moiety. It is the most widely used second-line drug in Europe. The dosage is generally 1,000 to 2,000 mg twice daily. Toxicities include gastrointestinal distress, rash, and "salicylism".

Penicillamine interferes with the binding of sulfhydryl groups, and is thought to possibly interfere with the binding of rheumatoid factor. In most cases it is used with a "go low, go slow" approach, beginning with 125 mg/day and increasing to 200, 500, or even 1000 mg/day. Toxicities include rash, nephritis, and hematologic depression, so that monthly monitoring of blood counts and urine is appropriate. Although occasional patients have excellent responses to penicillamine, its use has been largely supplanted by methotrexate.

Azathioprine is an immunosuppressive drug, which is thought to act through destruction of activated lymphocytes. It is given in dosages of 50 to 200 mg/day. Hematologic monitoring, initially at least monthly and later every 2 months, is indicated to check for bone marrow suppression. There is also some concern that azathioprine may contribute to increased susceptibility to malignancy, but this remains unusual in the doses used to treat RA (in contrast to doses used for immunosuppression in patients with transplants).

Cyclophosphamide is used primarily in patients with rheumatoid vasculitis. Although effective, it is not used in most patients because of the severe toxicities associated with long-term use, including leukemia and hemorrhagic cystitis leading to neoplasia of the bladder endothelium. The documented increases in long-term malignancies seen with cyclophosphamide are marked in contrast to methotrexate, which has little, if any, oncogenic potential in the doses used for patients with RA. Hematologic monitoring, including white blood cell counts and platelet counts, is indicated at least monthly in patients treated with cyclophosphamide.

Principles of Pharmacologic Management

The doses required for drugs such as methotrexate or azathioprine to be effective in treatment of RA are considerably lower than doses used to treat cancer or to suppress rejection in transplant patients. Patients with RA may experience substantial clinical improvement even if only 50% of activated lymphocytes are destroyed. Therefore, the margin of benefit to toxicity is considerably better in patients with RA treated with cytotoxic or immunosuppressive drugs than in other types of patients treated with these drugs.

Inflammatory activity is reversible, while resulting damage is irreversible (13). Therefore, the traditional paradigm that second-line drugs should not be used until there is evidence of severe disease, such as radiographic erosions, has been revised (1,30). It is now recognized that any patient is a candidate for second-line drugs as soon as the diagnosis of RA is established. Also, individual patients respond differently to different second-line drugs. There is no single drug that is optimal for all patients. Although all drugs used in RA have been documented to be quite effective in clinical trials, in clinical use, only methotrexate and corticosteroids are continued by more than 50% of patients for longer than 2 years, and by more than 20% for longer than 5 years (27,28). This means that each drug other than methotrexate and corticosteroids is effective for about one in five individuals but not effective for four of five individuals over long periods.

Recognition of severe outcomes in RA and limited effectiveness of current therapies in the long term suggest that an optimal treatment strategy is to control inflammation as aggressively as possible with combinations of several drugs, that are added or changed as needed (1,30,33). A decision as to whether an individual has Type I self-limited, or Type II or III progressive RA may require more than one visit, but can generally be made within 1 to 3 months of the first visit. Considerations of aggressive treatment may leave the health professional with a serious conundrum: the care of a patient with RA may be optimal only when both the professional and patient are concerned that treatment may be too aggressive or involve too many drugs. When it is obvious to all that aggressive treatment is needed, some irreversible progressive damage has likely already occurred, and it is probably too late to gain optimal benefit of treatment. The validity of an aggressive approach can be determined only through long-term studies, which should include a patient self-report questionnaire completed at each visit. The rethinking of treatment approaches to RA does appear to be leading to improved results to the benefit of people with this disease.

REFERENCES

1. Pincus T, Wolfe F, Callahan LF: Updating a reassessment of traditional paradigms concerning rheumatoid arthritis. In, Rheumatoid Arthritis: Pathogenesis, Assessment, Outcome, and Treatment. Edited by F Wolfe, T Pincus. New York, Marcel Dekker, Inc., 1994, pp. 1–74
2. Harris ED Jr: Rheumatoid arthritis: pathophysiology and implications for therapy. N Engl J Med 322:1277–1289, 1990
3. Nelson JL, Hughes KA, Smith AG, Nisperos BB, Branchaud AM, Hansen JA: Maternal-fetal disparity in HLA class II alloantigens and the preg-

nancy-induced amelioration of rheumatoid arthritis. N Engl J Med 329: 466–471, 1993

4. Pincus T, Callahan LF: How many types of patients meet classification criteria for rheumatoid arthritis (editorial)? J Rheumatol 21:1385–1389, 1994

5. O'Sullivan JB, Cathcart ES: The prevalence of rheumatoid arthritis: follow-up evaluation of the effect of criteria on rates in Sudbury, Massachusetts. Ann Intern Med 76:573–577, 1972

6. Fuchs HA, Brooks RH, Callahan LF, Pincus T: A simplified twenty-eight-joint quantitative articular index in rheumatoid arthritis. Arthritis Rheum 32:531–537, 1989

7. Felson DT, Anderson JJ, Boers M, et al: The American College of Rheumatology preliminary core set of disease activity measures for rheumatoid arthritis clinical trials. Arthritis Rheum 36:729–740, 1993

8. Hawley DJ, Wolfe F: Sensitivity to change of the Health Assessment Questionnaire (HAQ) and other clinical and health status measures in rheumatoid arthritis: results of short-term clinical trials and observational studies versus long-term observational studies. Arthritis Care Res 5:130–136, 1992

9. Olsen NJ, Callahan LF, Brooks RH, et al: Associations of HLA-DR4 with rheumatoid factor and radiographic severity in rheumatoid arthritis. Am J Med 84:257–264, 1988

10. Pincus T, Callahan LF, Brooks RH, et al: Self-report questionnaire scores in rheumatoid arthritis compared with traditional physical, radiographic, and laboratory measures. Ann Intern Med 110:259–266, 1989

11. Wolfe F, Pincus T: Data collection in the clinic. Rheum Dis Clin North Am 21:321–358, 1995

12. Pincus T, Callahan LF: Rheumatology Function Tests: grip strength, walking time, button test and questionnaires document and predict long-term morbidity and mortality in rheumatoid arthritis. J Rheumatol 19: 1051–1057, 1992

13. Pincus T, Callahan LF: Prognostic markers of activity and damage in rheumatoid arthritis: why clinical trials and inception cohort studies indicate more favorable outcomes than studies of patients with established disease. Br J Rheumatol 34:196–199, 1995

14. Fuchs HA, Kaye JJ, Callahan LF, et al: Evidence of significant radiographic damage in rheumatoid arthritis within the first 2 years of disease. J Rheumatol 16:585–591, 1989

15. Pincus T, Callahan LF, Sale WG, et al: Severe functional declines, work disability, and increased mortality in seventy-five rheumatoid arthritis patients studied over nine years. Arthritis Rheum 27:864–872, 1984

16. Sherrer YS, Bloch DA, Mitchell DM, et al: The development of disability in rheumatoid arthritis. Arthritis Rheum 29:494–500, 1986

17. Scott DL, Symmons DPM, Coulton BL, et al: Long-term outcome of treating rheumatoid arthritis: results after 20 years. Lancet 1:1108–1111, 1987

18. Yelin E, Meenan R, Nevitt M, et al: Work disability in rheumatoid arthritis: effects of disease, social, and work factors. Ann Intern Med 93:551–556, 1980

19. Pincus T, Callahan LF: Taking mortality in rheumatoid arthritis seriously—predictive markers, socioeconomic status and comorbidity. J Rheumatol 13:841–845, 1986

20. Pincus T, Callahan LF, Vaughn WK: Questionnaire, walking time and button test measures of functional capacity as predictive markers for mortality in rheumatoid arthritis. J Rheumatol 14:240–251, 1987

21. Fuchs HA, Pincus T: Radiographic damage in rheumatoid arthritis: description by nonlinear models (editorial). J Rheumatol 19:1655–1658, 1992

22. Mitchell JM, Burkhauser RV, Pincus T: The importance of age, education, and comorbidity in the substantial earnings losses of individuals with symmetric polyarthritis. Arthritis Rheum 31:348–357, 1988

23. Gordon DA, Stein JL, Broder I: The extra-articular features of rheumatoid arthritis: a systematic analysis of 127 cases. Am J Med 54:445–452, 1973

24. Pincus T, Brooks RH, Callahan LF: Prediction of long-term mortality in patients with rheumatoid arthritis according to simple questionnaire and joint count measures. Ann Intern Med 120:26–34, 1994

25. Pincus T, Marcum SB, Callahan LF, et al: Longterm drug therapy for rheumatoid arthritis in seven rheumatology private practices. I. Nonsteroidal antiinflammatory drugs. J Rheumatol 19:1874–1884, 1992

26. Wolfe F, Hawley DJ: Remission in rheumatoid arthritis. J Rheumatol 12:245–252, 1985

27. Pincus T, Marcum SB, Callahan LF: Long-term drug therapy for rheumatoid arthritis in seven rheumatology private practices. II. Second line drugs and prednisone. J Rheumatol 19:1885–1894, 1992

28. Wolfe F, Hawley DJ, Cathey MA: Termination of slow acting antirheumatic therapy in rheumatoid arthritis: a 14-year prospective evaluation of 1017 consecutive starts. J Rheumatol 17:994–1002, 1990

29. Morgan S, Baggott J, Vaughn W, et al: The effect of folic acid supplementation on the toxicity of low-dose methotrexate in patients with rheumatoid arthritis. Arthritis Rheum 33:9–18, 1990

30. Wilske KR: Inverting the therapeutic pyramid: observations and recommendations on new directions in rheumatoid arthritis based on the author's experience. Semin Arthritis Rheum 23 (suppl 1):11–18, 1993

31. Wolfe F, Pincus T, editors. Rheumatoid Arthritis: Pathogenesis, Assessment, Outcome, and Treatment. New York, Marcel Dekker, Inc., 1994, pp. 1–521

32. McCarty DJ, Harman JG, Grassanovich JL, et al: Combination drug therapy of seropositive rheumatoid arthritis. J Rheumatol 22:1636–1645, 1995

33. Tugwell P, Pincus T, Yocum D, et al: Combination therapy with cyclosporine and methotrexate in severe rheumatoid arthritis. N Engl J Med 333:137–141, 1995

Rheumatic Diseases in Childhood

DIANE M. ERLANDSON, RN, MS, MPH

The rheumatic diseases of childhood comprise a wide variety of acute but mostly chronic illnesses occurring before the age of 16 and affecting connective tissues. They range from single organ to multisystem diseases. Although some are short-term or self-limiting, the majority are chronic and can result in lifelong functional limitations. The rheumatic diseases of childhood are classified into clusters based on the nature of the disease or systems involved (1) (Table 1). These clusters include inflammatory rheumatic diseases of childhood, noninflammatory disorders, skeletal dysplasias, heritable disorders of connective tissue, storage diseases, metabolic disorders, systemic diseases with musculoskeletal manifestations, and hyperostosis. This chapter will focus on select inflammatory diseases, juvenile rheumatoid arthritis (JRA), and the spondylarthropathies.

Most of the epidemiologic data on childhood rheumatic diseases have been generated from the National Health Interview Survey (NHIS) and university-based clinic populations. Variations in prevalence, from 160,000 to 290,000 U.S. children (2), are largely the result of differences in data collection methodologies.

The age of onset is disease specific. In general, rheumatic diseases of childhood are more common among females, with the exceptions of systemic onset juvenile rheumatoid arthritis, the seronegative spondylarthropathies, some of the vasculitides, and septic arthritis (3). There is a racial predilection for some rheumatic diseases of childhood, which supports the possibility of genetic or environmental influence on etiology. For example, African-Americans have a higher incidence rate of systemic lupus erythematosus when compared to Caucasians (4).

JUVENILE RHEUMATOID ARTHRITIS

Juvenile rheumatoid arthritis is characterized by exacerbations and remissions and is the most common of the chronic inflammatory rheumatic diseases of childhood. The diagnosis is made only after all other disease entities are ruled out and the arthritis persists in one or more joints for at least 6 weeks (5). It is important for a pediatric rheumatologist to confirm the diagnosis early so that treatment can be started immediately. Other serious illnesses such as leukemia, which can also present with joint symptomatology, should be ruled out.

The diagnosis of JRA is based on clinical criteria with the support of laboratory tests and radiographs. The erythrocyte sedimentation rate (ESR) is usually elevated and can sometimes be used as a guide in the modification of treatment strategies, but it is not a diagnostic indicator. Active synovitis will yield an inflammatory synovial fluid; however, arthrocentesis is usually avoided in children because of its trauma. In early disease, radiographs may be of little diagnostic value but should be considered to establish a baseline. Magnetic resonance imaging, ultrasound, and computed to-

mography all play a valuable role in determining early joint and tissue changes (1).

There are three classifications of JRA based on the presentation at onset (first 6 months of disease): oligoarticular (40% to 50%), polyarticular (approximately 30%), and systemic onset (approximately 20%). The prognostic indicators for JRA are type, rheumatoid factor (RF) status, the course of disease, and the response to and side effects of treatments. It is essential to recognize that JRA is *not* adult rheumatoid arthritis in children. The clinical manifestations, pathophysiology, and approach to treatment are distinctly different.

The majority of children with JRA achieve permanent remission and, therefore, have no active symptomatology in the adult years. However, effects of the disease may cause long-term disability. Uncorrected flexion contractures, growth retardation, bone deformity, limb length discrepancies, visual impairment, and developmental delay may cause a lifetime of functional impairment (6). The treatment program *must always* incorporate regularly scheduled visits to a pediatric rheumatologist, physical and/or occupational therapy, regular ophthalmologic evaluations, and health teaching. In addition, the child's growth, development, nutritional status, and psychosocial function must be carefully monitored. Assessment and intervention in these areas will help prevent unnecessary problems and ensure the foundation for optimal function into the adult years.

The cause of JRA is unknown. Researchers continue to investigate possible etiologies such as infection, trauma, and genetic links. The initial presentation varies depending on the type of JRA and may include one, some, or all of the following signs and symptoms: joint pain and/or swelling, fever, stiffness, rash, fatigue, loss of appetite, irritability, altered mobility, and a change in or difficulty with activities of daily living, such as play. Impaired mobility, self-care deficit, and altered growth and development are common problems associated with JRA. Remissions may occur as part of the natural course of the disease or may be induced by treatment. Exacerbations may be an expression of the natural course of the disease, but frequently are a response to trauma, infection, or the withdrawal of anti-inflammatory drugs.

Oligoarticular Juvenile Rheumatoid Arthritis

Oligoarticular JRA is characterized by synovitis in four or fewer (asymmetric) joints, almost no systemic features, and a negative rheumatoid factor. Joints most commonly affected include the knee, ankle, or elbow. Children with this type of JRA and a positive test for antinuclear antibody are at very high risk for developing *uveitis*, which is usually asymptomatic and detected only by a slit-lamp exam performed by an ophthalmologist. If left untreated, uveitis (or its complications) can result in visual impairment, including complete blindness. Later onset oli-

Table 1. Classification of rheumatic diseases in childhood (RDC) (1).

Inflammatory RDC

- **Chronic Arthropathies**
  - Juvenile Rheumatoid Arthritis
    - Oligoarticular Onset
    - Polyarticular Onset
    - Systemic Onset
  - Spondylarthropathies
    - Juvenile-onset ankylosing spondylitis
    - Juvenile-onset psoriatic arthritides
  - Arthritides with inflammatory bowel disease
  - Reiter's syndrome
- Arthritis Associated with Infectious Agents
  - Infectious arthritis
    - Bacterial
    - Spirochetal (Lyme disease)
    - Viral
    - Other
  - Reactive
    - Acute Rheumatic Fever
    - Post-enteric infection
    - Post-genitourinary infection
    - Other
- **Connective Tissue Disorders**
  - Systemic Lupus Erythematosus
  - Juvenile Dermatomyositis
  - The Sclerodermas
    - Systemic sclerosis
    - Localized sclerodermas
    - Mixed connective tissue disease
    - Eosinophilic fasciitis
    - Other

Vasculitis

- Polyarteritis
  - Polyarteritis nodosa
  - Kawasaki disease
  - Microscopic polyarteritis nodosa
  - Other
- Leukocytoclastic vasculitis
  - Henoch-Schönlein purpura
  - Hypersensitivity vasculitis
  - Other
- Granulomatous vasculitis
  - Allergic granulomatosis
  - Wegener's granulotomatosis
  - Other
- Giant cell arteritis
  - Takayasu's arteritis
  - Temporal arteritis
  - Other
- **Arthritis and Connective Tissue Diseases Associated with Immunodeficiencies**
  - Complement Component Deficiencies
  - Antibody Deficiency Syndromes
  - Cell-mediated Deficiencies
- *Noninflammatory Disorders*
  - Benign Hypermobility Syndromes
    - Generalized
    - Localized
  - Pain Amplification Syndromes and Related Disorders
    - Growing Pains
  - Primary Fibromyalgia Syndrome
  - Reflex Sympathetic Dystrophy
  - Acute Transient Osteoporosis
  - Erythromelalgia

Overuse Syndromes

- Chondromalacia Patellae
- Plica Syndromes
- Stress Fractures
- Shin Splints
- Tennis Elbow, Little Leaguer's Elbow, Tenosynovitis
- Trauma
  - Osteochondritis Dissecans
  - Traumatic Arthritis, Non-accidental Trauma
  - Congenital Indifference to Pain
  - Frostbite Arthropathy
- Pain Syndromes Affecting Back, Chest or Neck
  - Spondylolysis and Spondylolisthesis
  - Intervertebral Disc Herniation
  - Slipping Rib
  - Costochondritis
  - Torticollis
  - Aneuralgic Amyotrophy
- *Skeletal Dysplasias*
  - Osteochondrodysplasias
    - Generalized
      - Achondroplasia
    - Diastrophic dwarfism
      - Metatrophic dwarfism
    - Epiphyseal Dysplasias
      - Spondyloepiphyseal dysplasias
      - Multiple epiphyseal dysplasias
  - Osteochondroses
    - Legg-Calvé-Perthes Disease
    - Osgood-Schlatter Disease
    - Thiemann's Disease, Köhler's Disease
    - Scheurmann's Disease
    - Freiberg's Infraction

Heritable Disorders of Connective Tissue

- Osteogenesis Imperfecta
- Ehler's Danlos Syndromes
- Cutis Laxa
- Pseudoxanthoma Elasticum
- Marfan's Syndrome
- *Storage Diseases*
  - Mucopolysaccharidoses
  - Mucolipidoses
  - Sphingolipidoses
- *Metabolic Disorders*
  - Osteoporosis
  - Amyloidosis
  - Rickets
  - Scurvy
  - Hypervitaminosis A
  - Gout
  - Ochronosis
  - Kashin-Beck disease
  - Mseleni disease
  - Fluorosis
- *Systemic Diseases with Musculoskeletal Manifestations*
  - Hemoglobinopathies
  - Hemophilia
  - Diabetes Mellitus
  - Hyperlipoproteinemias
  - Pseudohyperparathyroidism
  - Secondary Hypertrophic Osteoarthropathy
  - Sarcoidosis
- *Hyperostosis*
  - Infantile Corticla Hyperostosis (Caffey's Disease)
  - Other

---

goarticular JRA (age 10–12) is more common among boys and is often associated with the HLA–B27 genetic type.

Children with oligoarticular JRA are frequently stiff but may not always complain of pain. The level of discomfort is usually manifested by other findings such as irritability or holding the involved joint(s) in flexion or extension. Children are self-protective and change behaviors to avoid the discomforts of the disease.

Polyarticular Juvenile Rheumatoid Arthritis

Polyarticular JRA occurs more commonly in girls and is characterized by five or more joints with synovitis, occasional systemic features, and in some circumstances, positive test for rheumatoid factor. The joints affected are usually symmetric and may include the small joints of the hands and/or feet, wrists, elbows, shoulders, cervical spine, temporomandibular joints, hips, knees, and ankles. Because the bursae and tendons are also lined with synovial tissue, bursitis and tendinitis are not uncommon in children with polyarticular disease. Systemic features can include fever, anemia, leukocytosis, splenomegaly, hepatomegaly, and lymphadenopathy. Pericarditis and uveitis are rare (7). A positive test for rheumatoid factor in children with JRA is uncommon (approximately 20%), but when present it is usually seen in children who develop disease after the age of 11 (8), especially girls. These children tend to have more aggressive, erosive disease with subcutaneous nodules and more severe deformities. They very often require joint replacements and other surgical interventions during the young adult years or later adulthood.

Polyarticular JRA takes its toll on growth and development. Fatigue, pain, stiffness, and depression all play a role in limiting self-care, socialization, recreation, and participation in sports.

Systemic Onset Juvenile Rheumatoid Arthritis

Systemic onset JRA occurs at any age and is seen with equal frequency in boys and girls. It is characterized by daily high spiking fevers, synovitis in one or more joints, and a rash that is salmon pink, 2–5 mm in diameter, and macular with an erythematous perimeter (7). The fever may precede all other symptoms by months, so these children are often seen initially for fever of unknown origin. Other commonly observed signs and symptoms include malaise, irritability, serositis, anemia, leukocytosis, thrombocytosis, lymphadenopathy, hepatomegaly, splenomegaly, pericarditis, and/or pleuritis.

Systemic features of the disease, such as fever and fatigue, frequently impair function simply because the child feels too ill to do anything. Participation in play, recreational, or school activities may be dependent on the timing of the fever spike. Other functional limitations relate to the degree of involvement of the joints and other organ systems. As children get older it is possible for them to shed the systemic characteristics of the disease and develop more classic features of polyarticular JRA. These children are more likely to develop long-term disabilities.

Impact of Disease

Physical Impact. Juvenile rheumatoid arthritis presents special growth problems because of the hyperemia that arises with joint inflammation. Hyperemia around the joint provides excess nourishment to the bones, leading to overgrowth. When this overgrowth occurs in an extremity or a phalange, a discrepancy in length and size becomes apparent. If the hyperemia subsides in a short period of time, the rate of growth normalizes and the *catch up growth* phenomenon allows the unaffected side to reduce or eliminate the discrepancy. Stature may be stunted as a result of prolonged disease duration (9) and treatment, such as steroid use. The use of corticosteroids affects stature secondary to slow bone growth and vertebral crush fractures. When long bone growth is chronically delayed, permanent damage may be done. For example, when mandibular growth is retarded, *micrognathia* occurs, causing a recessed jaw. Cosmetically, this can be devastating to a child or teen. The associated dental problems include crowding of teeth, abnormal bite, and abnormal location of tooth eruption (10), all of which exaggerate the personal and financial repercussions of the disease.

Joint abnormalities include loss of motion in any and all planes, contractures, subluxation, and instability (6,11). Abnormalities usually occur when disease progression cannot be slowed or halted, or when physical and/or occupational therapy modalities fail. Ongoing synovitis can destroy not only the joint but the surrounding tendons and ligaments as well.

The gait of the child with JRA is disrupted because of insults to the lower extremities and the spine. Pain, stiffness, fatigue, active synovitis, joint abnormalities, spinal aberrations, foot callosities, discrepancies in length of the long bones, muscle weakness, and atrophy all contribute to an abnormal gait. Posture is also altered. Whatever the reasons for the aberrations in posture or gait, they should be evaluated and corrected as soon as possible to avoid or minimize long-term repercussions.

Psychosocial Impact. The psychosocial impact of JRA is very individual and requires initial and ongoing assessment by skilled professionals. Developing JRA is a stressful life event and causes further stressful life events such as frequent school absences (12) and change in financial status. The ability to cope with the stress of a chronic disease is influenced by personal skills, strengths and experience with coping, presence of concurrent stresses, availability and access to support systems, and response to treatment (13), all of which are dependent on the child's and family's stage of development. Severity

of illness does not seem to have the serious impact on the child psychologically or socially that one may expect (14). Problems that warrant assessment include impaired self-image, altered interpersonal and family relationships, dependency, anxiety, and feelings of powerlessness (14).

The child's or teen's perception of what is happening to his or her body, why it is happening, whether it will improve, whether the disease will ever go away, and what other people think are all based on stage of cognitive development. This is best demonstrated at the age of 13 or 14, when a child is cognitively able to understand the concept of conservation. Only then can a child understand the concept of *chronic*. It always comes as a surprise to the parent of a teen who has had JRA since early childhood that it is necessary to explain again that JRA is a chronic disease.

Families of children with JRA often experience grief not only at the time of diagnosis but also when exacerbations occur. The sense of loss of their "normal" child is overwhelming and recurrent. Not all family members go through the grieving cycle at the same time.

It is not uncommon for children and family members to require additional psychological support, such as professional, group, or family services, to assist them with coping. These options should always be recommended to families as part of their care plan. Children and families are usually much more receptive to psychological support if they are made to feel that referrals for such services are routine.

Function in the Developing Child

Because children are continuously growing and developing, using only one method for assessing function in children is not possible. The Washington Guide to Promoting Development in Young Children (15) provides reference on the necessary components of a functional evaluation at each stage of development. Function in the home, at play, recreation, school, and out of doors should always be assessed subjectively and, when possible or necessary, objectively. Pain, immobility, stiffness, weakness, and malaise associated with JRA can impair the achievement of developmental tasks or cause a regression in development. Parents can also play a role in impeding progress when they do things for the child because he or she takes too much time or elicits sympathy. Competency at each stage of development provides the foundation for positive self-esteem, confidence in independent function, and an affirmation of identity. Thus, health care providers should devote the time required not only to perform a functional assessment but provide the treatments and teaching needed to assure competency building. Parents should be actively involved in working with their child's competency program and providing the necessary guidance, encouragement, and reinforcement. Because school provides a strong medium for learning new skills, school personnel should be involved in the process, when possible, to provide continuity.

Treatment

The treatment program for a child with JRA is multifaceted. A medication-only program is not standard practice. All children with joint involvement should receive a physical and/or occupational therapy program and ongoing education tailored to individual and family needs. Other essential treatment program components include regular ophthalmologic exams and psychological support. Some children may also benefit from the services of an orthopedic surgeon, physiatrist, podiatrist, dentist, or nutritionist.

The treatment program should provide the necessary direction for the overall plan of care. Even though goals should be child- and family-specific, the following goals should always be a part of the plan: 1) alleviate or eradicate the inflammation and pain; 2) prevent physical abnormalities, disability, and psychosocial problems; and 3) ensure achievement of developmental competencies. These goals are best achieved through the efforts of an interdisciplinary team of professionals, the child, and the family. The use of health professionals with experience in the rheumatic diseases is key to the success of the plan. Even though the child's pediatrician should be an integral part of the team, the pediatrician does not usually have long-term experience in managing rheumatic diseases. Given the restrictions on approvals for specialty services, it will be a challenge for even the pediatric rheumatologist to continue developing long-term follow-up experience. It is not uncommon for case managers to allow reimbursement for a pediatric rheumatologist and other specialty services only if the child has a special problem or is in crisis. Health professionals must provide convincing evidence to case managers as to the potential short- and long-term outcomes for the child if their services are not provided.

Medications. There are no curative drugs for JRA. Instead the clinician must rely on anti-inflammatory and/or cytotoxic medications to alleviate inflammation. Recently, the standard approach to drug therapy for the child with JRA (initial course of aspirin before adding other drugs) has been questioned. There are numerous, well-documented studies that suggest the need for more aggressive anti-inflammatory treatment to suppress disease activity early in the disease process to limit erosive disease and, hopefully, disability (16). Children with active polyarticular JRA are now more commonly started with nonsteroidal anti-inflammatory drugs (NSAIDs) other than aspirin because of their ease in administration and low side effect rate. Methotrexate is another option (1).

Nonsteroidal anti-inflammatory drugs are short-acting drugs that can reduce the stiffness, pain, swelling, and sometimes the fevers associated with JRA. However, they have no impact on the disease process. Aspirin (75–90 mg/kg/day) is recommended in 4 divided doses daily, to achieve a therapeutic salicylate level of 20–25 mg/dL. Side effects of aspirin and other salicylates include stomach upset, tinnitus, behavior changes, constipation, bleeding, and hepatitis. Salicylates should be taken with food to prevent stomach upset; chewing should be avoided, when possible, because of the association with dental caries. Parents should be instructed about the association between Reye's syndrome and aspirin use while children are infected with influenza or varicella. It is customary for the clinician to discontinue aspirin if the child is exposed to varicella without immunity or if symptoms of influenza are suspected.

Other NSAIDs approved for use in children, such as tolmetin, naproxen, and ibuprofen, have been shown to be as effective as aspirin but are more costly. All can cause stomach upset and should be taken on a full stomach. The advantages of using NSAIDs other than aspirin include fewer daily doses and no risk associated with Reye's syndrome.

Disease-modifying antirheumatic drugs (DMARDs) are usually thought of as the second line of defense in the treatment of JRA. However, methotrexate is now recommended early in the course of polyarticular JRA because of its potential to reduce the pathological impact of disease. The DMARDs include methotrexate, antimalarials, gold, D-penicillamine, and sulfasalazine. These drugs are slow acting and, other than the antimalarials, have a high rate of toxicity. They are most often used in conjunction with NSAIDs.

Methotrexate (10–15 mg/M^2/week orally, up to 1mg/kg week parenterally) is given weekly. Tablets are often used first. If absorption becomes a problem, intramuscular or intravenous administration may be considered. The drug should be given on an empty stomach early in the morning. The Pediatric Rheumatology Study Group has established guidelines for the use of methotrexate (17).

Corticosteroids are used as infrequently as possible in the treatment of JRA due to significant side effects and the difficulty of weaning some children from their use, thus increasing the risk of the long-term side effects. They can be used as a last resort or in life-threatening situations that may occur with systemic JRA. Side effects of greatest concern are growth cessation, weight gain, Cushing's syndrome, osteoporosis with fractures, cataract formation, glaucoma, adverse effect on body image, and decreased immune response. Deflazacort may eventually prove to be less hazardous than prednisone and medrol (18). Occasionally pulse therapy is used in severe, unrelenting disease. Steroid drops are commonly used in the treatment of uveitis. On rare occasions when drops fail to reduce the inflammation, oral corticosteroids may be indicated. Intra-articular steroid injections in children are used occasionally when one or two severely inflamed joints are unresponsive to other treatment and infection has been ruled out.

Physical and Occupational Therapy. All children with joint disease should be evaluated by a physical and/or occupational therapist and provided with appropriate teaching and a treatment program. The goals of therapy are to improve motion and strength, preserve or enhance function, prevent disability, eliminate pain, and promote competency building consistent with developmental stage. Assessment should include careful interviews with the child and parent, musculoskeletal examination, and subjective and objective functional evaluations. An effective treatment plan is developed in collaboration with the child and parent, because they know best how a therapy program will fit into their daily lives. The plan should, therefore, be incorporated into the usual family schedule.

Most therapy programs for children include range of motion exercises, strengthening exercises, and pain relieving modalities. The therapist should start with baseline measures of overall function, muscles and joints, endurance, posture, gait, stair climbing, level of pain, and degree of stiffness.

All involved joints should be put through their full range of motion on a daily basis and ideally, range of motion should be accomplished twice a day. Parents and children find daily exercise difficult to adhere to when results are not immediate and when the program becomes a source of conflict. When possible, the therapeutic program should be fun and interesting. When joints are actively inflamed, therapy continues but becomes passive or active assisted. Therapists need to teach children and parents about the need to avoid forced or deep flexion in an inflamed joint. Prone lying is recommended for children with hip and knee contractures; this can be done with a pleasant distraction such as while listening to music, reading a book, or watching television.

When stiffness occurs during the day, the therapist can show the child methods to work it out using unobtrusive movements. Hydrotherapy and play exercises make therapy more palliative and help the child feel more normal. Education on gait and posture should be provided with each visit, and techniques for improvement should be incorporated into the child's day.

Splinting may be used to maintain alignment, relieve inflammation, and reduce flexion contractures (see Chapter 14, Splinting). Cervical collars can be helpful in preventing forward flexion and in stabilizing the head in the presence of cervical subluxation. Properly fitted footwear can reduce lower extremity pain and improve both posture and gait. Walking aids such as crutches and walkers (with or without platforms) are used only when necessary to limit weight bearing. Wheelchairs, scooters, and strollers are used only as a last resort. Use of artificial mobility can lead to flexion contractures in the hips and the knees, cause muscle atrophy and osteopenia, and make the child more dependent.

Heat and cold therapies are commonly used to reduce pain and stiffness and relax muscles for treatment. These modalities must be used with discretion in children, because they may not be able to adequately articulate discomforts. Heat modalities include warm water, hydrocollator packs, paraffin wax, heating pads, hot water bottles, whirlpools (with continuous professional supervision), electric blankets, and heat-retaining gloves. Ultrasound is not commonly used in children because of safety issues. Cold modalities include ice, commercial chemical cold packs, and ethyl chloride spray (19). Cold is usually applied until numbness occurs, or for up to 10 minutes for the young child who cannot communicate numbness.

Joint protection and energy conservation take on a different meaning in children. When children feel well or when they are determined, they will do what they want regardless of the disease. Most pediatric rheumatology teams try not to limit the child. Pediatric occupational therapists are especially skilled in teaching children how to alter tasks so that the joints are protected without attracting notice. As a rule, children should be cautioned to avoid repetitive movements (jumping, running, playing interactive video games) and aggressive sports (contact sports, karate) that could affect involved joints.

Surgery. Surgery in small children with JRA is rarely necessary. Synovectomy was once popular but the long-term outcomes of the procedure have not been significant. It is now used primarily as a palliative measure, after all else has failed. When performed, it is usually done through an arthroscope, thus expediting rehabilitation (20). Tenosynovectomy may be indicated when hand function is deteriorating or to avoid tendon rupture.

Joint replacements are only advisable when the growth plates have closed. Children with polyarticular JRA who have unrelenting disease may reach a time in the late teen or young adult years when the pain and loss of function prompt the need for arthroplasty. Usually a single joint, such as a hip or knee, is replaced. However, the need for multiple serial arthroplasties over many years is not uncommon especially in those who are rheumatoid factor positive (21). Prior to surgery, the appropriate therapists should evaluate the child and introduce the postoperative rehabilitation program.

Ophthalmologic Exams. All children with JRA should have a baseline slit-lamp exam by an ophthalmologist to determine if uveitis is present. The American Academy of Pediatrics recommends the schedule of exams outlined in Table 2

Table 2. Frequency of slit lamp exams by ophthalmologist in juvenile rheumatoid arthritis.*

Level of Risk	Risk Characteristics	Frequency of Exam
High Risk	Pauciarticular, onset <7 years, + ANA Polyarticular, onset <7 years, +ANA	No less than every 3–4 months
Medium Risk	Pauciarticular, onset ≥7 years, +ANA Pauciarticular, onset any age, −ANA Polyarticular, onset ≥7 years, +ANA Polyarticular, onset any age, −ANA	Every 6 months
Low Risk	Systemic, onset any age	Every year

* ANA = antinuclear antibodies.

(22) based on the identified risk factors. Frequent exams are also important for those children on drugs such as steroids or antimalarials and for children already diagnosed with cataracts or glaucoma. Ophthalmologic care and treatment must be individualized to meet the child's needs.

Nutrition. Diet has only recently received the attention it deserves in children with chronic diseases. Parents are particularly concerned about their children's dietary intake, with the hope that dietary changes will relieve disease. Nutritional screening is now recommended for children with JRA because 35% are noted to have protein-energy malnutrition (23). Nutritional consultation is recommended in children with weight gain or loss that is not consistent with their predicted growth curve and when steroids or cytotoxic drugs are prescribed. Because JRA impairs mobility, low energy expenditure in a child can cause rapid weight gain. Children and parents need the expert advice of a nutritionist to keep weight consistent with height and to prevent excessive strain on the weight-bearing joints.

SPONDYLARTHROPATHIES

The spondylarthropathies of childhood include juvenile ankylosing spondylitis, juvenile psoriatic arthritis, Reiter's syndrome, and inflammatory bowel disease. Even though these diseases may appear to be quite different from one another clinically, there are several important similarities. Each of the spondylarthropathies can cause peripheral arthritis, iritis, sacroiliitis and/or spondylitis, and are always rheumatoid factor negative. All of them may present with the signs and symptoms of JRA (usually oligoarticular) at onset, sometimes long before other disease manifestations emerge to help finalize the diagnosis. For example, children with psoriatic arthritis may develop oligoarthritis years before psoriatic lesions appear. Similarly, children with juvenile ankylosing spondylitis frequently will be diagnosed with oligoarticular JRA, but they will later develop other less characteristic symptoms of JRA, such as low back stiffness.

Table 3 provides an overview of each of the spondylarthropathies. Apart from juvenile ankylosing spondylitis, these diseases may appear at times to have nothing to do with arthritis. For example, a child with psoriatic arthritis may only have symptoms of psoriasis, while a child with inflammatory bowel disease may only complain of stomach cramps and diarrhea. Even though many of the treatments outlined in Table 3 are similar, treatment for the arthritis and other organ involvement may not only be intermittent but may be employed at different times.

Physical therapy is a mainstay for any treatment program for a child with spondylitis and sacroiliitis, especially juvenile

Table 3. Spondylarthropathies in children* (1, 7).

	Usual Age at Onset†	M:F	RF	ANA	HLA-B27	Sacroilitis	Spondylitis	Peripheral Arthritis	Enthesitis	Iritis	Systemic	Usual Treatment
Juvenile ankylosing spondylitis	8>	8:1	−	−	+	+	More so in adults	+	+	+	Rare	Tolmetin Indocin Sulfasalazine Physical therapy Occupational therapy
Juvenile psoriatic arthritis	<16	F>M	−	+	Low	+	Low	+	Low	Chronic	Psoriasis *Other – uncommon*	NSAIDs Gold Sulfasalazine Prednisone Topical steroids and coal tar (skin) Physical therapy Occupational therapy
Reiter's syndrome	<16	M>F	−	−	+	+	+	+	+	+	Urethritis Conjunctivitis Mucocutaneous lesions	NSAIDs Physical therapy
Inflammatory bowel disease	<16	Varies based on signs	−	−	+	+	Uncommon	+	+	+	Crohn's or ulcerative colitis Pyoderma gangrenosum Erythema nodosum	NSAIDs Sulfasalazine Steroids

*M = male; F = female; RF = rheumatoid factor; ANA = antinuclear antibody; NSAIDs = nonsteroidal anti-inflammatory drugs.
†In years.

ankylosing spondylitis. It is imperative that the child exercise daily, preferably at least twice, to maintain back motion and posture. Lying prone, stretching, and swimming are important components of a physical therapy program. Children with peripheral arthritis require an evaluation by a physical and/or occupational therapist, and often follow a therapeutic program similar to children with JRA. All children with inflammatory bowel disease must be evaluated by an experienced nutritionist with the benefit of ongoing follow-up during and after flares to ensure proper nutrition. Dermatologic consultation may be necessary for children with psoriasis. Treatment program methods, such as coal tar, are tedious and time consuming making adherence to the plan very difficult for the child and parents.

The impact of disease on children with a spondylarthropathy is very similar to that seen with JRA. Children with Reiter's syndrome may be embarrassed by and anxious about the urethritis and mucocutaneous lesions, just as flatulence and diarrhea can be upsetting for children with inflammatory bowel disease. The skin and nail lesions of psoriatic arthritis often have a significant impact on self-image. The lesions can be very difficult to hide and, therefore, leave the child open to ridicule from other children. Psoriatic lesions on the scalp cause severe flaking and scaling, which both adults and other children may perceive as the result of dirty hair. It is important to seek professional psychological screenings for these children and to make the necessary referrals for treatment when indicated.

THE SCHOOL SETTING

School participation is a child's work. It provides opportunities to develop intellectual and social competencies and motor skills. The health care team plays a role in helping the child

with school attendance and performance. This is accomplished by promoting collaboration between the school staff, the parent, and the team, by providing input to the school program (i.e., the individualized education plan) recommending physical and/or occupational therapy services during the school day, and offering ideas to modify school activities that are too difficult to accomplish or endure (24).

REFERENCES

1. Cassidy J, Petty R: Textbook of Pediatric Rheumatology. Third edition. Philadelphia, WB Saunders Company, 1995
2. Newacheck P, Taylor W: Childhood chronic illness: prevalence, severity, and impact. Am J Public Health 82:364–371, 1992
3. Maddison P, et al: Oxford Textbook of Rheumatology. New York, Oxford University Press, 1993
4. McCarty DJ, Manzi S, Medsger TA Jr, Ramsey-Goldman R, LaPorte RE, Kwoh CK: Incidence of systemic lupus erythematosus: race and gender differences. Arthritis Rheum 38:1260–1270, 1995
5. Brewer EJ Jr, Bass J, Baum J, et al: Current proposed revision of JRA criteria. Arthritis Rheum 20:195–199, 1977
6. Erlandson D: Juvenile rheumatoid arthritis. In, Pediatric Rehabilitation: A Team Approach for Therapists. Edited by M Logigian, J Ward. Boston, Little Brown and Co., 1989
7. Jacobs J: Pediatric Rheumatology for the Practitioner. New York, Springer-Verlag, 1982
8. Schaller JG: Juvenile rheumatoid arthritis: series 1. Arthritis Rheum 20:165–170, 1977
9. Allen RC, Jimenez M, Cowell CT: Insulin-like growth factor and growth hormone secretion in juvenile chronic arthritis. Ann Rheum Dis 50:602–606, 1991
10. Alepa R: Juvenile rheumatoid arthritis. In, Rheumatic Diseases: Rehabilitation and Management. Edited by G Riggs, E Gall. Boston, Butterworths, 1984
11. Athreya BH: The hand in juvenile rheumatoid arthritis. Arthritis Rheum 20:573–574, 1977
12. Lovell D, Levinson J: Health care services, school performance and needs

in pediatric rheumatology—results of a nationwide survey (abstract). Arthritis Rheum 30 (suppl 4):S35, 1987

13. Erlandson D: Helping the patient and family cope with systemic lupus erythematosus. In, Coping with Arthritis. Springfield, IL, Charles C. Thomas Publisher, 1988
14. McAnarney E, Pless IB, Satterwhite B, Friedman SB: Psychological problems of children with chronic juvenile arthritis. Pediatrics 53:523–528, 1974
15. Glanze W, Anderson K, Anderson L: The Mosby Medical Encyclopedia. New York, CV Mosby, 1992
16. Giannini E, Cassidy J: Methotrexate in juvenile rheumatoid arthritis: do the benefits outweigh the risks? Drug Saf 9:325–339, 1993
17. Gianinni EH, Lovell DJ, Hepburn B: FDA draft guidelines for the clinical evaluation of antiinflammatory and antirheumatic drugs in children: executive summary. Arthritis Rheum 38:715–718, 1995
18. Emery H: Treatment of juvenile rheumatoid arthritis. Curr Opin Rheumatol 5:629–633, 1993
19. Banwell B: Therapeutic heat and cold. In, Rheumatic Diseases: Rehabilitation and Management. Edited by G Riggs, E Gall. Boston, Butterworths, 1984
20. Vilkki P, Virtanen R, Makela A: Arthroscopic synovectomy in the treatment of patients with juvenile rheumatoid arthritis. Acta Univ Carol [Med] (Praha) 37:84–86, 1991
21. Scott R, Sledge C: The surgery of juvenile rheumatoid arthritis. In, Textbook of Rheumatology. Second edition. Edited by W Kelley, E Harris, S Ruddy. Philadelphia, Saunders, 1985
22. American Academy of Pediatrics Section on Rheumatology and Section on Ophthalmology: Guidelines for ophthalmologic examinations in children with juvenile rheumatoid arthritis. Pediatrics 92:295–296, 1993
23. Henderson CJ, Lovell DJ, Gregg DJ: A nutritional screening test for use in children and adolescents with juvenile rheumatoid arthritis. J Rheumatol 19:1276–1281, 1992
24. Wetherbee L, Neill A: Educational Rights for Children with Arthritis. Atlanta, Arthritis Foundation, 1989

Connective Tissue Diseases

JOHN H. KLIPPEL, MD

The term *connective tissue disease* describes a group of systemic rheumatic syndromes associated with antinuclear antibodies and immune-mediated tissue damage. The connective tissue diseases share a defect of the immune system characterized by a loss of tolerance to self-antigens resulting in the development of antibodies that are directed at nucleic acids and other intracellular proteins. The connective tissue diseases are often referred to as autoimmune diseases. The basic cause of the defective immunity in these diseases is uncertain, but likely involves an interaction between genetic factors and presumed, as yet unidentified, environmental agents. The prevalence, sex, and peak age distributions, and primary organ systems affected in the major connective tissue diseases are displayed in Table 1.

SYSTEMIC LUPUS ERYTHEMATOSUS

Systemic lupus erythematosus (SLE) is the most common of the connective tissue diseases (1–3). The clinical spectrum of SLE is wide and ranges from a benign, easily treated disease with rash, arthritis, and fatigue to a very severe and life-threatening illness with progressive nephritis leading to renal failure or irreversible central nervous system damage (Table 2).

Skin Rashes

Acute inflammatory rashes occur over the malar regions of the face (known as the "butterfly rash") (Figure 1, left) and between the interphalangeal joints of the fingers; however similar erythematous rashes may appear on areas of the trunk or the upper extremities that are exposed to sun. Chronic, scarring rashes, termed *discoid lupus*, may develop and have a predilection for the face, scalp, ears, and upper extremities (Figure 1, right).

Most lupus rashes are photosensitive. Patients should be advised to avoid intense sun exposure and to regularly use sunscreens. Topical applications of corticosteroid preparations are often helpful, and discoid lesions may be injected directly with long-acting corticosteroid suspensions. Antimalarial drugs, particularly hydroxychloroquine, are recommended in patients with generalized lupus rashes or rashes that fail to fully respond to topical corticosteroids. Options for drug therapy for patients with refractory rashes include antimalarial combinations (hydroxychloroquine, chloroquine, quinacrine), dapsone, retinoids, azathioprine, and low-dose oral corticosteroids.

Musculoskeletal Disease

The most frequent patterns of arthritis seen in SLE are a symmetric polyarthritis that resembles rheumatoid arthritis and a migratory oligoarthritis. A persistent monoarthritis, particularly of the shoulders, hips, or knees, suggests osteonecrosis

(avascular necrosis), or less commonly, septic arthritis. About 10% of SLE patients develop a deforming, rheumatoid-like arthropathy of the hands referred to as *Jaccoud's arthropathy*. The arthropathy develops as a consequence of recurrent inflammation of tendons and other supporting structures of the joints. The deformities are easily reducible, and bone erosions are not evident on radiographs of the hands. These findings are helpful in distinguishing the arthropathy from rheumatoid arthritis.

The arthritis of SLE typically responds well to nonsteroidal anti-inflammatory drug (NSAID) therapy; low-dose corticosteroids, hydroxychloroquine, or oral weekly methotrexate may be needed to control joint symptoms in patients with chronic arthritis. Early physical and occupational therapy is important in patients with Jaccoud's arthropathy to prevent progression of the malalignments and minimize functional disabilities (Figure 2). There are limited options for the medical management of patients with osteonecrosis. Patients should be referred to an experienced physical and occupational therapist for recommendations to reduce forces across the joint surfaces. Decompression core biopsy should be considered in patients in the early stages of the disease, as detected by magnetic resonance imaging scans. Patients with advanced osteonecrosis are candidates for total joint replacements.

Hematologic Disorders

Hematologic manifestations of SLE include anemia, leukopenia, and thrombocytopenia. Mild hematologic features typically respond to moderate-dose oral corticosteroids. Acute hemolytic anemia or aplastic anemia and severe thrombocytopenia with platelet counts less than 50,000/mm^3 are rare but serious complications that require aggressive treatment with high-dose corticosteroids combined with intravenous cyclophosphamide (see below). Additional treatment options for patients with severe thrombocytopenia include dapsone, immune globulin, and splenectomy.

Renal Involvement

In most patients, the presence of lupus nephritis or lupus nephropathy is first detected on routine screening studies with the finding of abnormalities on urinalysis and/or elevations of the blood urea nitrogen (BUN) or serum creatinine. The extent of the evaluation required depends on the type and degree of abnormalities found. For example, the finding of low-grade proteinuria on dipstick (Trace to 1+) and occasional red blood cells or white blood cells is generally a sign of mild renal disease that can be closely followed without the need for extensive evaluation or change in drug therapy. On the other hand, the finding of higher levels of proteinuria, greater numbers of cellular elements (particularly cellular casts) in the spun

Table 1. Epidemiology of the connective tissue diseases.

	Prevalence (Female:Male)	Peak Ages (yrs)	Primary Organs Affected
Systemic lupus erythematosus	15–50* (10:1)	15–40	Skin, kidneys, central nervous system
Scleroderma	10–20 (5:1)	30–50	Skin, lungs, kidneys
Inflammatory myopathy	5–10 (3:1)	5–15 and 30–50	Muscle, lungs, skin
Sjögren's syndrome	10–40 (9:1)	30–50	Exocrine glands

* Per 100,000 population.

urinary sediment, or clinical signs of renal disease such as peripheral edema or hypertension clearly indicate the need for a thorough evaluation to determine appropriate drug treatment.

Drug therapy for lupus nephritis/nephropathy is determined by factors related to the prognosis and severity of the renal disease. In general, a renal biopsy is required to determine whether proliferative changes are mild (mesangial or focal proliferative nephritis) or severe (diffuse proliferative nephritis) or whether membranous nephropathy is present. From a prognostic standpoint, the biopsy is particularly helpful in documenting glomerular sclerosis or tubulointerstitial disease, so-called chronicity features associated with an increased risk of end-stage renal failure (4).

In all patients with lupus nephritis/nephropathy, it is extremely important to aggressively control hypertension, use diuretics for fluid overload states, and treat hyperlipidemia with diet or drug interventions. Corticosteroids, typically mod-

erate-to-high dose oral prednisone given in the morning, are the mainstay of initial drug therapy. Bolus intravenous methyl-prednisolone is often given at the start of therapy to more rapidly control kidney inflammation, particularly in patients who are massively nephrotic or have an extremely active urinary sediment with red blood cell casts. The dose of oral prednisone is gradually reduced after 4 to 6 weeks; the rate of reduction (tapering) varies depending on how well the patient has responded and whether residual symptoms of SLE are present or not. In patients with diffuse proliferative glomerulonephritis, studies have shown that bolus intravenous cyclophosphamide reduces the risk of end-stage renal failure (5). Patients who develop end-stage renal failure are treated with hemo- or peritoneal dialysis and become candidates for renal transplantation.

Neurologic or Psychiatric Disease

The range of potential neurologic or psychiatric manifestations in patients with lupus is extensive (6). Clinical findings of central nervous system involvement predominate, and may include seizures, stroke syndromes, and transverse myelopathies. Minor psychiatric disorders, such as depression or dis-

Table 2. Clinical and laboratory findings in systemic lupus erythematosus.

Constitutional Signs	Musculoskeletal
Fever	**Arthritis***/Arthralgia
Fatigue	Subcutaneous nodules
Anorexia	Myositis
Weight loss	Osteonecrosis
Myalgias	Deforming arthropathy (Jaccoud's)
Mucocutaneous	Cardiopulmonary
Photosensitivity*	**Pleuritis/pericarditis***
Malar rash*	Endocarditis (Libman-Sacks)
Discoid rash*	Pneumonitis
Oral/nasal ulcers*	Raynaud's phenomenon
Alopecia	Thrombophlebitis
Xerostomia/xerophthalmia	
Renal	Neurologic/Psychiatric
Active urine sediment (nephritis)*	**Seizures***
Proteinuria (nephropathy)*	Stroke syndromes
Renal vein thrombosis	Movement disorders
	Psychosis*
Hematology	Immunologic Studies
Lymphopenia or leukopenia*	**Antinuclear antibody***
Anemia/**hemolytic anemia***	**Positive LE cells***
Thrombocytopenia*	**Anti-DNA and Anti-Sm***
False positive STS*	Antiphospholipid antibodies
Increased PTT	Depressed serum complement levels

* Criteria for classification of systemic lupus erythematosus developed by the American College of Rheumatology are indicated in bold print (Arthritis Rheum 25:1271–1277, 1982). Diagnosis requires presence of four criteria during any period of observation.

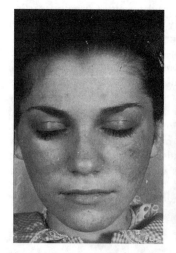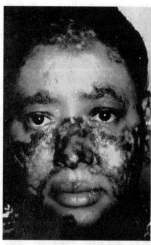

Figure 1. Lupus rashes. At left, erythematous eruption on the malar regions of the cheek extending across the bridge of the nose (the "butterfly rash"). At right, scarring discoid rash involving malar distribution (reprinted from the Clinical Slide Collection on the Rheumatic Diseases, copyright 1995. Used by permission of the American College of Rheumatology).

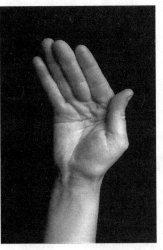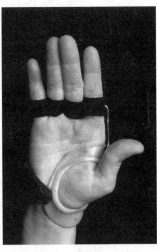

Figure 2. Correction of Jaccoud's arthropathy in systemic lupus erythematosus with orthoses (courtesy of Bonnie Thornton).

turbances of mental function, are frequent, yet in many patients it may be difficult to determine that they are secondary to underlying SLE as opposed to the stresses associated with chronic illness. The evaluation of patients with neurologic or psychiatric illnesses is complicated by the frequent failure to detect any abnormalities on routine testing with lumbar puncture, electroencephalograms, and magnetic resonance or computerized tomography scans.

Management of patients with neurologic and psychiatric manifestations is complex, with few therapeutic studies to guide treatment. The benefits of counseling, particularly in SLE patients with psychological disorders, has been clearly demonstrated in several studies (7–9). Attention to standard neurologic practices including anticonvulsant therapy for patients with seizures, anticoagulants for transient ischemia episodes, and acute and chronic stroke care are important. Aggressive drug management with high-dose corticosteroids or bolus intravenous cyclophosphamide as used in lupus nephritis is indicated in acute settings in which vasculitis is suspected. Thrombotic thrombocytopenic purpura is a rare but important cause of neurologic disease in lupus patients and represents the only clear, unequivocal indication for plasmapheresis.

SCLERODERMA

Scleroderma is divided into diffuse and limited subsets based on the extent of skin and visceral organ involvement, autoantibodies, and prognosis (Table 3) (10). In patients with diffuse scleroderma, there is a rapidly progressive, generalized skin thickening affecting the distal and proximal extremities and trunk. In contrast, the skin thickening in patients with limited scleroderma is confined to the distal extremities and the face. Limited scleroderma is often referred to as the CREST syndrome, which stands for typical clinical findings of <u>C</u>alcinosis, <u>R</u>aynaud's, <u>E</u>sophageal dysmotility, <u>S</u>clerodactyly, and <u>T</u>elangiectasis.

Skin and Calcinosis

Skin changes are first noted in the fingers in most patients. The skin goes through phases of early edema in which the skin is

Table 3. Comparison of diffuse and limited idiopathic scleroderma.

	Diffuse %	Limited (CREST*) %
Skin findings		
Telangiectasis	30	90
Calcinosis	5	50
Raynaud's	90	99
Musculoskeletal		
Arthralgias/arthritis	95	95
Tendon friction rubs	70	5
Myopathy	40	10
Gastrointestinal		
Esophageal hypomotility	80	80
Pulmonary		
Pulmonary fibrosis	70	30
Pulmonary hypertension	5	25
Renal crisis	20	0
Antinuclear antibodies	95	95
Anticentromere antibody	5	50
Anti-topoisomerase I (Scl-70)	40	10
Cumulative survival		
5 year	70	90
10 year	50	75

* CREST = **C**alcinosis, **R**aynaud's phenomenon, **E**sophageal dysmotility, **S**clerodactyly, and **T**elangiectasis.

swollen, shiny, and taut, followed by a slowly progressive hardening; both hypo- and hyperpigmentation may be seen. Ulcerations on the tips of the fingers from minor trauma are a nagging problem in many patients. Regular soaking of the ulcers in an antiseptic solution, topical application of antibiotic ointment, and use of occlusive dressing is helpful; however, it may take weeks before ulcers fully heal. Joint contractures result from fibrotic changes within tendon sheaths and should be aggressively treated with physical therapy. D-penicillamine is considered to be beneficial in patients with diffuse, progressive skin involvement (11).

Treatment options for subcutaneous calcium deposits that develop on the hands and in periarticular tissues along bony eminences are limited. Nonsteroidal anti-inflammatory drugs or oral colchicine may be helpful in reducing inflammation around the deposits; diltiazem, warfarin, and diphosphonates have been used in patients with severe, progressive calcinosis with occasional success. Calcific deposits frequently ulcerate, yielding a white, chalky drainage with secondary infection, typically with staphylococcal species, which require antibiotic treatment. Surgical excision and drainage of large deposits should be reserved for patients with massive accumulations because of problems with wound healing and the high likelihood of recurrence.

Raynaud's Phenomenon

All patients with scleroderma experience Raynaud's phenomenon (12). Mild symptoms are easily controlled with attention to practical measures such as adjusting the thermostat upward, avoiding exposure to cold, dressing warmly, and using insulated mittens or gloves. Patients who smoke should be strongly encouraged to quit. Battery-operated or chemical hand and foot warmers sold in sporting goods stores may help some patients. Warming hands in tepid water is usually an effective way to abort an attack. Biofeedback training may be helpful in patients who fail to respond to traditional conservative measures (13).

Drug therapy should be reserved for patients with severe symptoms. Calcium channel blocking agents are often effective. However, in many patients the dosage needed to improve symptoms is associated with intolerable vasodilatory side effects such as headaches, flushing, dizziness, palpitations, or fluid retention. Other drugs helpful in patients with severe, recalcitrant Raynaud's include prazosin or nitroglycerine preparations, used either as a paste applied to the digits or as a transdermal patch.

Gastrointestinal Disturbances

Gastrointestinal complaints are extremely common in patients with scleroderma. Dysphagia and symptoms of gastroesophageal reflux require attention to simple practical measures such as elevating the head of the bed, avoiding alcohol and caffeinated beverages, and eating smaller more frequent meals. Reflux esophagitis is managed with antacids, proton-pump inhibitors such as omeprazole or H2-receptor antagonists, and sucralfate used as a thick slurry prior to meals and at bedtime. Strictures of the esophagus may develop and necessitate periodic dilatation. Reducing the fiber and fat content of the diet helps minimize abdominal symptoms caused by dysmotility of the small bowel. Advanced involvement of the bowel leads to malabsorption and the need for oral liquid supplements or, in severe instances, intravenous hyperalimentation. Bacterial overgrowth may contribute to abdominal symptoms, including malnutrition, and should be treated with short, rotating courses of broad spectrum antibiotics.

Pulmonary Involvement

Several different types of lung pathologies are seen in patients with scleroderma, including diffuse inflammatory alveolitis, interstitial fibrosis, and pulmonary hypertension. In addition, scleroderma patients are at increased risk for the development of lung cancer. General measures of pulmonary care are important and include prevention of aspiration through the use of anti-reflux regimens, use of bronchodilators in patients with wheezing, yearly influenza vaccinations, early treatment of respiratory infections, and strong encouragement for smokers to quit. Recent studies suggest that intravenous cyclophosphamide may prevent progressive loss of lung function in patients with interstitial pulmonary fibrosis (14). Supplemental oxygen should be used as needed, and patients with advanced, end-stage disease are candidates for lung or heart–lung transplantation.

Renal Crisis

Renal crisis with malignant hypertension, microangiopathic hemolytic anemia, thrombocytopenia, and rapidly progressive renal failure is a serious, life-threatening complication of scleroderma. Prompt and aggressive treatment of the hypertension using angiotensin-converting enzyme (ACE) inhibitors is

Table 4. Differential diagnosis of inflammatory myopathies.

Drug- and toxin-induced	Corticosteroids, colchicine, cimetidine, zidovudine (AZT), lovastatin, D-penicillamine, chloroquine, alcohol, heroin, cocaine
Endocrinopathies	Hyper- and hypothyroidism, acromegaly, Cushing's syndrome, Addison's disease
Electrolyte disturbances	Hypokalemia, hypercalcemia, hypocalcemia, hypomagnesemia
Neurologic diseases	Myasthenia gravis, amyotrophic lateral sclerosis, muscular dystrophy, Guillain–Barré syndrome, periodic paralysis
Infections	Viruses (influenza, coxsackie, HIV, adenovirus, hepatitis B, rubella), toxoplasmosis, trichinella, Rickettsia, bacterial toxins (staphylococcal, streptococcal, clostridia)

critical. There is no role for corticosteroids, plasmapheresis, or immunosuppressive drugs in scleroderma renal crisis. Intravenous enalapril or short-acting oral ACE inhibitors may be used to acutely titrate the blood pressure to normal levels. Minoxidil is indicated in patients who fail to respond to ACE inhibitors in maximum dosage. Blood transfusions and diuretics may be used to manage symptoms of congestive heart failure. Patients who progress to end-stage renal failure should be treated with hemodialysis (or peritoneal dialysis). The experience with renal transplantation in these patients is promising.

INFLAMMATORY MYOPATHIES

Two major forms of inflammatory myopathy are recognized: polymyositis and dermatomyositis (15,16). The syndromes differ clinically on the basis of whether rashes are present or absent. Differences in pathophysiology of the two disorders are thought to exist, with *polymyositis* regarded as a cellular-mediated immune process against muscle myofibrils and *dermatomyositis* as an antibody-mediated injury of muscle capillaries. A third variant termed *inclusion body myositis* has slightly different clinical features and unique findings on electron microscopy of muscle biopsy sections showing microtubular or filamentous inclusions. The inflammatory myopathies may develop in patients with other connective diseases (mixed or overlap syndromes). In addition, there is an extensive differential diagnosis that must be considered in patients with proximal muscle weakness and suspected inflammatory myopathies (Table 4).

Routine studies helpful in the evaluation of patients with suspected inflammatory myopathies include measurement of levels of various enzymes in the serum, electromyography, and muscle biopsy. Levels of creatinine kinase and aldolase are sensitive markers of muscle inflammation; in addition, many patients have elevations of LDH, SGOT, and SGPT and often mistakenly undergo assessments for liver disease. The electromyogram is helpful in discriminating between pure neurologic and myopathic disorders. However, muscle biopsy remains the only means to establish the diagnosis with certainty.

Muscle Weakness

Patients with inflammatory muscle disorders often present with complaints of weakness of the proximal muscles of the upper and lower extremities. These commonly involve difficulties in performing simple everyday functions like rising from a chair, climbing stairs, dressing, or grooming. The weakness may be of abrupt or insidious onset. Other muscle groups commonly affected include the neck flexors (such that the patient is unable to lift the head against gravity), muscles of the oropharynx or esophagus causing dysphagia, and diaphragmatic and intercostal muscles leading to dyspnea. Involvement of distal muscles is a late finding; impairment of distal muscles early in the disease course suggests inclusion body myositis. Ocular and facial muscles are essentially never involved in the inflammatory myopathies.

Physical and occupational therapy play a very important role in the evaluation and treatment of patients with inflammatory muscle disease. In addition to providing assessments of muscle strength and functional assessments to help guide and monitor the response to therapy, active rehabilitation programs are a critical component of clinical care (17).

In most forms of inflammatory myopathy, therapy is initiated with high-dose corticosteroids, typically oral prednisone in doses of 1 mg/kg/day. The response to corticosteroids is often slow, and several weeks or more of therapy may be required before muscle strength begins to improve. In patients with very severe, acute disease, particularly those in whom constitutional signs such as fever, anorexia, and weight loss are prominent, intravenous bolus methylprednisolone in doses of 1 gram or 15 mg/kg often provides more immediate benefit. Methotrexate, either orally or intramuscularly, given weekly and/or azathioprine is recommended in patients who fail to completely respond to corticosteroids. Treatment failures with combined corticosteroid and antimetabolite drugs are a problem. Preliminary studies suggest there may be a role for gammaglobulin (18) or cyclosporin A (19) in such patients. Patients with inclusion body myositis tend to respond poorly to drug therapy (20).

Rashes

Several distinctive rashes occur in patients with dermatomyositis. Scaly violaceous patches (*Gotron's papules*) form over the extensor surfaces of joints, most commonly over the knuckles, elbows, and knees. The radial surfaces and pads of the fingers may become dry and cracked with black pigmentary changes (mechanic's hands). Erythematous, often photosensitive rashes occur on the neck, shoulder, and upper chest (V sign or shawl sign), and the malar region of the face. The facial rash can easily be confused with the butterfly rash of SLE; crossing of the nasolabial fold is a helpful physical finding that occurs in dermatomyositis. The upper eyelids may become edematous and develop a purplish (heliotrope) hue. Subcutaneous calcifications may develop within muscle planes, particularly in childhood-onset dermatomyositis, and these may ulcerate, drain, and become secondarily infected.

In most patients, specific therapies directed at the skin disease is not required, and rashes improve as the muscle inflammation comes under control. Hydroxychloroquine should be considered in patients with severe or progressive

Table 5. Diseases associated with parotid enlargement.

Viral infections (mumps, HIV, Epstein-Barr, others)
Sarcoidosis
Amyloidosis
Hyperlipoproteinemia
Endocrine disorders (acromegaly, diabetes mellitus, hypogonadism)
Chronic pancreatitis
Alcoholism/hepatic cirrhosis
Uremia
Tumors (especially lymphoma)

skin disease, particularly of the erythematous, photosensitive variety. There are no satisfactory treatments for calcinosis.

Pulmonary Disease

Dyspnea in patients with inflammatory muscle disease may result from several different causes. Myositis of the diaphragm or intercostal muscles directly interferes with the mechanics of respiration, dysfunction of the pharyngeal muscles may result in aspirations, and involvement of the myocardium or cardiac conduction systems leads to congestive heart failure. Interstitial alveolitis and progressive fibrosis occur in a subset of patients with antibodies to transfer-RNA synthetases, the most common antibody found is directed against histadyl t-RNAase (Jo-1). Therapeutic approaches to interstitial lung disease in inflammatory myopathies is identical to that described for pulmonary involvement in scleroderma.

SJÖGREN'S SYNDROME

Sjögren's syndrome is characterized by an immune-mediated inflammatory process of the exocrine glands (21,22). It is generally divided into primary and secondary forms based on whether or not another rheumatic disorder is present, such as rheumatoid arthritis or any of the other connective tissue diseases.

In most patients, the presenting complaint is dryness, typically of the eyes (*xerophthalmia*) or mouth (*xerostomia*). Tenderness or swelling of the parotid glands may also be seen. Evaluation of patients with suspected Sjögren's syndrome may include biopsy of the minor salivary glands of the lip, functional tests of ocular or oral glands, and testing for autoantibodies. Sjögren's syndrome must be differentiated from other disorders that affect the salivary glands (Table 5). Minor salivary gland biopsy is the only reliable method to diagnose the disease with certainty. Typical pathology consists of focal aggregates of lymphocytes, plasma cells, and macrophages adjacent to and replacing the normal acini. Larger foci often exhibit formation of germinal centers.

The Schirmer's tear test is used to assess tear secretion by the lacrimal glands. *Keratoconjunctivitis sicca*, the sequelae of decreased tear secretion, is diagnosed using an aniline dye (Rose Bengal) that stains the damaged epithelium of both the cornea and conjunctiva. Slit lamp examination after Rose Bengal staining shows a punctate or filamentary keratitis. Autoantibodies are commonly detected in patients with Sjögren's syndrome, in particular rheumatoid factors, antinuclear antibodies, and antibodies to extractable nuclear antigens, termed Ro (SS-A) and La (SS-B). These autoantibodies are not specific for Sjögren's syndrome and may be found in other autoimmune diseases, especially SLE.

The treatment of Sjögren's syndrome is largely symptomatic with the goal of keeping the conjunctivae and mucosal surfaces moist. Artificial tears should be used regularly. Available preparations differ primarily in viscosity and preservative. The thicker, more viscous drops require less frequent application, although they can cause blurring and leave residue on the lashes. Less viscous drops require more frequent applications. Soft contact lenses may help protect the cornea, especially in the presence of filimentary keratitis; however, patients must be followed very carefully because of the increased risk of infection. Avoiding windy or low humidity environments is helpful. Cigarette smoking and drugs with anticholinergic side effects such as phenothiazines, tricyclic antidepressants, antispasmodics, and anti-Parkinsonian agents should be avoided whenever possible.

Treatment of xerostomia is difficult. Most patients learn on their own the importance of taking small sips of water frequently and carrying bottles of water with them at all times. Stimulation of salivary flow by chewing sugar-free gum or using lozenges is often helpful. Patients should be instructed to avoid dry food, smoking, or the use of drugs with anticholinergic side effects that decrease the salivary flow. Periodontal disease and tooth decay are serious problems in patients with xerostomia; thus, patients should be reminded of the importance of brushing their teeth after meals. Topical treatment of the teeth with stannous fluoride enhances dental mineralization and retards damage. In cases of rapidly progressive dental disease, fluoride can be directly applied to the teeth from plastic trays that are used at night. Vaginal dryness is treated with lubricant gels and dry skin with moisturizing lotions.

Systemic and major organ manifestations of Sjögren's syndrome are infrequent, but include interstitial pneumonitis, glomerulonephritis, vasculitis, and peripheral neuropathy. Corticosteroids and immunosuppressive drugs such as oral or intravenous cyclophosphamide are used for patients with severe, progressive extraglandular disease. Sjögren's patients are at increased risk for the development of lymphoma. Decisions regarding chemotherapy and/or radiation depend on the histologic type, location, and extension of the tumor and should be guided by experienced oncologists.

REFERENCES

1. Mills JA: Systemic lupus erythematosus. N Engl J Med 330:1871–1890, 1994
2. Boumpas DT, Austin HA, Fessler BJ, Balow JE, Klippel JH, Lockshin MD: Systemic lupus erythematosus: emerging concepts. Part 1. Renal, neuropsychiatric, cardiovascular, pulmonary, and hematologic disease. Ann Intern Med 122:940–950, 1995
3. Boumpas DT, Fessler BJ, Austin HA, Balow JE, Klippel JH, Lockshin MD: Systemic lupus erythematosus: emerging concepts. Part 2. Dermatologic and joint disease, the antiphospholipid antibody syndrome, pregnancy and hormonal therapy, morbidity and mortality, and pathogenesis. Ann Intern Med 123:42–53, 1995
4. Esdaile JM, Abrahamowicz M, MacKenzie T, Hayslett JP, Kashgarian M: The time-dependence of long-term prediction in lupus nephritis. Arthritis Rheum 37:359–368, 1994
5. Boumpas DT, Austin HA, Vaughan EM, Klippel JH, Steinberg AD, Balow JE: Severe lupus nephritis: controlled trial of pulse methylprednisolone versus two different regimens of pulse cyclophosphamide. Lancet 340:741–744, 1992
6. West SG: Neuropsychiatric lupus. Rheum Dis Clin North Am 20:129–158, 1994
7. Peterson MGE, Horton R, Engelhard E, Lockshin MD, Abramson T: Effect of counselor training on skills development and psychosocial status of volunteers with systemic lupus erythematosus. Arthritis Care Res 6:38–44, 1993
8. Braden CJ, McGlone K, Pennington F: Specific psychosocial and behavioral outcomes from the systemic lupus erythematosus self-help course. Health Educ Q 20:29–41, 1993
9. Maisiak R, Austin JS, West SG, Heck L: The effect of person-centered counseling on the psychological status of persons with systemic lupus erythematosus or rheumatoid arthritis: a randomized, controlled trial. Arthritis Care Res 9:60–66, 1996
10. Seibold JR: Systemic sclerosis: clinical features. In, Rheumatology. Edited by JH Klippel, PA Dieppe. London, Mosby-Year Book, 1994
11. Pope J: Treatment of systemic sclerosis. Curr Opin Rheumatol 5:792–801, 1993
12. Klippel JH: Raynaud's phenomenon: the French tricolor. Arch Intern Med 151:2389–2393, 1991
13. Yocum DE, Hodes R, Sundstrom WR, Cleeland CS: Use of biofeedback training in treatment of Raynaud's disease and phenomenon. J Rheumatol 12:90–93, 1985
14. Steen VD, Lanz JK Jr, Conte C, Owens GR, Medsger TA Jr: Therapy for severe interstitial lung disease in systemic sclerosis: a retrospective study. Arthritis Rheum 37:1290–1296, 1994
15. Dalakas MC: Polymyositis, dermatomyositis, and inclusion-body myositis. N Engl J Med 325:1487–1498, 1991
16. Plotz PH, Rider LG, Targoff IN, O'Hanlon TP, Miller FW: NIH conference: myositis: immunologic contributions to understanding cause, pathogenesis, and therapy. Ann Intern Med 122:715–724, 1995
17. Hicks JE: Rehabilitation of patients with myositis. In, Rheumatology. Edited by JH Klippel, PA Dieppe. London, Mosby-Year Book, 1994
18. Dalakas MC, Illa I, Dambrosia JM, Soueidan SA, Stein DP, Otero C, Dinsmore ST, McCrosky S: A controlled trial of high-dose intravenous immune globulin infusions as treatment for dermatomyositis. N Engl J Med 329:1993–2000, 1993
19. Grau JM, Herrero C, Casademont J, Fernández-Solà J, Urbano-Márquez A: Cyclosporine A as first choice therapy for dermatomyositis (letter). J Rheumatol 21:381–382, 1994
20. Leff RL, Miller FW, Hicks J, Fraser DD, Plotz PH: The treatment of inclusion body myositis: a retrospective review and a randomized, prospective trial of immunosuppressive therapy. Medicine (Baltimore) 72:225–235, 1993
21. Fox RI, Saito I: Criteria for diagnosis of Sjögren's syndrome. Rheum Dis Clin North Am 20:391–407, 1994
22. Vitali C, Moutsopoulos HM, Bombardieri S: The European Community Study Group on diagnostic criteria for Sjögren's syndrome: sensitivity and specificity of tests for ocular and oral involvement in Sjögren's syndrome. Ann Rheum Dis 53:637–647, 1994

Spondylarthropathies

VICTORIA GALL, PT, MEd

ETIOLOGY AND PATHOGENESIS

The spondylarthropathies are a group of inflammatory disorders that share a number of common features, the most important being sacroiliitis (1). The prototype of spondylarthropathies is ankylosing spondylitis. Other spondylarthropathies include reactive arthritis (Reiter's syndrome), enteropathic arthritis (arthritis associated with inflammatory bowel disease), psoriatic arthritis with a spinal component, juvenile onset spondylarthropathy, and a variety of less clearly defined conditions (2). An increased prevalence of the histocompatibility antigen HLA–B27 is noted in most of the spondylarthropathies. The precise role of HLA–B27 in the pathogenesis of these diseases is under intense investigation. The fact that not all individuals with HLA–B27 develop a spondylarthropathy suggests that another factor such as an environmental or infectious agent is necessary to trigger the disease.

Periarticular structures and the associated entheses (or attachment sites) are the structures which become inflamed in spondylarthropathies. Prolonged inflammation may lead to osseous erosion and bony proliferation limiting motion and possibly leading to fusion. After the sacroiliac joints, the most commonly involved areas are the costovertebral, manubriosternal discovertebral, and apophyseal joints; the paravertebral ligaments; plantar fascia; and the achilles tendon (1). When present, peripheral joint involvement is similar to the synovitis of rheumatoid arthritis (RA).

DIFFERENTIAL DIAGNOSIS

Skeletal and extraskeletal manifestations differentiate ankylosing spondylitis and the related diseases. Table 1 compares ankylosing spondylitis with other spondylarthropathies. Inflammatory back pain, the hallmark of these diseases, differs from mechanical back pain. The onset of inflammatory back pain is insidious, occurs before age 40, is persistent, is associated with morning stiffness, and improves with exercise. Each disorder has a set of diagnostic criteria, but they are thought to be too restrictive, particularly in early disease where there may not be radiographic evidence of sacroiliitis. A broader classification system is being developed by the European Spondylarthropathy Study Group (3).

Laboratory tests do not confirm spondylarthropathy, nor do they correlate well with disease activity. History and physical findings are key to the correct diagnosis. Tissue typing for HLA-B27 should not be done routinely but may be helpful where the history and exam suggest a disease but radiographs are inconclusive. This is also true for the use of complex imaging studies.

PHYSICAL AND FUNCTIONAL ASSESSMENT

Assessment by a health professional establishes a baseline for treatment. The goal of treatment is the prevention of disability and/or the adaptation to already established functional limitations. Some of the commonly used assessment measures are the Schöber test (lumbosacral flexion), Smythe test (thorocolumbar flexion/extension), lateral trunk flexion, tragus to wall distance (Figure 1), chest expansion (Figure 2), height, forward finger to floor distance, and hip and shoulder range of motion (4). The Bath Ankylosing Spondylitis Metrology Index is reproducible and sensitive to change across a wide disease spectrum (5). The Bath Ankylosing Spondylitis Functional Index (BASFI; Table 2) has a greater sensitivity than the Functional Index of Dougados and the Health Assessment Questionnaire for Spondylarthropathies (HAQ-S) (6). A disease activity index is also available (7).

DISEASE COURSE

The spondylarthropathies have variable courses. Early diagnosis and intervention help the majority of people diagnosed with spondylarthropathy to remain physically active. Persons who are able to alter their tasks and avoid prolonged bending, sitting, and jarring activities have a better chance of maintaining employment. There are differences in disease expression in men and women, particularly in the degree of radiologic changes and severity of cervical symptoms.

In a retrospective study of 151 patients with spondylarthropathies, having three of the following seven factors before the second year of disease were predictive of poorer long-term outcome (8). The factors predicting poorer outcome were hip disease, oligoarthritis, disease onset before age 16, poor efficacy of nonsteroidal anti-inflammatory medications (NSAIDs), limited lumbar motion, erythrocyte sedimentation rate greater than 30, and presence of sausage fingers or toes. Complications from NSAIDs and cervical spinal rigidity (risk of fracture or dislocation) may slightly decrease life expectancy.

TREATMENT

There are no known cures for the spondylarthropathies. The aims of disease management are to control pain and inflammation and minimize disability. Inactivity increases stiffness and leads to a flexed posture, which further increases the biomechanical stresses on the spinal support structures.

Table 1. Comparison of ankylosing spondylitis and related spondylarthropathies.

Characteristic	Disorder				
	Ankylosing Spondylitis	Reactive Arthritis (Reiter's Syndrome)	Juvenile Spondylarthropathy	Psoriatic Arthropathy*	Enteropathic Arthropathy†
Usual age at onset	Young adult age <40	Young to middle age adult	Childhood onset, ages 8 to 18	Young to middle age adult	Young to middle age adult
Sex ratio	3 times more common in males	Predominantly men	Predominantly men	Equally distributed	Equally distributed
Usual type of onset	Gradual	Acute	Variable	Variable	Gradual
Sacroiliitis or spondylitis	Virtually 100%	<50%	<50%	≈20%	<20%
Symmetry of sacroiliitis	Symmetric	Asymmetric	Variable	Asymmetric	Symmetric
Peripheral joint involvement	≈25%	≈90%	≈90%	≈95%	Frequent
Eye involvement‡	25–30%	Common	20%	Occasional	Occasional
Cardiac involvement	1–4%	5–10%	Rare	Rare	Rare
Skin or nail involvement	None	Common	Uncommon	Virtually 100%	Uncommon
HLA–B27 (in whites)	~90%	~75%	~85%	<50%§	~50%
Role of infectious agents as triggers	Unknown	Yes	Unknown	Unknown	Unknown

* About 5–7% of patients with psoriasis develop arthritis, and psoriatic spondylitis accounts for about 5% of all patients with psoriatic arthritis.
† Associated with chronic inflammatory bowel disease.
‡ Predominantly conjunctivitis in reactive arthritis and acute anterior uveitis in the other disorders listed above.
§ HLA–B27 is higher in those with spondylitis or sacroiliitis (adapted with permission from: Khan MA, Wilkens RF: A new look at ankylosing spondylitis. Patient Care 23(19):82–101, 1989).

Pharmacologic Management

Nonsteroidal anti-inflammatory drugs provide the foundation for pharmacologic management of the peripheral and spinal symptoms associated with spondylarthropathy. Indomethecin and naproxen are the most widely used. No second-line agent is considered to be superior, nor is there evidence that any are truly disease modifying. Short courses of sulfasalazine may be effective in ankylosing spondylitis, but it is more commonly used in patients with an inflammatory bowel component. Methotrexate is used in psoriatic arthritis and Reiter's syndrome, and occasionally in cases of severe progressive ankylosing spondylitis (9). Intra-articular injections of cortisone are often helpful in persistent peripheral enthesopathies (10). Pharmacologic agents for the extraskeletal symptoms are numerous and may include antimicrobials.

Rehabilitation

Knowledge about the disease and appropriate treatment, participation in a regular exercise program, and activity modifications are key components of a self-management program for persons with spondylarthropathy. Rehabilitation efforts must be centered on patient-generated goals and strategies.

Exercise

Exercise is the most important aspect of the management of ankylosing spondylitis. Exercise as well as self-assessment must be taught by a skilled health professional. Significant changes in mobility and function have been recorded in both supervised individual programs and group exercise programs (11–13).

There is growing consensus that a fitness program for people with spondylarthropathies should be vigorous and include stretching, strengthening, and a cardiovascular component. All

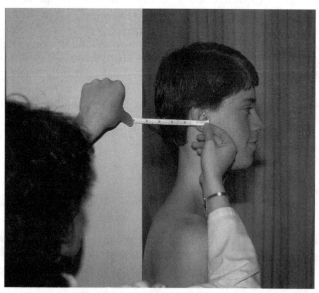

Figure 1. Tragus to wall distance.

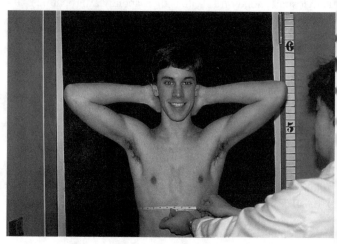

Figure 2. Chest expansion measurement.

spinal and peripheral joints, along with soft tissues, should be included in the flexibility program. Special attention should be given to spinal extension, lateral flexion, pelvic mobility, hip and shoulder motion, and stretching of the pectorals, hamstrings, and iliopsoas muscles. The contract–relax technique has been successful in stretching painful soft tissues, as have applications of heat or cold (14). A strengthening component should be included when flexibility has been maximized. Postural muscles especially in the thoracic spine and the gluteal and quadriceps muscles should be emphasized. A cardiovascular component is needed because of the restrictive pulmonary nature of the disease. Such exercises have resulted in significant improvements in both vital capacity and exercise tolerance, mainly due to the compensation by the diaphragm (15). Sedentary patients, particularly those with cardiac abnormalities, should have an exercise tolerance test and/or approval of their rheumatologist before beginning an aerobic program. Exercising in water offers the most benefit, because buoyancy can assist with stretching, offers resistance for strengthening, and decreases joint stresses during the endurance component (16). Table 3 lists components for a weekly fitness program.

Sports

Sports as forms of exercise are enjoyable but should not replace the therapeutic exercise program. Sports that emphasize spinal extension and rotation such as volleyball and basketball are preferable to flexion sports such as biking and bowling (17). Using a mask and snorkel for swimming is an alternative for the person with restricted thoracic or cervical

Table 3. Components of a weekly fitness program.

Daily	Gentle morning stretching
	Frequent position changes
	A few brief stretching sessions to problem areas (determined by weekly self-assessment)
	Relaxation techniques
	Heat or cold as needed
2–3 times per week	Total body flexibility and strengthening program
3–4 times per week	Cardiovascular exercises and recreational sports

motion. Because of the decreased shock absorbing abilities of the spine, contact and high-impact sports are discouraged for patients with rigid spines. Ankle and foot enthesopathies may require orthotics and guidance in footwear selection.

Modalities

Modalities are used for relaxation and pain relief with the goal of facilitating movement. Superficial heat and cold are the most often used due to ease of application. Warm water (84° to 92°) exercise is recommended. Some data show that transcutaneous electrical nerve stimulation (TENS) is helpful. Ultrasound or phonophoresis may also have some benefit in treatment of peripheral enthesopathies such as achilles tendonitis and plantar fasciitis (10). Pain relief from biofeedback and relaxation has not been studied in the spondylarthropathies.

Table 2. Bath Ankylosing Spondylitis Functional Index (reprinted from 7, with permission).

Please place a mark on each line below to indicate your level of ability with each of the following activities during the <u>past week</u>. (An aid is a piece of equipment that helps you perform an action or movement.)

1. Putting on your socks or stockings without help or aids (e.g., sock aid).

    easy _____ impossible

2. Bending forward from the waist to pick up a pen from the floor without an aid.

    easy _____ impossible

3. Reaching up to a high shelf without help or aids.

    easy _____ impossible

4. Getting up out of an armless dining room chair without using your hands or any other help.

    easy _____ impossible

5. Getting up off the floor from your back without help.

    easy _____ impossible

6. Standing unsupported for 10 minutes without discomfort.

    easy _____ impossible

7. Climbing 12–15 steps without using a hand rail or walking aid—**one foot on each step.**

    easy _____ impossible

8. Looking over your shoulders without turning your body.

    easy _____ impossible

9. Doing physically demanding activities (e.g., physical therapy exercises, gardening, or sports).

    easy _____ impossible

10. Doing a full day's activities whether it be at home or at work.

    easy _____ impossible

Mobilization

Inflammatory conditions of the spine have been a contraindication to manipulation. Patients go to chiropractors because they feel the need for some type of soft tissue traction or joint mobilization. If passive treatments are indicated, they should be done by a physical therapist, chiropractor, or osteopath with knowledge and experience in ankylosing spondylitis. The patient should be instructed in safe independent maneuvers such as low-weight static cervical traction, use of a thoracic wedge, and partner-assisted gentle soft tissue distraction techniques.

Postural Guidelines

Flexion is a position that can reduce pain, but it also may inhibit the ability of the extensor muscles. When the spine is even slightly forward, the supporting muscle must fight gravity to prevent further bending. This is fatiguing. Although exercise can help improve and maintain posture, it is not enough. Attention to all tasks and positions is necessary. Principles of good body mechanics should be followed, and work (in or out of the home), leisure, sleeping, and driving positions should be discussed (see also Chapter 15, Enhancing Functional Ability). Changing positions and stretching should be done frequently.

MODIFICATIONS

Techniques and devices may be needed to accommodate the lack of spinal, cervical, hip, or shoulder movement, but should not be used if the motion is still present. Safety techniques for maintaining balance in a person with a forward rigid spine are essential. A self-report or observed spinal-specific activities of daily living (ADL) assessment will help the therapist identify problems. Devices considered very useful include long-handled dressing aids, swivel chairs, reading stands, portable inclined writing boards, and elongated rear view mirrors (17,18). Lumbar back supports for sitting can provide feedback to correct posture. Lumbar corsets and cervical collars should be used only for exacerbation of acute pain or instability.

Sleep disturbances have been shown to affect pain, fatigue, and stiffness (see Chapter 21, Sleep Disturbance). Therefore, sleep hygiene is an important component of patient education. One should use as few pillows as possible, but at least one is needed to support the head and cervical lordosis. Mattress type and firmness are personal choices. A compromise may be necessary to maintain extension and yet be comfortable. Frequent position changes are advised.

Information on positioning during sexual activities is available from several sources, including the Arthritis Foundation and the National Ankylosing Spondylitis Society. Problems may be multifactoral and additional counseling may be useful.

ADHERENCE STRATEGIES

The patient with a spondylarthopathy is asked to comply with many recommendations, including medication use, exercise, modifying the environment, and implementing stress-reducing strategies. The effectiveness of these recommendations cannot be determined unless they are implemented. It has been sug-gested that "cooperation with a regimen is mediated by the patient's belief system and requires a therapeutic process of mutual inquiry, problem solving, and negotiation between the health care provider and patient" (19). Having a chronic disease requires self-management skills. One bridge from formal medical care to self-management is through participation in self-help groups.

Self-help groups in ankylosing spondylitis differ from other arthritis self-help groups because the primary focus is on exercise. Weekly exercise groups are common in Europe—over 80 programs are ongoing in the United Kingdom alone. In these groups, vigorous land and water exercise sessions are led by physical therapists under the direction of the National Ankylosing Spondylitis Society. Studies of these groups show that members are less reliant on health care providers, have a greater belief in the value of exercise, adhere better to exercise programs, and have greater satisfaction with medical supports (20). Developing disease-specific exercise groups may be unrealistic, so patients should be encouraged to join community fitness programs. Health professionals should offer guidelines to the community instructors.

SURGICAL INTERVENTION

Surgery is performed to improve function. The most common procedure is hip arthroplasty (see Chapter 17, Pre- and Post-surgical Management of the Hip and Knee). A decrease in hip motion is more functionally limiting than a fused spine. Both short- and long-term outcomes (greater than 7 years) are very good (21). In patients where formation of heterotopic ossification is probable, a course of indomethecin or prophylactic radiation may be given postoperatively.

Spinal osteotomy is an extremely complex procedure and is only performed to correct a severe deformity. It is more often done in the lumbar region, with the goals being restoration of the ability to see horizontally, improvement in respiration, and decrease in the abnormal stresses on a flexed spine. Spinal fusion may be necessary in cases of a painful pseudoarthrosis that has not responded to conservative management, or to stabilize an atlantoaxial subluxation.

The postoperative rehabilitation team must be sensitive to transfers and ADL adaptations that people with ankylosing spondylitis have had to make because of limited spinal motion. Patients should have input in the rehabilitation process, including bed positioning, supine-to-stand techniques, dressing, and maintaining balance with assistive walking devices.

COMPLEMENTARY CARE

Nontraditional remedies are appealing because there are no known cures for the spondylarthropathies. Frequently, they offer a more holistic approach to care. Most frequently tried interventions by people with ankylosing spondylitis are acupuncture, Tai Chi, spa treatments, massage, chiropractic, and various body awareness methods. All of these options typically result in decreased pain but none have been subjected to strict clinical trials (22).

REFERENCES

1. Khan MA: Ankylosing spondylitis: clinical features. In, Rheumatology. Edited by JH Klippel, PA Dieppe. St. Louis, Mosby, 1994
2. Taurog JD: Seronegative spondyloarthrophies: epidemiology, pathology, and pathogenesis. In, Primer on the Rheumatic Diseases. Tenth edition. Edited by HR Schumacher, JH Klippel, WJ Koopman. Atlanta, Arthritis Foundation, 1993
3. Dougados M, van der Linden S, Juhlin R, Huitfeldt B, Amor B, Calin A, Cats A, Dijkmans B, Olivieri I, Pasero G, Veys E, Zeidler H, the European Spondylarthropathy Study Group: The European Spondylarthropathy Study Group preliminary criteria for the classification of spondylarthropathy. Arthritis Rheum 34:1218–1227, 1991
4. Gall V: Patient evaluation. In, Physical Therapy in Arthritis. Edited by BF Banwell, V Gall. New York, Churchill Livingston, 1988
5. Jenkinson TR, Mallorie PA, Whitelock HC, Kennedy LG, Garrett SL, Calin A: Defining spinal mobility in ankylosing spondylitis (AS). The Bath AS Metrology Index. J Rheumatol 21:1694–1698, 1994
6. Calin A, Garrett S, Whitelock H, Kennedy LG, O'Hea J, Mallorie P, Jenkinson T: A new approach to defining functional ability in ankylosing spondylitis: the development of the Bath Ankylosing Spondylitis Functional Index. J Rheumatol 21:2281–2285, 1994
7. Garrett S, Jenkinson T, Kennedy LG, Whitelock H, Gaisford P, Calin A: A new approach to defining disease status in ankylosing spondylitis: the Bath Ankylosing Spondylitis Disease Activity Index. J Rheumatol 21: 2286–2291, 1994
8. Amor B, Santos RS, Nahal R, Listrat V, Dougados M: Predictive factors for the longterm outcome of spondyloarthropathies. J Rheumatol 21:1883–1887, 1994
9. Espinoza LR, Cuéllar ML: Psoriatic arthritis management. In, Rheumatology. Edited by JH Klippel, PA Dieppe. St. Louis, Mosby, 1994
10. Haslock I: Ankylosing spondylitis: management. In, Rheumatology. Edited by JH Klippel, PA Dieppe. St. Louis, Mosby, 1994
11. Viitanen JV, Suni J: Management principles of physiotherapy in ankylosing spondylitis—which treatments are effective? Physiotherapy 81:322–329, 1995
12. Hidding A, van der Linden S, Boers M, Gielen X, de Witte L, Kester A, Dijkmans B, Moolenburgh D: Is group physical therapy superior to individualized therapy in ankylosing spondylitis? A randomized controlled trial. Arthritis Care Res 6:117–125, 1993
13. Kraag G, Stokes B, Groh J, Helewa A, Goldsmith C: The effects of comprehensive home physiotherapy and supervision on patients with ankylosing spondylitis—a randomized controlled trial. J Rheumatol 17: 228–233, 1990
14. Bulstrode S, Barefoot J, Harrison R, Clarke AK: The role of passive stretching in the treatment of ankylosing spondylitis. Br J Rheumatol 26:40–42, 1987
15. Fisher LR, Cawley MID, Holgate ST: Relation between chest expansion, pulmonary function, and exercise tolerance in patients with ankylosing spondylitis. Ann Rheum Dis 49:921–925, 1990
16. Gall V: Exercise in the spondyloarthropathies. Arthritis Care Res 7:215–220, 1994
17. Spondylitis Association of America: Straight Talk on Spondylitis. Second edition. Sherman Oaks, CA, Spondylitis Association of America, 1993
18. Melvin JL: Rheumatic Disease in the Adult and Child: Occupational Therapy and Rehabilitation. Third edition. Philadelphia, FA Davis Co., 1989
19. Jensen GM, Lorish CD: Promoting patient cooperation with exercise programs: linking research, theory, and practice. Arthritis Care Res 7:181–189, 1994
20. Barlow JH, Macey SJ, Struthers GR: Health locus of control, self-help and treatment adherence in relation to ankylosing spondylitis patients. Patient Educ Couns 20:153–166, 1993
21. Calin A, Elswood J, Rigg S, Skevington SM: Ankylosing spondylitis—an analytical review of 1500 patients: the changing pattern of disease. J Rheumatol 15:1234–1238, 1988
22. Champion GD: Unproven remedies: alternative and complementary medicine. In, Rheumatology. Edited by JH Klippel, PA Dieppe. St. Louis, Mosby, 1994

Additional Recommended Reading

1. Calin A, Edmunds L, Kennedy LG: Fatigue in ankylosing spondylitis—why is it ignored? J Rheumatol 20:991–995, 1993
2. Daltoy LH, Larson MG, Roberts WN, Liang MH: A modification of the Health Assessment Questionnaire for the spondyloarthropathies. J Rheumatol 17:946–950, 1990
3. Dougados M, Gueguen A, Nakache J–P, Nguyen M, Mery C, Amor B: Evaluation of a functional index and articular index in ankylosing spondylitis. J Rheumatol 15:302–307, 1988
4. Resnick D: Inflammatory disorders of the vertebral column: seronegative spondyloarthropathies, adult-onset rheumatoid arthritis, and juvenile chronic arthritis. Clin Imaging 13:253–268, 1989
5. Tomlinson MJ, Barefoot J, Dixon AST: Intensive inpatient physiotherapy courses improve movement and posture in AS. Physiotherapy 5:238–241, 1986
6. Spondylitis Association of America (quarterly newsletter). P.O. Box 5872, Sherman Oaks, CA 91413
7. Walker JM, Helewa A, editors: Physical Therapy in Arthritis. First edition. Philadelphia, WB Saunders, 1996

Osteoarthritis

C. MICHAEL STEIN, MBCHB, MRCP; MARIE R. GRIFFIN, MD, MPH; and
KENNETH D. BRANDT, MD

Osteoarthritis (OA) is the most common of all joint diseases and results in considerable pain, disability, and substantial health care expenditure. No treatment is curative for OA, and increased appreciation of the risks associated with the use of nonsteroidal anti-inflammatory drugs (NSAIDs) has resulted in an approach to therapy that emphasizes nonpharmacologic measures.

ETIOLOGY AND PATHOGENESIS

Osteoarthritis is a heterogeneous condition and is not due to a single cause. Abnormal biomechanical properties of joint tissues such as articular cartilage or subchondral bone, abnormal or excessive biomechanical loading (such as may occur after trauma to a joint), or a combination of these play a role in the pathogenesis. Increased release of matrix-degrading enzymes in the articular cartilage may lead to morphologic changes such as pitting, fibrillation, and thinning of the tissue with diminished ability to dissipate mechanical load (1). Further contributions to the process may be made by associated low-grade inflammation, release of cytokines, and changes in subchondral bone.

INCIDENCE AND RISK

Estimates of the prevalence of OA vary depending on the criteria used for diagnosis. The prevalence of both radiographic and symptomatic OA increases with age (2,3). Radiographic evidence of OA is seen in less than 1% of the population in their 20s but in more than 50% of people in their 70s and 80s. Female gender, obesity, trauma, and genetic factors increase the risk of OA. Among these risk factors, obesity is modifiable, and weight loss reduces the risk of symptomatic OA (4).

Although radiographic signs of OA can be detected in most people in their 70s, symptoms occur in less than one-half (5). It is unclear why some individuals, but not others, are symptomatic. Osteoarthritis is often thought of as a minor problem of little importance; however, hip and knee OA are a major cause of disability in the elderly. The percentage of patients with OA who are limited in their activities because of musculoskeletal symptoms (60% to 80%) is similar to that for rheumatoid arthritis (6).

CLINICAL ASPECTS

The joints most commonly involved are the knees, hips, interphalangeal joints, the first carpometacarpal (CMC) joint, and the spine. Involvement of the elbows, shoulders, and metacar-pophalangeal (MCP) joints is relatively unusual in the absence of predisposing trauma, a predisposing metabolic abnormality (such as hemochromatosis), or calcium pyrophosphate crystal deposition disease. Pain after use, which is relieved by rest, is classical. With more advanced disease, pain at rest and nocturnal pain may occur. Morning stiffness is usually less than 30 minutes in duration and is restricted to involved joints. This contrasts with the more prolonged and generalized morning stiffness that characterizes rheumatoid arthritis.

Physical findings include joint tenderness and pain on motion, sometimes with audible or palpable crepitus and joint swelling. A synovial effusion may be present but more often the joint swelling is firm, due to overgrowth of bone and cartilage. Markers of inflammation, such as the erythrocyte sedimentation rate, are normal; systemic features of illness, such as weight loss or fever, are absent. There is no diagnostic laboratory test for OA. Instead, diagnosis is based on the history, physical examination, and radiographs. The radiographic features of OA include joint space narrowing (often asymmetric within a joint), sclerosis of bone, marginal osteophytes, and bony remodelling.

COURSE AND PROGNOSIS

The pathologic changes associated with established OA are presumably irreversible, but the symptoms often have a relapsing and remitting course with periods during which patients may be relatively asymptomatic. Although OA often progresses, it does so at highly variable rates in different patients, and in some people it may not progress at all.

TREATMENT

The goals of treatment are to relieve pain and improve or maintain function. No drug has been shown to modify the course of OA in clinical trials. The diagnosis of OA often results in the uncritical institution of long-term NSAID therapy. Patients may be unaware that their "arthritis medicine" is, in fact, a treatment for pain which has little effect on the underlying disease. An increased appreciation that the use of NSAIDs is associated with a risk of potentially serious adverse effects has led to a re-examination of the use of NSAIDs and a shift in emphasis to other therapeutic strategies. Steps in the management of a patient with OA may include: 1) determine if OA is the likely cause of pain; 2) implement interventions to alleviate pain and/or maintain function; 3) use appropriate drug therapy; and 4) consider referral for surgery.

Determine if Osteoarthritis is the Likely Cause of Pain

A common, unsatisfactory clinical sequence of events is that a patient complains of pain in the vicinity of a joint, a radiograph of the joint reveals changes of OA, a diagnosis of OA consequently results, and long-term treatment with an NSAID is instituted. The prevalence of radiographic changes of OA, particularly in the elderly, and the poor correlation between the severity of x-ray findings and clinical symptoms mean that the attribution of a patient's pain to OA, on the basis of radiographic evidence, will lead to diagnostic and therapeutic errors.

Extensive diagnostic testing for OA is unnecessary and unhelpful. A careful history and physical examination are required to exclude other causes of musculoskeletal pain, including referred pain, bursitis, and inflammatory rheumatic diseases such as gout or rheumatoid arthritis. Often trochanteric bursitis is misdiagnosed as OA of the hip and anserine bursitis as OA of the knee. Disease of the hip joint commonly causes pain anteriorly, in the inguinal region, or in the buttocks. A patient who localizes the site of "hip" pain to the area of the greater trochanter may therefore have symptoms related to trochanteric bursitis rather than to hip OA. Treatment of soft tissue pain with a local corticosteroid injection may rapidly and effectively relieve symptoms.

Implement Interventions to Alleviate Pain and/or Maintain Function

Several interventions that do not require systemic administration of a drug have been used to treat OA. Evidence regarding the efficacy of interventions such as the use of local heat and cooling, local applications of creams, exercise, weight loss, orthotics, transcutaneous electrical nerve stimulation, and pulsed electromagnetic fields has been reviewed (7). There are relatively few randomized, controlled clinical trials of these interventions. Study of these therapies is complicated both by difficulty in designing a true placebo intervention (for example: exercise or acupuncture) and by the high placebo response that characterizes most interventions for OA. Practical management of OA, which has evolved from clinical observations and controlled trials, involves patient education and support, unloading and protecting involved joints, strengthening the muscles around joints, local pain relief measures, and drug therapy.

Patient Education and Support. The long-term management of OA is primarily in the hands of the patient. The role of health care professionals is to provide guidance and support. A rational approach to disease management is based on patient education and continuing support. However, because this is more time consuming and challenging than providing a prescription for the newest NSAID, it may be neglected. It is helpful to have the key points, which form the basis for discussion with the patient, outlined on a single-sheet patient handout. The front page of the handout (Figure 1A) is designed to allow a personalized approach for each patient, and the back page (Figure 1B) summarizes discussion points about the risks and benefits of drug therapy. Telephone contact is an efficient and effective means of providing patient support between visits and has been shown to improve outcomes (8).

Unloading Joints. For patients who are overweight and suffer from hip and/or knee OA, a weight loss program should be instituted. Even modest weight loss is therapeutically useful; however, perfunctory advice to lose weight will not be effective. Specific planned efforts must be directed at the weight problem. It should be clearly explained to patients that, as they age, maintenance of function and mobility become increasingly important. This is more difficult to achieve in obese patients. The problem can be made more immediate and comprehensible by characterizing excess weight as an extra load the joints must carry (use an example that the patient can relate to, such as carrying a 30-lb child all day). A lifelong alteration in eating habits with realistic goals and behavior modification, accompanied by a low-impact aerobic exercise program, is more likely to be effective than popular diets that cannot be sustained.

The load on weight-bearing joints can be reduced by the use of a cane in the opposite hand. Patients are often reluctant to use a cane but may be persuaded to continue use if symptoms improve after a trial period. Short periods of rest during the day can relieve pain, but it must be emphasized that both rest and exercise have a role in management of OA (see Chapter 12, Rest and Exercise). The prescription of short periods of rest interspersed through the day should not be considered a prescription for inactivity. Prolonged standing may cause as much or more pain than walking. Frequent changes in posture or activity will also prevent the pain and stiffness that often occur when an affected joint has been immobile in one position too long (gelling).

Joint malalignment may place additional biomechanical stress on symptomatic joints. Pronation of the foot and varus or valgus knee deformities are common and can be countered with appropriate orthotics. A simple wedged insole may benefit some patients. In patients who have knee OA with involvement of the patellofemoral joint, tape applied to pull the patella medially can provide pain relief (9). The use of a splint for short periods of time can be useful for exacerbations of symptoms or for stressful activities. For example, in patients with involvement of the first CMC joint, a working hand splint that immobilizes this joint and the first MCP joint but allows mobility of the other MCP joints may provide symptomatic relief. However, as a general principle, joints should not be immobilized for prolonged periods or muscle atrophy and contractures will result.

Protecting Joints. Joints can be protected by avoiding activities that cause unwarranted stress. Kneeling and squatting, both of which aggravate knee symptoms, can usually be circumvented by modification of leisure and employment-related activities. The use of firm, high chairs, rather than soft low ones; raising the height of the toilet seat; and providing handles to grip will help in rising from the seated position. For patients with hand involvement, the use of devices such as jar openers, electric can openers, and electric scissors is useful, as are light-weight or large-handled utensils. Patients with lumbar spine involvement should avoid lifting heavy loads. If lifting is necessary, it should be performed with the knees bent, the back straight, and with the load held close to the body. Postures that aggravate back symptoms such as prolonged leaning over a desk or child's crib, should be avoided. A knee brace will provide support for patients with instability of that joint. Referral to an occupational therapist for selected patients, particularly those with severe OA affecting the hands, is useful. (See also Chapter 14, Splinting, and Chapter 15 Adaptive and Assistive Aids.)

Strengthening Muscles and Maintaining Range of Motion. Patients should be encouraged to maintain daily activities

PRESCRIPTION: DECREASE PAIN, IMPROVE FUNCTION

Take the load off your joints
1. Try brief periods of rest.
2. A cane in the opposite hand can relieve painful knees and hips.
3. Changing positions frequently takes the strain off the back.
4. Weight loss greatly lessens the load on the back, knees, and hips.
5. Wrist splints as tolerated.
6. Soft Thomas collar (neck), sling (shoulder), corset (back) for brief periods.

Protect your joints
1. Do not squat, kneel, or sit cross-legged (knees/hips).
2. Be careful when lifting and bending.
3. Use aids to open jars, fasten clothing, hold utensils (hands).
4. Use aids to reach for objects; keep work close, so that elbows remain next to your body (shoulders).

Strengthen the muscles around your joints
1. Stay active; try to walk 20 to 30 minutes daily (start with 5 minutes/day).
2. Use jogging shoes or orthotics on a level surface or walk in a warm pool.
3. Do stretching and strengthening exercises.

Other ways to relieve pain
1. Apply heat to painful joints: use warm water (bath, whirlpool, running water) or paraffin bath (hands).
2. Some people find cold helpful: use a bag of frozen vegetables.
3. Try topical creams.
4. Wear thin gloves to keep hand joints warm.

Pills
1. If pills don't improve your pain, don't take them.
2. Acetaminophen (Tylenol) 500 mg (1-2 pills 3-4 times/day is the first choice most of the time.

Special Instructions: _____

_____

_____

New Ways of Treating Joint and Muscle Problems: Recommendations of an Expert Panel

1. The Role of Pills

Pills don't cure joint and muscle problems.

Pills usually give only partial relief of pain.

New research has shown that anti-inflammatory pills (e.g., aspirin, ibuprofen) have a high rate of serious side effects like stomach pains and ulcers, especially in older patients.

Ulcers may cause serious problems in some patients who have taken these pills for years, even in those without stomach pains.

2. If Pills are Used, Acetaminophen (Tylenol) is our First Choice

Acetaminophen is a strong medicine at high doses.

When taken properly, it works as well as anti-inflammatory drugs for many people.

It has fewer side effects than anti-inflammatory pills.

3. Remember:

Pills and alcohol don't mix; talk to your doctor about your alcohol use.

Consult your doctor before taking other pain pills (including those you can buy without a prescription).

Write questions for your doctor here and bring this paper with you to your next visit: _____

_____

_____

Figure 1. Examples of a prescription sheet (A) that can be used to personalize a management program for a patient with osteoarthritis (left), and a patient information sheet (B) that can be used as a basis for discussing the role of medications in the management of osteoarthritis (right). Courtesy of the Vanderbilt University School of Medicine.

within the limitations of their pain; however, a specific exercise program should be prescribed for patients with hip and knee OA. Exercise improves strength, improves function, decreases pain, and results in increased feeling of well-being. Stretching and mobility exercises maintain the range of motion and prevent joint contractures. The major benefit of exercise in OA of the knees is related to improved quadriceps strength. This can be achieved by isometric (without joint motion) exercises or resistive exercises. An aerobic exercise program such as walking or pool exercises may reduce pain and improve function in patients with hip or knee OA.

The exercise program should be tailored to the patient. Isometric or resistive exercises such as those described in Table 1 and Figure 2 are convenient because they require no special equipment and are easy to perform. An aerobic exercise may have additional benefits, such as facilitating weight loss, that are useful for particular patients. The data from studies suggest that suitable low-impact aerobic exercise, such as walking or pool exercises, does not result in disease flares or increase joint damage and, in fact, improves function and pain. Referral to a physical therapist may be helpful for patients who are unable to undertake the exercise programs outlined above.

Local Pain Relief Measures. Many patients find that application of heat or cold results in an improvement in joint symptoms. Heat may be applied locally in the form of a heating pad or warm cloth or more generally by means of a hot bath or hot tub. Local application of cold may be performed using ice or, more conveniently, a bag of frozen vegetables.

The local application of rubifacients, many of which contain methylsalicylate, may provide symptomatic relief, although their efficacy in controlled clinical trials has been variable. Capsaicin, the alkaloid that makes chili peppers hot, applied to symptomatic joints four times daily in patients with OA was found to be more effective than application of placebo. However, the initial burning sensation following application makes it difficult to perform true placebo-controlled studies. The frequency of application and the initial burning sensation felt

Table 1. Quadriceps exercises for osteoarthritis of the knee.* (Developed by Indiana University Multipurpose Arthritis and Musculoskeletal Diseases Center.)

Straight Leg Raising

1. Lie flat on your back on the floor or in bed with your legs straight out in front of you.
2. To exercise the right leg, first bend the left knee with the left foot flat on the floor or bed.
3. Tighten the big muscle above the right knee and lift the right leg straight up as far as it will go, then lower it slowly and hold it just off the bed or floor for 5 seconds. Repeat 5–10 times. Exercise the other leg in the same way.
4. Begin this strengthening program with 5–10 repetitions for each leg and increase the number of repetitions by 1/day until you are up to 15 per set. Do these exercises 2–4 times daily starting with a low number of repetitions but eventually working up to a goal of 200 straight leg raises per day per leg.

* In most patients these exercises will not cause an increase in joint pain. However, if you have significant pain during the exercise or pain lasting more than 20 minutes after the exercise, temporarily decrease the number of repetitions by one-half.

by many patients limit the current clinical applicability of capsaicin (10), but it may be useful in selected patients with limited joint involvement.

Response to intra-articular injection of corticosteroids for flares of symptoms is highly variable. Controlled clinical trials

---

PROTECT YOUR KNEES

1. Sit on a firm surface or lie flat in bed (see figures below).

2. Cross your ankles with legs straight and right leg above the left.

3. With heels on the floor or bed, push down with right leg and push up with left leg, squeezing ankles together. (Pretend you are crushing a walnut between your ankles.) There should be little movement except for muscle tightening.

4. Hold for 5 seconds.

5. Relax the muscles.

6. Reverse so that left leg is now on top.

Repeat steps 1 through 5

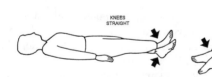

Begin this strengthening program with 10 repetitions for each leg. Do this seven times each day. Increase the number of repetitions by 1 per day until you are up to 15 per set. By the end of one week you should be able to do 15 per set, seven times a day.

If you are having knee pain, try applying heat for 15 to 20 minutes before doing these exercises.

Caution: In most patients, these exercises will not cause or increase joint pain. If, however, you have significant pain lasting more than 20 minutes after you do these exercises, decrease the number of repetitions by 5 per set. Gradually work up to 15 per set when knee comfort improves.

Figure 2. Crossed ankles resistive isometric quadriceps exercise (developed by Indiana University Multipurpose Arthritis and Musculoskeletal Diseases Center).

indicate a modest response of 1–4 weeks' duration (11). The knee joint is most frequently injected, particularly in patients with moderate or large effusions. Occasional patients have a significant clinical response that may last months. To limit potential local adverse effects of intra-articular corticosteroids, the number of injections administered to any one joint is generally restricted to two or three per year. A lack of clinical response following two intra-articular injections indicates that further injections in that joint are unlikely to be beneficial. Soft tissue injections of local corticosteroids will often improve symptoms caused by subacromial, anserine, or trochanteric bursitis. The role of intra-articular injections of hyaluronic acid or potentially disease-modifying drugs remains experimental (11).

Use Appropriate Drug Therapy

Drug therapy, which is not curative and does not alter the outcome of OA, is ancillary to the more general measures used to control pain. Long-term studies emphasize the modest clinical benefits of all types of drug therapy in OA (12). Therefore, patients and physicians must have realistic expectations of pharmaceutical interventions. Acetaminophen is usually the drug of first choice.

Acetaminophen. Several clinical trials suggest that acetaminophen (3–4 g/day) provides symptom relief equivalent to that obtained with NSAIDs (13,14). In therapeutic doses, acetaminophen has few adverse effects and is safer than NSAIDs for most patients. Hepatotoxicity occurs most commonly after accidental or intentional overdose with doses usually in excess of 10 g/day. However, hepatotoxicity with therapeutic use of acetaminophen, although unusual, has occurred. It is most common in alcoholics; therefore, caution is indicated if the drug is used in this patient population. Patients may not recognize that many brand name over-the-counter and prescription analgesics contain acetaminophen. They should be cautioned against the unsupervised use of other analgesics while taking therapeutic doses of acetaminophen so that they are not inadvertently exposed to the dangers of a daily dose of acetaminophen higher than that recommended.

Long-term use of acetaminophen has been associated with chronic renal toxicity, as has been the case with NSAIDs. The data are controversial but indicate that a small increased risk probably exists. Nevertheless, acetaminophen in therapeutic doses remains the safest analgesic available, even in patients with known renal impairment.

The safety and cost of acetaminophen, and its efficacy in clinical trials, suggest that it should be the first drug tried in OA patients who require drug therapy. Some patients with episodic, mild pain may take acetaminophen as needed, rather than regularly, with good effect. Patients with severe symptoms are more likely to respond to a fixed dose of acetaminophen (1 g, 3–4 times daily). The addition of opioids in the form of acetaminophen/codeine or acetaminophen/dextropropoxyphene preparations for long-term use clearly increases the frequency of adverse effects such as dizziness, nausea, and constipation, without increasing efficacy significantly. In patients whose joint pain is unsatisfactorily controlled with acetaminophen, combination therapy with an analgesic dose of an NSAID, taken as needed, may be effective.

Nonsteroidal Anti-inflammatory Drugs. Frequently, NSAIDs are prescribed for OA. They are more effective than placebo but have only modest efficacy and are not curative. There is no evidence that any one NSAID is more effective than another, although patient responses may vary. Several studies suggest that ibuprofen in analgesic doses (<1800 mg/day) has a lower frequency of gastrointestinal toxicity than other NSAIDs. If an NSAID is indicated, particularly at higher doses to achieve an anti-inflammatory effect, different toxicity profiles should be considered.

Potential adverse effects include renal impairment, skin rashes, antagonism of the hypotensive effect of some antihypertensive drugs, and ulceration of small and large bowel. However, the most common adverse effect resulting in serious morbidity or mortality is upper gastrointestinal toxicity (15). Elderly patients are at greatest risk from NSAID-induced upper gastrointestinal tract ulceration, hemorrhage, and death (16,17). The annual rate of hospitalization for peptic ulcer complications in persons 65 years and older currently using NSAIDs was 16 per 1,000 persons per year (four times higher than persons not taking NSAIDs) and rose to 40 per 1,000 persons per year in those taking the highest doses of NSAIDs (18). The excess risk of hospitalization for ulcer complications in elderly NSAID users is 1% to 2% per year, which is similar to the risk of serious bleeding while on chronic oral anticoagulant therapy. Gastrointestinal toxicity from NSAIDs is more likely to occur in patients concurrently taking corticosteroids or anticoagulants.

Misoprostol is the only drug approved for the prophylaxis of NSAID-associated gastropathy. Selecting patients for such prophylactic "gastroprotective" therapy from the population of patients receiving NSAIDs chronically is a problem, because serious gastrointestinal effects may occur in the absence of any warning symptoms. Misoprostol should be considered in patients receiving an NSAID who are at a high risk of gastrointestinal bleeding. These include elderly patients, patients with prior gastrointestinal bleeding, and patients taking corticosteroids. The addition of a second drug to prevent gastrointestinal side effects associated with NSAIDs increases the complexity and cost of treatment and introduces the risk of additional adverse drug reactions. The optimal clinical use of the drug remains to be defined.

Nonsteroidal anti-inflammatory drugs have a role in the management of OA in patients who do not respond to acetaminophen and the nonpharmacologic measures described above. In these patients, after explanation of the risks and potential benefits, NSAID therapy—either in combination with acetaminophen or alone—can be tried. The aim of therapy is to control symptoms using the lowest effective dose of NSAID. Ibuprofen in analgesic doses (<1800 mg/day) has the advantages of a lower rate of gastrointestinal side effects and the availability of a variety of formulations that allow flexibility of dosing regimens. In patients requiring regular NSAID therapy, the use of a longer-acting NSAID that can be taken once or twice daily may be more convenient.

For patients with OA who have been receiving NSAIDs chronically, the risks and benefits of such therapy should be discussed. When appropriate, a trial of acetaminophen therapy together with non-drug interventions should be tried. Studies indicate that 60% to 70% of such patients can be switched to acetaminophen (19). However, these data also indicate that there are patients for whom NSAIDs are more effective. Because adverse effects of NSAIDs increase with higher doses, the minimum effective dose should be used. The degree of pain from OA varies, so a flexible dosing regimen is useful. When used as needed rather than regularly, NSAIDs may provide adequate symptom control in many patients. The need for continuing drug therapy should be reviewed periodically; indefinite drug therapy is not always required.

Consider Referral for Surgery

Surgical interventions that have been useful in selected patients with more severe disease include arthroscopic debridement/joint lavage, osteotomy, and joint replacement. The major indications for referral to an orthopedist are pain, loss of function, and disability unresponsive to the measures described above. The patient's age, attitude toward surgery, and expectations from surgery are also important considerations. Uncontrolled studies of patients undergoing arthroscopic debridement/surgical repair have reported that 50% to 70% improve after the procedure. However, a comparison of closed needle joint lavage and arthroscopic surgery suggests that joint lavage, rather than the arthroscopic repair of intra-articular abnormalities, may account for much of the benefit (20). Osteotomy, which alters joint alignment, may provide improvement in symptoms for some years and is useful in younger patients with moderately advanced disease of the knee in whom delaying the need for total joint arthroplasty is a consideration.

The greatest improvement in quality of life for a patient with severe, functionally incapacitating OA of the hip or knee may result from joint replacement. Hip and knee replacement surgery results in excellent pain relief and improved function. There is, however, a morbidity and mortality associated with joint replacement surgery, and best results are obtained in appropriately selected patients. Considerations in the selection of patients for surgery include previous pharmacologic and nonpharmacologic interventions, the severity of pain and disability, the age and general health of the patient, and patient expectations.

REFERENCES

1. Brandt KD, Mankin HJ: Pathogenesis of osteoarthritis. In, Textbook of Rheumatology. Fourth edition. Edited by WN Kelley, ED Harris, S Ruddy, CB Sledge. Philadelphia, WB Saunders Co., 1993
2. Davis MA, Ettinger WH, Neuhaus JM, Mallon KP: Knee osteoarthritis and physical functioning: evidence from the NHANES I epidemiologic followup study. J Rheumatol 18:591–598, 1991
3. Felson DT, Naimark A, Anderson J, Kazis L, Castelli W, Meenan RF: The prevalence of knee osteoarthritis in the elderly: the Framingham osteoarthritis study. Arthritis Rheum 30:914–918, 1987
4. Felson DT, Zhang Y, Anthony JM, Naimark A, Anderson JJ: Weight loss reduces the risk for symptomatic knee osteoarthritis in women. Ann Intern Med 116:535–539, 1992
5. Bagge E, Bjelle A, Eden S, Svanborg A: Osteoarthritis in the elderly: clinical and radiological findings in 79–85 year olds. Ann Rheum Dis 50:535–539, 1991
6. Yelin EH, Felts WR: A summary of the impact of the musculoskeletal conditions in the United States. Arthritis Rheum 33:750–755, 1990
7. Puett DW, Griffin MR: Published trials of nonmedicinal and noninvasive therapies for hip and knee osteoarthritis. Ann Intern Med 121:133–140, 1994
8. Weinberger M, Tierney WM, Cowper PA, Katz BP, Booher PA: Cost-effectiveness of increased telephone contact for patients with osteoarthritis. Arthritis Rheum 36:243–246, 1993
9. Cushnaghan J, McCarthy C, Dieppe P: Taping the patella medially: a new treatment for osteoarthritis of the knee joint. BMJ 308:753–755, 1994
10. Zhang WY, Li Wan Po A: The effectiveness of topically applied capsaicin: a meta-analysis. Eur J Clin Pharmacol 46:517–522, 1994

11. Menkes CJ: Intraarticular treatment of osteoarthritis and guidelines to its assessment. J Rheumatol 21 (Suppl 41):74–76, 1994
12. Williams HJ, Ward JR, Egger MJ, Neuner R, Brooks RH, Clegg DO, Field EH, Skosey JL, Alarcón GS, Willkens RF, Paulus HE, Russel IJ, Sharp JT: Comparison of naproxen and acetaminophen in a two-year study of treatment of osteoarthritis of the knee. Arthritis Rheum 36:1196–1206, 1993
13. Bradley JD, Brandt KD, Katz BP, Kalasinski LA, Ryan SI: Comparison of an antiinflammatory dose of ibuprofen, an analgesic dose of ibuprofen, and acetaminophen in the treatment of patients with osteoarthritis of the knee. N Engl J Med 325:87–91, 1991
14. Griffin MR, Brandt KD, Liang MH, Pincus T, Ray WA: Practical management of osteoarthritis: integration of pharmacologic and non-pharmacologic measures. Arch Fam Med 4:1049–1055, 1995
15. Brooks PM, Day RO: Nonsteroidal anti-inflammatory drugs—differences and similarities. N Engl J Med 324:1716–1725, 1991
16. Griffin MR, Piper JM, Daugherty JR, Snowden M, Ray WA: Nonsteroidal anti-inflammatory drug use and increased risk for peptic ulcer disease in elderly persons. Ann Intern Med 114:257–263, 1991
17. Guess HA, West R, Strand LM, Helston D, Lydick EG, Bergman U, Wolski K: Fatal upper gastrointestinal hemorrhage or perforation among users and non-users of nonsteroidal anti-inflammatory drugs in Saskatchewan, Canada 1983. J Clin Epidemiol 41:35–45, 1988
18. Smalley WE, Ray WA, Daugherty J, Griffin MR: Nonsteroidal anti-inflammatory drugs and the incidence of hospitalizations for peptic ulcer disease in elderly persons. Am J Epidemiol 141:539–545, 1995
19. Swift GL, Rhodes J: Are nonsteroidal antiinflammatory drugs always necessary? A general practice survey. Br J Clin Pract 46:92–94, 1992
20. Chang RW, Falconer J, Stulberg SD, Arnold WJ, Manheim LM, Dyer AR: A randomized, controlled trial of arthroscopic surgery versus closed-needle joint lavage for patients with osteoarthritis of the knee. Arthritis Rheum 36:289–296, 1993

Additional Recommended Reading

1. Scott DL, on behalf of the Joint Working Group: Guidelines for the diagnosis, investigation and management of osteoarthritis of the hip and knee. J Royal Coll Phys London 27:391–396, 1993
2. Hochberg MC, Altman RD, Brandt KD, Clark BM, Dieppe PA, Griffin MR, Moskowitz RW, Schnitzer TJ: Guidelines for the medical management of osteoarthritis. Part I. Osteoarthritis of the hip. Arthritis Rheum 38:1535–1540, 1995
3. Hochberg MC, Altman RD, Brandt KD, Clark BM, Dieppe PA, Griffin MR, Moskowitz RW, Schnitzer TJ: Guidelines for the medical management of osteoarthritis. Part II. Osteoarthritis of the knee. Arthritis Rheum 38:1541–1546, 1995

Acute Inflammatory Arthritis

H. RALPH SCHUMACHER, JR, MD

Patients often think of arthritis as a chronic, slowly progressive disorder. However, it can also first present as a new, acute symptom (1–3). This should raise consideration of infection, crystal disease, and trauma, although it can also be the first sign of many other joint and systemic diseases.

CLINICAL FINDINGS

History

Taking the patient's family history can help, because gout, rheumatoid arthritis (RA), systemic lupus erythematosus (SLE), and the spondylarthropathies often run in families.

Symptoms that precede the acute arthritis may provide important clues. Back pain that is worse in the morning may suggest spondylarthropathy. Pharyngitis suggests rheumatic fever, Neisseria or viral infection, or Still's disease. Urethritis or pelvic inflammatory disease may indicate gonococcal arthritis or Chlamydia- or Ureaplasma-related "reactive arthritis". Diarrhea may suggest Reiter's syndrome, other reactive arthritis, or the arthritis of inflammatory bowel disease. Any preceding infection can be the origin of an organism causing infectious arthritis. A previous joint procedure also suggests possible infection. Lyme disease may be suspected when there is a history of recent tick exposure, rash, palpitations, or Bell's palsy.

A history of trauma can suggest the occurrence of a fracture or an internal derangement of tendon or cartilage, but minor trauma can also precipitate acute gout or introduce infection. Medications used may also provide clues, as they can affect the results of tests and influence the choice or outcome of therapy.

Physical Examination

The physical examination must distinguish an arthritis, which is an inflammation in the articular space, from processes that affect the periarticular area such as a bursitis, tendinitis, or cellulitis. Deep, axial joints such as the hips and sacroiliac joints are particularly difficult to evaluate.

An effort should be made to look for signs at extra-articular sites suggesting specific causes, such as pustules in gonococcemia, and mouth ulcers in Behcet's syndrome, Reiter's syndrome, and SLE. Small patches of psoriasis may be found between the buttocks or behind the ears. The keratoderma blennorrhagicum of Reiter's syndrome can be subtle and often affects only the feet. Erythema nodosum may suggest the presence of SLE, sarcoidosis, or inflammatory bowel disease. Skin ulcerations can be a source of infection. Splinter hemorrhages suggest bacterial endocarditis. Tophi of gout usually do not antedate arthritis, but they can be seen over joints, at Achilles tendons, and over the extensor surface of the fore-

arms. Fever occurs with several types of arthritis but raises concern about infection.

On careful physical examination of the joint, tenderness, some limitation of function, and soft-tissue swelling can virtually always be detected in true arthritis. Characteristics may not match a textbook-defined type of arthritis, so making a definitive diagnosis can be difficult in the early days or weeks after onset. However, early attempts at classification of the arthritis are essential. An important early step is differentiating the joint inflammation of arthritis from symptoms caused by periarticular disease or degenerative or mechanical problems. Most often, inflammation localized at one side of the joint raises concerns of tendinitis, bursitis, bone disease, or cellulitis. Pain on a single motion such as abduction at the shoulder suggests bursitis.

Sometimes, inflammatory arthritis is only a minor feature of a potentially serious systemic disease; thus, arthritis should prompt a full and careful general evaluation even if mild. Among systemic diseases that may have mild inflammatory arthritis as the first clue are SLE, Wegener's granulomatosis and other types of vasculitis, polymyositis, scleroderma, subacute bacterial endocarditis, sarcoidosis, hemochromatosis, hyperparathyrodism, leukemia, lymphoma, and other malignant tumors. Classifying the pattern of joint swelling, as described below, may narrow the diagnostic possibilities.

Monarthritis. Swelling and pain in a single joint is the most common presentation of infectious arthritis and requires evaluation without delay. Monarthritis is also a common presentation of crystal-induced arthritis, hemarthrosis from trauma or other causes, exacerbations of osteoarthritis, and occasionally of foreign bodies, tumors, avascular necrosis, Lyme disease, or other systemic diseases.

Oligoarthritis. Involvement of several joints can occasionally occur with any infection, but this is more likely in immunosuppressed hosts, persons with antecedent joint disease, and abusers of intravenous drugs. Oligoarthritis is a characteristic presentation of Lyme disease, Reiter's syndrome, reactive arthritis, and other seronegative spondylarthropathies and is not uncommon in crystal diseases especially after the early bouts. Lower extremity, asymmetric, and large-joint involvement is often most prominent in the spondylarthropathies. Tuberculosis involves two or three joints in 10% to 15% of cases.

Gonococcal arthritis is especially likely to produce migratory arthritis and tendinitis before lodging in one joint. Rheumatic fever and Lyme disease can also cause migratory arthritis. Palindromic rheumatism involves a series of joints in sequence, with symptom-free intervals between attacks.

Polyarthritis. Rheumatoid arthritis is the most common cause of persistent polyarthritis, but viral arthritis and other systemic diseases must be considered early. Distinguishing early RA from viral arthritis, SLE, and other systemic rheumatic diseases may be impossible unless other clues are detected on history and physical examination. Inflammation of many joints, symmetric joint involvement, involvement of metacarpophalangeal joints, and long duration of morning stiffness tend to predict RA. Subcutaneous nodules also are strong evidence for RA, but they usually do not occur early and occasionally require aspiration or biopsy for definitive diagnosis.

Up to 25% of patients with recent onset polyarthritis have a transient disease, which resolves without diagnosis. The more acute the onset and the fewer prognostic factors for RA that are present, the more likely that the polyarthritis is not RA and that resolution will occur.

RADIOGRAPHIC FINDINGS

Radiographs of the involved joint are often not helpful in establishing the cause of acute arthritis. However fractures, tumors, or signs of antecedent chronic disease such as osteoarthritis can be seen on plain radiographs. Chondrocalcinosis in the involved joint suggests but does not prove that the acute arthritis is pseudogout. Periarticular calcification can suggest apatite crystal disease. In suspected acute septic arthritis, there are usually no radiologic findings other than soft-tissue swelling, but a film can help exclude other causes and provide a baseline for future comparisons. Magnetic resonance imaging is probably overused but may help identify early sacroiliac involvement. Magnetic resonance imaging can help localize an infectious or inflammatory process to the joint, its surrounding tissue, or bone; it may also be useful in diagnosing joint infections during pregnancy.

LABORATORY TESTING

The use of cultures and Gram's stains of blood, skin lesions or ulcers, cervical or urethral swabs, urine, or any other possible sources of microorganisms is important in suspected infectious arthritis. This is especially true for gonococcal arthritis, because synovial fluid cultures are positive in only approximately 25% of patients. Testing for HIV antibodies and Lyme antibodies may be appropriate, but no single serologic test can establish the cause of any acute arthritis. The test for rheumatoid factor can be positive not only in RA but in many diseases associated with arthritis, including sarcoidosis and subacute bacterial endocarditis. Measurements of serum uric acid during the acute phase of arthritis are notoriously misleading, and results must be interpreted with caution. Other tests should be done as indicated by each specific disease under consideration. Analysis of synovial fluid is often considered the single most useful test (4,5).

Arthrocentesis and Synovial Fluid Analysis

Arthrocentesis provides crucial information and can be performed at the bedside or in the office with almost no complications as long as sterile techniques are used. Arthrocentesis should be performed in virtually every patient with acute arthritis and certainly with monarthritis (6), especially if infection is suspected. It may be difficult to aspirate fluid from some joints, such as the hips or the sacroiliac joints, and the procedure may need to be done under the guidance of ultrasonography, computed tomography, or fluoroscopy. Most of the

important information from synovial fluid analysis is obtained through the total leukocyte count and differential count, cultures, Gram's stain, and examination of a wet preparation for crystals and other microscopic abnormalities. All these studies can be performed with only 1 to 2 ml of fluid; often, only a few drops are needed. Failure to use synovial fluid analysis was one of the major factors that led to misdiagnoses and prolonged hospital stays in one recent study (2).

Gross Examination. Important clues can be obtained from gross examination of the joint fluid. Bloody fluid suggests fracture, tumor, coagulation abnormalities, destructive arthritis of any kind, or rare problems such as scurvy. Cloudy yellow fluid indicates one of the inflammatory arthritides and must be investigated further. Absolutely clear transparent fluid with no color or pale yellow is most often due to non-inflammatory causes of effusion. Opaque material may be pus, but may also occasionally be due to urate or apatite crystals.

Leukocyte Counts and Differentials. Normal synovial fluid contains fewer than 180 cells/mm^3, most of which should be mononuclear. Fluid is considered to be "noninflammatory" if it contains fewer than 2,000 cells/mm^3, although most samples of synovial fluid from patients with osteoarthritis contain fewer than 500 cells/mm^3. In general, as the leukocyte count increases, so does the suspicion of infection. Effusions containing more than 100,000 leukocytes/mm^3 are considered septic until proven otherwise. The wide spectrum of leukocyte counts in both sterile and septic inflammatory arthritis makes strict classification imprudent. Differential leukocyte counts can help; a finding of more than 90% polymorphonuclear cells should prompt concern about infection or crystal-induced disease.

Wet Drop Preparation and Crystal Identification. Careful examination of a single drop of synovial fluid under a cover slip to identify crystals can establish a diagnosis early and avoid unnecessary hospital admissions for the treatment of suspected infectious arthritis (5,7). Although most easily seen as brightly negatively birefringent needles on compensated polarized light microscopy, monosodium urate crystals can also be seen and tentatively identified using normal light microscopy. Calcium pyrophosphate dihydrate (CPPD) crystals are less intensely birefringent than monosodium urate crystals and are more rod-shaped or rhomboid with positive birefringence on compensated polarized light microscopy. These crystals may be small and difficult to see on normal light microscopy. Other less common crystals should be considered if findings are atypical (5). Among those that can cause acute arthritis are the pyramidal oxalates or the maltese crosses of lipid liquid crystals. Wet preparations of all synovial fluids should be examined not only for crystals but also for other particles such as fat droplets and blood. Large fat droplets in synovial fluid suggest a fracture involving the marrow. Small lipid droplets, as can occur in pancreatic fat necrosis or fractures, can be misread by Coulter counters as leukocytes.

Cultures. The presence of crystals does not exclude infection, as antecedent abnormalities such as gout may increase the likelihood of septic arthritis. Cultures should be performed on samples of synovial fluid if there is any concern about infection, even if crystals are present. Cultures and Gram's stain are obligatory when infection is suspected. Gram-positive bacteria can be seen on a well-prepared slide of culture-positive fluids approximately 80% of the time. Gram-negative bacteria are seen less frequently, and *Neisseria gonorrhoea* and *Neisseria* *meningitides* are rarely seen. Special stains and cultures for mycobacteria and fungi are sometimes appropriate.

Synovial Biopsy, Arthroscopy, and Special Techniques. Needle biopsy of the synovial membrane or a biopsy obtained during arthroscopy is seldom practical as an initial step. However, culture of synovial tissue may have a greater yield than a synovial fluid culture in certain settings, such as when gonoccal or mycobacterial disease is suspected or when no fluid is available for culture. Biopsies can identify infiltrative diseases such as amyloidosis, sarcoidosis, or pigmented villonodular synovitis, although some studies suggest that early biopsy can be predictive. Recent use of polymerase chain reaction and immuno-electron microscopy may allow diagnosis of some difficult to identify infections (8).

SEPTIC ARTHRITIS

Etiology and Pathogenesis

Acute infections in joints can be caused by virtually any microbial agent (9). Entry into the joint can be via the circulation from a site of infection elsewhere or by direct penetration as after a wound, surgery, or infection. Gonococcal arthritis is probably the most common septic arthritis, although the frequency varies among populations. Women are affected two to three times as often as men. A migratory tendinitis or arthritis often precedes gonococcal monarthritis. The response to therapy is usually rapid and complete; thus, this form of infectious arthritis is much less destructive than staphylococcal arthritis.

Nongonococcal bacterial infections are the most serious (10). Large joints such as the knee or hip are the most frequently affected, but any joint can be involved. Sternoclavicular joint infection is more common among intravenous drug users.

Most (80% to 90%) of nongonococcal bacterial infections are monarticular. Polyarticular involvement may occur more often in the presence of a predisposing condition such as RA. The discovery of a primary site of infection can be an important clue to the infectious agent involved. By far the most common agents are gram-positive aerobes (approximately 80%). *Staphylococcus aureus* accounts for 60%, non-group A, B-hemolytic streptococci for 15%, and *Streptococcus pneumoniae* for 3%. Gram-negative bacteria (accounting for 18% of infections) and anaerobes are increasingly frequent causes due to drug use and the rising number of immunocompromised hosts. Anaerobic infections are also more common in patients who have wounds of an extremity or gastrointestinal cancers.

Although tuberculosis and fungal arthritis are more likely to be chronic, acute mycobacterial arthritis has been reported. Acute monarthritis associated with herpes simplex virus and other viruses has also been described.

The characteristic acute oligoarthritis of Lyme disease occurs months after the initial infection and may occur in as many as 60% of untreated patients. Large joints such as the knee are usually involved and tend to be more swollen than painful. Acute monarthritis can also be caused by other spirochetes such as *Treponema pallium,* and some subacute infectious synovitis can be due to chlamydia and ureaplasma that are especially difficult to culture.

Incidence and Risk

Although septic arthritis is less common than other types of acute inflammatory arthritis, its potential impact is greater. Thus, early diagnosis and treatment are essential. Risk factors that should increase concern about septic arthritis include infection elsewhere in the body, elderly age and childhood, other systemic diseases, recent arthrocentesis or surgery, prosthetic joints, immunosuppression, and intravenous drug abuse.

Clinical Aspects

Infected joints are painful, tender, and limited in motion; the classical hot, red, dramatic swelling is often but not invariably present and some signs may be masked by partial treatment or use of immunosuppressive drugs. Single joint involvement is most common, but multiple joints can be involved or a single joint can be infected in a patient with RA or other types of arthritis in other joints. Fever is usually present but may be low grade in up to 50% of cases or even absent in patients taking aspirin or acetaminophen. Shaking chills are especially suggestive of infection.

The most useful diagnostic test is arthrocentesis for cultures, Gram and/or acid fast staining, and full synovial fluid analysis as described above. Blood cultures and complete blood counts looking for leukocytes with left shift are required. Radiographs provide a baseline to compare for later evidence of erosions or osteomyelitis or to look for gas suggesting anaerobic infection or *Escherichia coli*. In joints that cannot be easily aspirated, gallium or indium scans can help suggest infection.

Course and Prognosis

Prognosis is excellent if diagnosis is established during the first several days and appropriate treatment is started. Acute gonococcal or streptococcal septic arthritis often resolve completely over 2 weeks. Resolution may be much slower with staphylococcal and gram-negative infections. Some improvement should be noted within 1 week with appropriate therapy. Prognosis is worse when previously diseased joints, late treatment, immunosuppression, polyarticular disease, and other high risk factors are present.

Treatment

Initial treatment includes prompt aspiration of the joint and repeated aspiration daily or more often to keep the joint free of destructive exudate. Guided by clinical and joint fluid clues, broad spectrum parental antibiotic coverage for gram-positive and (if any clues) for gram-negative organisms is usually needed until culture and sensitivity reports are obtained. Initial coverage should include a drug for methicillin-resistant staphylococci. If diagnosis or treatment are delayed, if the joint is less accessible to needle drainage, or if the patient is not responding, arthroscopic or surgical drainage may be needed. Splinting can reduce pain, but passive then active range of motion should be started as soon as tolerated to prevent contractures and loss of strength.

Duration of antibiotic therapy is determined by response and associated factors. Parenteral antibiotics are usually continued until the joint is virtually normal. Oral antibiotics are then used for an additional period. Staphylococcal infection in a RA joint may require at least 6 weeks of antibiotic treatment.

GOUT

Etiology and Pathogenesis

Gout is the deposition of monosodium urate crystals in joints and other connective tissues. This deposition is the result of hyperuricemia, with elevated serum uric acid levels causing supersaturation of extracellular fluids. As defined, gout can be asymptomatic when crystals are precipitated and detected only coincidentally. Most often gout is identified when urate crystal deposition causes acute or chronic arthritis, *tophi* (deposits visible over joints or in connective tissue or seen in radiographs on bones), gouty nephropathy, or renal stones.

Increased uric acid in the serum and in total body stores can result from overproduction or underexcretion of uric acid. Many genetic and environmental factors influence an individual's uric acid level. Some of the principal potentially treatable causes of hyperuricemia include underexcretion of uric acid due to diuretics, low-dose aspirin, cyclosporine, acidosis, or renal insufficiency. Overproduction of uric acid can be due to enzyme deficiencies but also occasionally to hematologic malignancies and psoriasis. Alcoholism contributes to gout both by increased production and decreased excretion of urate.

Whatever the cause of the hyperuricemia, when sufficient levels are present deposition of the monosodium urate (MSU) crystals can occur in joints and other connective tissues, including those of the kidney. If there is overexcretion, uric acid can precipitate in the renal collecting system and can cause stones.

Monosodium urate crystals in the joint can cause acute or chronic inflammation by stimulating the release of chemotactic factors and a variety of other mediators of inflammation. Crystals can also exist in the joint without causing inflammation; several groups are investigating how various proteins bound to the crystals and cytokines generated by the crystals affect the presence and pattern of inflammation.

Incidence and Risk

The prevalence of gout has increased over the last few decades in the U.S. and in a number of other countries with a high standard of living. Gout is predominantly a disease of adult men, with a peak incidence in the fifth decade. In 1986, the prevalence of self-reported gout in the U.S. was estimated at 13.6/1,000 men, and 6.4/1,000 women. Thus, gout is the most common cause of inflammatory arthritis in men over age 30, and probably the second most common form of inflammatory arthritis in the U.S. (11). In addition, gout frequently results in significant short-term disability, occupational limitations, and utilization of medical services, making the disease a significant public health problem.

Clinical Aspects

As with the other crystal diseases, gout can take several forms. Asymptomatic hyperuricemia is not strictly considered gout, as by no means all patients with hyperuricemia will develop clinical signs of gout.

The acute arthritis of gout is the most common early clinical manifestation. The metatarsophalangeal joint of the first toe is involved most often, and is affected at some time in 75% of patients. The ankle, tarsal area, and knee are also commonly involved. A wrist or finger joint is less often involved during early attacks. The first episode of acute gouty arthritis may begin fairly abruptly in a single joint, often during the night, so that the patient awakes with dramatic unexplained joint pain and swelling. Affected joints are usually warm, red, and tender. The diffuse periarticular erythema that often accompanies these attacks can be confused with cellulitis.

Early attacks tend to subside spontaneously over 3 to 10 days even without treatment. Desquamation of the skin overlaying the affected joint may occur when inflammation subsides. Patients are often completely free of symptoms after an acute attack. Subsequent episodes may occur more frequently, involve more joints, and persist longer. Polyarticular gout occasionally occurs in patients having their first attack. Usually, patients with more than one inflamed joint are those with more prolonged disease and suboptimal management. Acute attacks may be triggered by a specific event such as trauma, alcohol, drugs, swings in uric acid levels, surgical stress, or acute medical illness.

The intervals between attacks constitute the intercritical stage of gout. Even during an asymptomatic period, MSU crystals can often be aspirated from previously involved joints or from joints that have never been overly affected. Because crystal deposition persists between attacks, a definitive diagnosis can still be made even during this asymptomatic period (12).

Clinically evident subcutaneous MSU crystal-containing tophi occur only in fairly advanced gout, although microtophi appear to be present in the synovial membrane even at an early stage. On average, tophi are generally first noted 10 years after the initial episode of arthritis. Deforming arthritis can develop as a result of the erosion of cartilage and subchondral bone caused by crystal deposition and the chronic inflammatory reaction. Chronic gouty arthritis can mimic RA, although it tends to be less symmetric than typical rheumatoid disease and it can involve any joint.

Radiographs are usually normal except for soft tissue swelling with early acute gout. The bony erosions that can also occur in chronic gout are round or oval and are surrounded with a sclerotic margin.

The demonstration of MSU crystals is now generally considered to be mandatory for establishing the diagnosis of gout as an explanation to acute arthritis, because serum urate levels can be misleading. Only a single drop of fluid is necessary for the detection of crystals, and even the small amount of synovial fluid obtainable from the first metatarsophalangeal joint suffices in many cases. The crystals, which are either intra- or extracellular and are typically rod- or needle-shaped (3–20 μ), are usually visible with a light microscope. A polarizing microscope shows the characteristic negative birefingence.

The value of serum uric acid levels in diagnosis of the acute attack is limited. Serum uric acid levels can be normal at the time of acute gouty arthritis. Some normal levels are explained by high doses of aspirin or recent institution of a uricosuric agent. In almost all patients, serum uric acid levels will be elevated at some time. Serum urate measurements are important in following treatment. Some patients may have elevated serum uric acid due to drugs or other causes and do not have gout.

Course and Prognosis

Initial acute attacks subside spontaneously over days to a week. If gout is inadequately treated, episodes become more frequent and chronic tophaceous gout can develop. Over 20 years, more than 50% of untreated patients would develop overt chronic disease.

Treatment

Acute gout can be managed with one of several drugs, but resting the acutely inflamed joint will make any regimen more effective. Use of a nonsteroidal anti-inflammatory drug (NSAID) in doses at or near the maximum recommended is probably the most common regimen in patients with no contraindications to these agents. Colchicine is used less often, but 2 to 3 tablets (0.5 mg each) can be dramatically effective if given at the first sign of an attack. When given in the often recommended regimen of 0.5 mg every hour until 8 pills or intolerance, side effects such as nausea, vomiting, or diarrhea are common. Because many patients with gout have contraindications to NSAIDs or colchicine, or have severe attacks that are less responsive, adrenocorticosteroids or adrenocorticotrophic hormone (ACTH) have been increasingly used. Prednisone can be given at 20–40 mg/day and then gradually tapered as the attack subsides; ACTH can be given as 40–80 i.u. subcutaneously. If only one or two joints are involved, depot (or locally retained) corticosteroids can be injected intra-articularly once infection has been excluded. Intravenous colchicine is also a useful alternative in patients who are not taking medication orally.

If patients have recurrent attacks or tophi, plans must be made for long-term treatment with urate lowering agents, such as the uricosuric probenecid, or with allopurinol.

CALCIUM PYROPHOSPHATE DIHYDRATE DEPOSITION DISEASE

Etiology and Pathogenesis

Calcium pyrophosphate dihydrate crystal deposition disease can be defined as illness related to the presence of these crystals in joints, bursae, or other periarticular tissues (13). Deposition primarily occurs in cartilage and menisci and is initially asymptomatic. Crystal deposition can also occur as a late result of osteoarthritis. In this situation, the role of the CPPD is not clear.

Acute inflammation is thought to result from a dose-related response to release of CPPD crystals from deposits in cartilage or other tissues into the joint space. Phagocytosis of crystals (as occurs with urates in gout) releases inflammatory mediators causing the acute symptoms.

Radiographs showing calcific densities in articular hyaline or fibrocartilaginous tissue are diagnostically helpful. The most characteristic sites for this chondrocalcinosis are the knees and wrists, so these may be radiographed for screening. Joints with extensive joint space narrowing may not show chondrocalcinosis but may still contain CPPD.

Incidence and Risk

Although common, clinically symptomatic CPPD-associated disease is about half as frequent as gout. Incidence is nearly equal in men and women, but CPPD deposition dramatically increases with age. Nearly 50% of people have radiographic evidence of chondrocalcinosis (almost always due to CPPD) in their 80s. Risk of CPPD-associated disease clearly increases with age. Some associated diseases in younger patients include hyperparathyroidism, hemochromatosis, ochronosis, myxedematous hypothyroidism, hypophosphatasia, hypomagnesemia, and familial hypocalciuric hypercalcemia.

Clinical Aspects

There are a variety of clinical presentations seen with CPPD, including acute arthritis often called "pseudogout", chronic RA-like inflammatory arthritis, osteoarthritis, and a very destructive arthritis (13). Acute arthritis is the pattern in about 25% of cases.

Acute attacks occur in one or more joints and can last for several days or weeks. Attacks are self-limited but can be as abrupt in onset and as severe as true acute gout. The average attack is less painful than in gout. The knee is the site of almost one-half of all attacks, although any other joint (including the first metatarsophalangeal joint) can be involved. Provocation of acute attacks by surgery or other acute illness is common. Patients are usually asymptomatic between acute attacks.

Definitive diagnosis is only by identification of the classical rod- or rhomboid-shaped crystals as described above. Infection can coexist with CPPD disease, so it should be excluded. Some patients with CPPD disease develop significant fevers that cause confusion. Younger patients identified with CPPD should be checked by a thorough examination and with iron, transferrin, thyroid stimulating hormone, calcium, phosphorus, and magnesium levels in serum. Some CPPD deposits result from previous traumatic arthritis or meniscectomy and are localized to one joint.

Course and Prognosis

There is no known treatment to eliminate CPPD crystal deposits. Deposition generally increases gradually unless an underlying metabolic cause is corrected. Recurrent attacks or chronic arthritis often develop, although disabling disease is uncommon. Associated diseases can be life-threatening if not detected and treated.

Treatment

Acute attacks in large joints can be treated by thorough aspiration alone or combined with injection of a depot corticosteroid. Nonsteroidal anti-inflammatory drugs are often effective. Colchicine given intravenously may be used in patients who cannot take NSAIDs. Colchicine (0.5 mg once to twice a day) is often successfully used to prevent attacks.

APATITE CRYSTAL DISEASE

Etiology and Pathogenesis

Apatite crystals and other associated calcium phosphates commonly deposit in tendons, other soft tissues around joints, and in synovia. Most cases are idiopathic, although local trauma may be a factor as may be some systemic diseases. As with urates and CPPD, these deposits can be asymptomatic until aggregates of crystals are released into joint or bursal spaces to be phagocytized and cause acute inflammation (14,15).

Incidence and Risk

There are no accurate studies of incidence of either periarticular calcifications or acute attacks. This cause of acute arthritis or bursitis may be even more common than gout but may be missed because of difficulty in diagnosis. One survey showed that 5% of all adult shoulders had periarticular calcifications. Calcifications can be transient and disappear after attacks. Adults of all ages can be affected and incidence increases with age. Important risk factors for apatite deposition are renal failure treated with chronic dialysis and associated with hyperphosphatemia, the renal phosphate retaining syndrome of tumoral calcinosis, local deposition from steroid injections, central nervous system insults, collagen disease, and milk alkali syndrome.

Clinical Aspects

Acute inflammation due to apatite crystals is often more localized to a bursa or tendon sheath suggesting this diagnosis, although the entire joint may also be involved. There may be erythema, swelling, and tenderness; fever can occur. Pain on motion stressing the involved structure may also be severe with less objective evidence of inflammation. Common sites include shoulders, fingers, wrists, hips, and even the first metatarsophalangeal joints.

Diagnosis depends on classic findings: radiographic evidence of calcification in soft tissue at the site of pain, and ideally, crystal identification by aspiration of synovial or bursal fluid as described above. Individual apatite crystals can be seen only by electron microscopy, but clumps of crystals can appear as shiny but non-birefringent 2–20 μ chunks.

Course and Prognosis

Unless an underlying cause of correctable hyperphosphatemia or hypercalcemia can be detected, most patients remain at risk of further attacks. Disabling chronic disease is generally rare in idiopathic cases.

Treatment

Acute attacks can be treated with NSAIDs or with oral or intravenous colchicine. Aspiration of the calcific deposit and injection of a depot corticosteroid can also be very effective. Rest during the most acute pain should be followed by range of motion exercise as symptoms improve to prevent residual stiffness.

MANAGEMENT OF UNDIAGNOSED ACUTE ARTHRITIS

Management decisions often must be made before all the results of tests are available. For instance, a patient with synovial fluid indicating a highly inflammatory process, a negative Gram's stain, and no obvious source of infection requires antibiotic coverage, though it is wise to obtain several cultures first. Needle aspiration at least once daily is mandatory in suspected cases of septic arthritis as long as fluid is present. If cultures are negative and the arthritis persists, antibiotics are often discontinued and more extensive tests are performed. Often, NSAIDs are best withheld for a few days to avoid obscuring the natural course and any fever. In culture-negative patients, all fluid removed should be examined for crystals even if no crystals were seen in the first specimen aspirated. Colchicine, although initially considered a diagnostic test for gout, does not prove this diagnosis.

Local heat or cold applications are usually not needed. However, cold packs may occasionally be helpful when carefully used over acute gouty joints. Local protection with a splint or wrap may alleviate symptoms during evaluation. Casting should not be done over an acutely inflamed joint.

Several new techniques suggest that synovial biopsy may be useful in undiagnosed cases. Increased availability of the polymerase chain reaction and immuno-electron microscopy on synovium may allow the identification of elusive etiologic agents such as *Borrelia burgdorferi* causing Lyme disease, gonococci, chlamydia, or ureaplasma.

EDUCATION

Brochures from the Arthritis Foundation about specific suspected diseases can be used to initiate patient education. Adherence to treatment regimens may be especially critical in suspected septic arthritis and gout. Using a team approach to patient education did make an important difference in compliance and outcome in one study in patients with gout (16). Reassurance is often in order as soon as it becomes apparent that one is dealing with a self-limited and less dangerous form of acute arthritis.

REFERENCES

1. Baker DG, Schumacher HR: Acute monarthritis. N Engl J Med 329:1013–1020, 1993
2. Panush RS, Carias K, Kramer N, Rosenstein ED: Acute arthritis in the hospital. J Clin Rheumatol 1:74–80, 1995
3. Schumacher HR: Arthritis of recent onset. A guide to evaluation and initial therapy for primary care physicians. Postgrad Med 97:52–63, 1995
4. Eisenberg JM, Schumacher HR, Davidson PK, et al: Usefulness of synovial fluid analysis in the evaluation of joint effusions: use of threshold analysis and likelihood ratios to assess a diagnostic test. Arch Intern Med 144:715–719, 1984
5. Schumacher HR, Reginato AJ: Atlas of synovial fluid analysis and crystal identification. Philadelphia, PA, Lea & Febiger, 1991
6. American College of Rheumatology Ad Hoc Committee on Clinical Guidelines: Guidelines for the initial evaluation of the adult patient with acute musculoskeletal symptoms. Arthritis Rheum 39:1–8, 1996
7. Paul H, Reginato AJ, Schumacher HR: Alizarin red S staining as a screening test to detect calcium compounds in synovial fluid. Arthritis Rheum 26:191–200, 1983

8. Rahman MU, Cheema MA, Schumacher HR, et al: Molecular evidence for the presence of Chlamydia in the synovium of patients with Reiter's syndrome. Arthritis Rheum 35:521–529, 1992

9. Goldenberg DL, Reed JI: Bacterial arthritis. N Engl J Med 312:764–771, 1985

10. Mahowald M: Infectious arthritis: A. Bacterial agents. In, Primer on the Rheumatic Diseases. Tenth edition. Edited by HR Schumacher, JH Klippel, WJ Koopman. Atlanta, Arthritis Foundation, 1993, pp. 192–197

11. Lawrence RC, Hochberg MC, Kelsey JL, et al: Estimates of the prevalence of arthritic and musculoskeletal diseases in the United States. J Rheumatol 16:427–441, 1989

12. Pascul EV: Persistence of monosodium urate crystals and low-grade inflammation in the synovial fluid of patients with untreated gout. Arthritis Rheum 34:141–145, 1991

13. McCarty DJ: Calcium pyrophosphate dihydrate crystal deposition disease. In, Primer on the Rheumatic Diseases. Tenth edition. Edited by HR Schumacher, JH Klippel, WJ Koopman. Atlanta, Arthritis Foundation, 1993, pp. 219–222

14. McCarty DJ, Gatter RA: Recurrent acute inflammation associated with local apatite deposition. Arthritis Rheum 9:804–819, 1966

15. Fam AG, Ruberstein J: Hydroxyapatite pseudopodagra. Arthritis Rheum 32:741–747, 1989

16. Murphy-Bielicki B, Schumacher HR: How does patient education affect gout? Clin Rheumatol Prac 2:77–80, 1984

Rheumatic Diseases of Aging: Osteoporosis and Polymyalgia Rheumatica

MICHAEL J. MARICIC, MD

Rheumatic diseases of the elderly may result in significant pain, functional disability, and loss of independence. Although the elderly are susceptible to a wide variety of musculoskeletal disorders (e.g., osteoarthritis and crystalline arthritis) and immunologic disorders (e.g., rheumatoid arthritis) that may also affect younger patients, the problems of osteoporosis with resultant fractures and polymyalgia rheumatica/giant cell arteritis are found most commonly in patients over the age of 60, where they may cause a dramatic decline in patient's quality of life.

OSTEOPOROSIS

Etiology, Pathogenesis, and Incidence

Osteoporosis is "a disease characterized by low bone mass and microarchitectural deterioration of bone tissue, leading to enhanced bone fragility and a consequent increase in fracture risk" (1). Osteoporosis is a major medical, economic, and social health problem in the U.S. It has been estimated that 1.2 million fractures attributable to osteoporosis occur each year in persons aged 45 years and older (2). This includes 600,000 vertebral crush fractures and 250,000 fractures of the hip. One-third of women over the age of 65 will have vertebral fractures. The risk of hip fracture begins to increase after age 45, then rises exponentially, doubling for every five years of age.

When hip fracture does occur in the elderly, there is a 12% to 20% excess mortality rate in the next year due to complications of immobilization, such as pneumonia and pulmonary embolus. Approximately 50% of elderly patients with hip fractures never regain the same level of functional independence, and 25% require long-term institutional care. The total direct and indirect annual costs for osteoporosis approach $10 billion per year.

The etiology of osteoporosis is multifactorial. Genetics accounts for 40% to 60% of variance in bone mass. Postmenopausal estrogen deficiency, calcium deficiency, chronic alcohol and nicotine use, immobilization, and medications such as corticosteroids, anticonvulsants, and excessive thyroid supplementation all may contribute to accelerated bone loss.

Clinical Aspects and Diagnosis

Although assessing a patient's clinical risk factors for osteoporosis should be a routine component of the history, these risk factors have been shown to be unreliable for predicting an individual's bone density—the most important predictor of future fracture risk. Therefore, an essential component of diagnosis, prediction of future fracture risk, and measurement of the response to treatment involves bone density measurement. Dual energy x-ray absorptiometry (DEXA) is currently the gold standard because of its high level of accuracy and precision. Bone density measurement is essential for the diagnosis of low bone mass (3) and is an excellent method for assessing future fracture risk (4) and determining efficacy of therapy.

Quality of Life Assessment

Assessment of quality of life and functional disability should be as important in osteoporosis as in any other rheumatic disorder, for interventional studies and for the individual patient. A number of generic health assessment tools such as the Nottingham Health Profile and the Sickness Impact Profile, as well as more arthritis-specific instruments such as the Arthritis Impact Measurement Scales (AIMS) and modified Health Assessment Questionnaire (MHAQ), have been utilized in studies on osteoporosis. However, the validity of these instruments in osteoporosis has not been firmly established.

Treatment

Calcium. Retrospective studies have correlated lifelong calcium intake to increased bone density and decreased risk of hip fracture in later life (5). Prospective studies have also demonstrated prevention of bone loss, especially in women with low daily calcium intakes of less than 400 mg/day.

Chapuy and colleagues (6) were able to show a 43% reduction in hip fractures and 32% reduction in nonvertebral fractures in elderly community-dwelling patients treated for 18 months with 1.2 grams of elemental calcium and 800 IU Vitamin D_3. This study, conducted in France, may have included a number of patients who were vitamin D "insufficient", decreasing the potential applicability of the calcium supplementation to other populations. Nevertheless, the results emphasize the importance of calcium and vitamin D supplementation in this elderly population.

Calcium supplementation to achieve a total of 1,500 mg/day should be considered prudent therapy. In the elderly, calcium should be given with meals to ensure proper absorption, because hypoacidity impairs calcium absorption.

Estrogen Replacement Therapy. Estrogen replacement therapy (ERT) has been shown to prevent bone loss and osteoporotic fractures in postmenopausal women (7). Best results are obtained when therapy is started within 5 years of menopause; however, a recent study revealed significant benefit on bone density of the hip and lumbar spine in women an average of 14.6 years after menopause (8).

How long estrogen should be continued is not clear, but studies suggest a minimum of 5 to 7 years to significantly reduce fracture risk. After stopping ERT, rapid trabecular bone loss ensues just as it would have had ERT not been started. The decision to continue ERT must be based on the risk/benefit ratio for the individual patient. Most studies have been done with 0.625 mg conjugated equine estrogen, although 0.3 mg has also been shown to be protective in some patients. If a woman has had a hysterectomy, she may take unopposed daily estrogen. If the uterus is intact, ERT should either be cycled with medroxyprogesterone or given in daily combination with small daily doses of progesterone (such as medroxyprogesterone 2.5 mg/day) to protect the uterus from endometrial hyperplasia and carcinoma.

Women should have yearly mammograms while on ERT, and all breakthrough bleeding should be thoroughly investigated. The only absolute contraindications to ERT are prior breast or uterine carcinoma. Relative contraindications such as phlebitis *may* be more safely managed with the use of the estrogen patch, as there is no first-pass hepatic metabolism with tendency to raise fibrinogen levels. Some patients with migraines prefer transdermal to oral estrogen due to the more constant serum estrogen levels. Transdermal estrogen has been shown to prevent postmenopausal bone loss and osteoporotic fractures.

New selective estrogen receptor modulators such as raloxifene may prove to have beneficial effects on bone density preservation without the potential for stimulating breast and uterine tissue. Clinical trials are currently underway.

Calcitonin. Synthetic injectable salmon calcitonin has been available since 1986 for the treatment of osteoporosis (9). The usual dose is 50–100 IU every other day. Nasal spray calcitonin was approved in 1995 for the treatment of osteoporosis, and due to the ease of administration and diminished frequency of side effects such as nausea and flushing, will likely replace the use of the injectable form. The dose for the nasal spray is 200 Units (1 puff) per day. Administration of nasal spray calcitonin has been shown to result in increases of 2% to 3% in lumbar spine bone density over 2 years (10). It has not yet been shown conclusively to decrease the incidence of osteoporotic-related fractures, however studies designed to examine the endpoint of vertebral fracture prevention are underway.

One study of postmenopausal women treated with injectable calcitonin separated patients into high and low turnover groups on the basis of serum osteocalcin levels, urinary hydroxyproline/creatine ratios, and whole body retention of ^{99m}Tc-methylene diphosphonate. Significant differences were demonstrated at one year in vertebral and hip bone densities, especially in the spine, where a 22% increase was noted in the high turnover group (11). This would suggest that measuring parameters of bone resorption might be helpful in preselecting candidates for calcitonin and other anti-resorptive therapy.

Vitamin D. The recommended daily allowance for vitamin D is 400 IU/day, which is usually readily achieved through diet or exposure to sunlight. There is no currently established indication for large doses of vitamin D, including corticosteroid-induced osteoporosis. Because high levels of vitamin D may stimulate bone resorption in addition to causing hypercalcemia and hypercalciuria, therapy with large doses is potentially harmful.

1-25 dihydroxyvitamin D levels have been shown to decline in the elderly, hence there is some rationale for examining the role of supplementation in this age group. Some studies have suggested stabilization of bone loss; however, other studies have not been encouraging. The use of this metabolite should still be considered experimental.

Sodium Fluoride. Interest in therapeutic use of fluoride was stimulated in the early 1980s by studies that showed dramatic decreases in the incidence of vertebral crush fractures. However, sodium fluoride has significant toxicity in the gastrointestinal (nausea, pain, and rarely bleeding) and musculoskeletal (insufficiency fractures) systems. A recent 4-year, prospective trial of sodium fluoride versus placebo in postmenopausal women with osteoporosis demonstrated increases in vertebral bone density but no decrease in the number of new vertebral fractures (12). The radial shaft bone density decreased, however, and the number of nonvertebral fractures (including hip fractures) was higher in the fluoride treatment group. Fluoride therapy increased cancellous but decreased cortical bone mineral density leading to increased skeletal fragility. Sodium fluoride must still be considered an experimental therapy and used only with caution.

Androgens. The use of androgens in postmenopausal osteoporosis continues to stimulate interest because of their potential for increasing muscle mass as well as bone. Nandrolone decanoate in doses of 25–50 mg every 3 to 4 weeks has recently been shown to significantly increase total body calcium and forearm bone density in women and may prove to be a useful therapy in selected patients. Virilizing adverse effects often limit patient adherence.

Gonadal insufficiency should be suspected in any male with osteoporosis, especially those with chronic disease and/or on corticosteroid therapy (13). Testosterone replacement may be achieved with testosterone cypionate (200 mg intramuscularly every 3 weeks).

Bisphosphonates. Disodium etidronate was shown in an early study to significantly increase bone density and decrease the rate of new vertebral fractures. However, continuation of this study revealed an increase in vertebral fractures in the treatment group compared to placebo during the third year (14). Overall, there were less vertebral fractures in the treatment group over 3 years, but this difference was not statistically significant. Significant increases in spinal and hip bone density were seen after 3 years.

Disodium etidronate is given in doses of 400 mg/day for the first 2 weeks of a 12-week cycle. It must be given at least 2 hours before or after meals, because absorption even on an empty stomach is less than 5%. Patients must be instructed not to take this drug continuously; prolonged continuous treatment may cause osteomalacia and spontaneous fractures. It is not FDA-approved for the prevention or treatment of osteoporosis. Third-generation bisphosphonates such as tiludronate, alendronate, and risedronate, which inhibit osteoclastic bone resorption but not mineralization, may prove to be safer and more effective than disodium etidronate. Alendronate disodium received FDA approval in 1995 on the basis of a recent 3-year study that showed increases of 8.2% and 7.2% in spinal and femoral neck bone mineral density, respectively, with a 48% decrease in new vertebral compression fractures in the treatment group (15). Alendronate disodium (10 mg) should be taken early in the morning with an 8-ounce glass of water at least 30 minutes before breakfast, because the concomitant ingestion of any food or fluids other than water completely inhibits absorption. The most frequent adverse effect of bisphosphonates is esophageal irritation, so patients must be warned to remain upright and not to go back to bed, which could result in prolonged contact of the pill with the esophagus.

Corticosteroid-induced Osteoporosis

Corticosteroids induce osteoporosis through a variety of mechanisms (16). They inhibit bone formation by osteoblasts (in part by reducing bone cell production of insulin-like growth factors), decrease calcium absorption by the gut, and increase calcium excretion by the kidney. This leads to a net negative calcium loss and resultant secondary hyperparathyroidism, and also appears to decrease sex steroid hormone production.

An early study seemed to indicate that vitamin D could reverse these effects; however, these results have never been duplicated. Calcitonin, in some small studies, has been shown to prevent bone loss due to corticosteroids. A larger definitive study is underway. Studies of alendronate and risedronate for the prevention of corticosteroid-induced osteoporosis are also underway.

At present, there is no known effective therapy for corticosteroid-induced osteoporosis. Unfortunately, alternate-day corticosteroid administration does not result in less bone loss.

Optimization of calcium intake, regular weight-bearing exercise, and replacement of sex steroid hormone if prematurely diminished, are conservative and prudent measures. Deflazacort, an oxazoline analogue of prednisone, may induce less bone loss than other corticosteroids. Further clinical trials of this compound are necessary.

Physical Therapy and Exercise

Exercise regimens are an essential component of the overall management of patients with osteoporosis. Exercise can be divided into three main categories: 1) weight-bearing exercise to maintain bone mass; 2) exercises to decrease back pain; and 3) exercises to maintain lower extremity strength and prevent falls.

Although walking to maintain bone mass should be considered prudent in patients with osteoporosis, studies demonstrating benefit in maintaining or improving bone mass have been hampered due to small sample size, short trial duration, and ascertainment bias of the participants. Therefore, the scientific demonstration of benefit should be approached with caution. Part of the difficulty in assessing bone density response to exercise lies in the measurement of physical activity by various questionnaires and interviews, most of which have not been tested for reliability or validity. Some studies have shown that walking a few times a week for short periods may increase lumbar bone density (17), whereas other more strenuous exercise trials have demonstrated little or no benefit.

Because much of the chronic back pain in patients with osteoporosis originates in the soft tissue, physical therapy to stretch and strengthen back muscles should be an integral part of the treatment plan. In patients with established osteoporosis, extension exercises help increase back extensor muscle strength, whereas flexion exercises may be harmful (18).

Risk Prevention

Other risk factors for fracture such as home health hazards, the use of sedative medications, and ocular and auditory deficits should be corrected. In addition, an exercise program designed to improve muscle strength, balance, ability to transfer, and gait should be given to elderly patients at risk for falling (19). This may make a much more significant impact on fracture risk than any pharmacologic intervention in this age group.

POLYMYALGIA RHEUMATICA

Etiology, Pathogenesis, and Incidence

Polymyalgia rheumatica (PMR) is a common rheumatic disorder of older persons (20). The main clinical manifestations are pain and morning stiffness in the proximal areas of the shoulder and hip girdle. This syndrome is rarely diagnosed before the age of 50. In those aged 50 and older, the annual incidence of PMR is approximately 50/100,000. One of the most important features of PMR is its association with giant cell arteritis (approximately 20%).

Clinical Aspects and Diagnosis

Polymyalgia rheumatica is most commonly diagnosed after the age of 60, with a mean age of 70 years at diagnosis. The onset of symptoms is usually quite abrupt, and patients are often able to date the exact onset of their problem. The chief complaints are severe pain and stiffness of the neck and shoulder region, lower back, and proximal thighs. Morning stiffness is pronounced, usually for hours. Patients notice some improvement in their pain and stiffness with exercise and/or heat, but often the stiffness returns when they sit again. Symptoms are usually symmetric, although they may begin on one side only.

Patients may describe their pain as being "muscular", even though inflammation is in the joints. Distal muscular pain is rare; however, peripheral synovitis of joints including the knees, wrists, and hands is not uncommon. Some patients have carpal tunnel syndrome. Constitutional symptoms such as fatigue, anorexia, or weight loss may be present.

Physical examination of the patient with PMR is usually normal except for tenderness of the proximal musculature. Although patients may complain of being "weak", true weakness is absent. Prolonged stiffness of the musculature may lead to adhesive capsulitis, especially in the shoulder, which should be evaluated on physical exam.

An elevated erythrocyte sedimentation rate (ESR) is usually the cardinal and sole abnormal laboratory finding. Mild anemia may also be present.

Due to the marked morning stiffness and occasional synovitis in these patients, PMR may be confused with rheumatoid arthritis, and in fact has been called "rheumatoid arthritis of the elderly". Up to 10% of patients in this age group may have a positive rheumatoid factor, further complicating the diagnosis. In general, patients with PMR usually have predominantly proximal symptoms, while patients with rheumatoid arthritis usually have predominant symptoms in the small joints of the hands or feet.

A viral syndrome with diffuse myalgias may simulate PMR; however, symptoms of viral myalgia would not be expected to last more than a few days to a week. Hypothyroidism, Parkinson's disease, and depression may present with symptoms of stiffness and should be excluded. Fibromyalgia usually has an onset in a younger age group and the ESR is normal.

Course and Prognosis

Approximately 20% of patients with PMR have or will develop giant cell arteritis (also called temporal arteritis). This is a systemic vasculitis that leads to inflammation and occlusion of the arteries involved. Patients diagnosed as having PMR should be carefully questioned about symptoms of giant cell arteritis, because the prognosis and treatment are dramatically different. Likewise, older patients presenting with headache or visual disturbances and suspected of having giant cell arteritis should be questioned about symptoms of proximal stiffness and pain. This may be an important clue to the diagnosis of giant cell arteritis, as 50% of patients with giant cell arteritis have PMR.

Headache is the most common symptom of giant cell arteritis and is characteristically throbbing in nature and predominantly in the temporal area. However, the quality of the pain may be dull or sharp, and the location may be occipital or diffuse. Ophthalmic features include blurred vision, double vision, or amaurosis fugax. Pain on chewing, secondary to claudication of the jaw muscles, or scalp tenderness or numbness may be present. Constitutional symptoms such as weight loss, malaise, and low-grade fever are common.

Physical examination of the patient with giant cell arteritis may reveal tenderness, nodularity, or pulselessness of the temporal artery, although these findings are rare. Decreased visual acuity or fundoscopic findings such as ischemia or cotton wool spots may be present.

Laboratory findings often overlap those seen in PMR. The ESR is usually markedly elevated, and the anemia of chronic disease is often present. An elevation of the serum hepatic alkaline phosphatase is occasionally present.

Treatment

In the patient in whom giant cell arteritis is not present, treatment of PMR with low-dose prednisone should be instituted (21). The usual starting dose of prednisone is 10–20 mg/day. Patients usually report a dramatic improvement and even resolution of symptoms within 2 days. Many rheumatologists, in fact, consider such a response important in confirming their clinical diagnosis, and might reconsider the differential diagnosis if the patient did not have a dramatic response in a few days.

The rate of reduction of prednisone thereafter is dependent on the individual's clinical response. Steroids should be tapered according to the amount of tolerable stiffness and pain experienced by the patient. Some clinicians also utilize the ESR in deciding when to taper, although in most cases this is a reflection of patient symptomatology. In general, prednisone should be reduced as slowly as 1 mg every month or two, recognizing that PMR is usually self-limited and lasts 2 years on average.

At this dose and duration of prednisone, patients usually do not develop intolerable side effects of the drug such as osteoporotic fractures, diabetes mellitus, and cataracts. Should side effects develop, steroid-sparing agents such as plaquenil or methotrexate could be added in an attempt to decrease the symptoms of synovitis. Their efficacy is unproven, however.

In the patient with PMR who also has signs or symptoms of giant cell arteritis, prednisone (in doses of 40–60 mg/day) should be instituted and a temporal artery biopsy performed. Because 25% of temporal artery biopsies may be negative in patients with giant cell arteritis, the clinical diagnosis and suspicion is of utmost importance.

In giant cell arteritis, the initial dose of prednisone can be tapered after 1 month, depending on the clinical response. One tapering schedule might be to reduce the amount of prednisone by 10% every 2 weeks; however, this must be individualized according to therapeutic response and adverse effects. Due to the higher doses of prednisone used in this disorder, more frequent and serious adverse effects of corticosteroids such as osteoporotic vertebral compression fractures should be expected, and must be explained to the patient. As in PMR, treatment of giant cell arteritis is required for an average period of 2 years.

Physical therapy is often an important component in the treatment of patients with PMR and giant cell arteritis. Although PMR itself does not cause muscle weakness, the combination of corticosteroid-induced myopathy and disuse myopathy may result in significant proximal weakness and a predisposition to falling. Another clinical problem encountered in patients with PMR is adhesive capsulitis of the shoulders due to chronic synovitis. Exercises to maintain joint range of motion and proximal muscle strength may play a significant role in preventing immobility and functional disability in these patients.

REFERENCES

1. Kanis JA, Melton LJ, Christiansen C, Johnston CC, Khaltaev N: Perspective: the diagnosis of osteoporosis. J Bone Min Res 8:1137–1141, 1994
2. Riggs BL, Melton LJ: The prevention and treatment of osteoporosis. N Engl J Med 327:620–627, 1992
3. Johnston CC, Slemenda CW, Melton LJ: Clinical use of bone densitometry. N Engl J Med 324:1105–1109, 1991
4. Wasnich RD: Bone mass measurement: prediction of risk. Am J Med 96:6–10, 1993
5. Matkovic V, Kostal K, Simunovic I, Buzina R, Brodarec A, Nordin BEC: Bone status and fracture rates in two regions of Yugoslavia. Am J Clin Nutr 36:540–549, 1979
6. Chapuy MC, Arlot ME, Duboeuf F, et al: Vitamin D_3 and calcium to prevent hip fractures in elderly women. N Engl J Med 327:1637–1642, 1992
7. Lindsay R, Hart, DM, Forrest C, Baird C: Prevention of spinal osteoporosis in oophorectomized women. Lancet 1:1151–1153, 1980
8. Lindsay R, Tohme JF: Estrogen treatment of patients with established postmenopausal osteoporosis. Obstet Gynecol 76:291–295, 1990
9. McDermott MT, Kidd GS: The role of calcitonin in the development and treatment of osteoporosis. Endocr Rev 8:377–390, 1987
10. Overgaard K, Hansen MA, Jensen SB, Christiansen C: Effect of salcaatonin given intranasally on bone mass and fracture rates in established osteoporosis: a dose-response study. BMJ 305:556–561, 1992
11. Civitelli R, et al: Bone turnover in postmenopausal osteoporosis: effect of calcitonin therapy. J Clin Invest 82:1268–1274, 1988
12. Riggs BL, et al: Effect of fluoride treatment on the fracture rate in postmenopausal women with osteoporosis. N Engl J Med 322:802–809, 1990
13. Seeman E: Osteoporosis in men: epidemiology, pathophysiology, and treatment possibilities. Am J Med 95:21–28, 1993
14. Harris ST, et al: Four-year study of intermittent cyclic etidronate treatment of postmenopausal osteoporosis: three years of blinded therapy followed by one year of open therapy. Am J Med 95:557–567, 1993
15. Liberman UA, Weiss SR, Bröll J, et al: Effect of oral alendronate on bone

mineral density and the incidence of fractures in postmenopausal osteoporosis. N Engl J Med 333:1437–1443, 1995

16. Libanati CR, Baylink DJ: Prevention and treatment of glucocorticoid-induced osteoporosis. Chest 102:1427–1435, 1992

17. Krolner B, Toft B, Neilsen SP, et al: Physical exercise as prophylaxis against involutional vertebral bone loss: a controlled trial. Clin Sci 64: 541–546, 1983

18. Sinaki M, Mikkelsen B: Postmenopausal spinal osteoporosis: flexion versus extension exercises. Arch Phys Med Rehabil 65:593–596, 1984

19. Tinetti ME, Baker DI, McAnvay G, et al: A multifactorial intervention to reduce the risk of falling among elderly people living in the community. N Engl J Med 331:821–827, 1994

20. Machedo EBV, Michet CJ, Ballard DJ, et al: Trends in incidence and clinical presentation of temporal arteritis in Olmestead County, Minnesota 1950-1985. Arthritis Rheum 31:745–749, 1988

21. Kyle V, Hazelman BL: Treatment of polymyalgia rheumatica and giant cell arteritis: steroid regimes in the first 2 months. Ann Rheum Dis 48:658–661, 1989

Common Soft Tissue Rheumatic Disorders:
Bursitis, Tendinitis, Carpal Tunnel, Myofascial Pain, and Fibromyalgia

SHARON R. CLARK, PhD, RN-C, FNP

There are 640 muscles in the human body, and in adults of normal weight the soft tissue muscle mass constitutes 40% of the total body mass. The majority of patients who present to their health care provider with a complaint of rheumatic pain have a soft tissue disorder rather than a true arthritis. Appropriate diagnosis is challenging; in most instances, diagnostic tests are unavailable and diagnosis requires correctly identifying the precise anatomical structures involved.

Effective management of common soft tissue conditions requires a structured history that includes identification of precipitating and aggravating factors. Injury may result from a single event or may be caused by repetitive overload. The practitioner should ask questions regarding repetitive activities that irritate the involved structures and evaluate for biomechanical dysfunction, such as unequal leg lengths, that may be contributing factors. It is not unusual for more than one syndrome to occur concomitantly.

In patients with a septic bursitis or tendinitis, there should be a history of a penetrating injury. In the absence of such history, look for a blood-borne sepsis such as gonococcemia.

PRINCIPLES OF MANAGEMENT

There are common strategies of management for bursitis, tendinitis, carpal tunnel, and myofascial pain. If possible, the aggravating factors should be identified. Then, counsel the patient on avoidance of the aggravating factors, which may include modification of the work environment. Prescribe appropriate aids to correct biomechanical disruption. Such aids can include slings, shoe lifts, splints, or canes. Relief of pain is another important principle. Prescribe nonsteroidal anti-inflammatory drugs (NSAIDs) when evidence of inflammation is present. If appropriate, consider the use of intra-lesional corticosteroid injections. Finally, a physical therapy program should be designed, including stretching and strengthening exercises to avoid recurrence.

BURSITIS

Inflammation of a bursa may be superficial (such as in the shoulder, knee, or elbow) or deep (such as those around the hip and the ischial tuberosity). The latter do not present with obvious swelling and thus the diagnosis must be inferred from eliciting local tenderness (Table 1) and exacerbation of pain by

activation of the associated muscles. Because bursitis seldom shows on imaging studies, these should not routinely be obtained. Aspiration of the bursa can be useful to differentiate between irritated, gouty, and infective bursitis.

For non-infective bursitis, the affected area should be rested by use of a sling, cane, or splint. After aspirating the bursa, inject a mixture of 1% procaine (about 3 ml) containing 1–2 ml of a long-acting corticosteroid preparation such as triamcinolone hexacetonide, prednisolone acetate, or dexamethasone acetate. The patient should experience pain relief within 10 minutes due to the local anesthetic. Warn the patient that this relief will wear off within an hour and that they may experience more pain over the next 12 to 24 hours. Pain should subside when the corticosteroid preparation takes effect. In some cases, the injection of a long-acting corticosteroid preparation may invoke an acute inflammatory reaction similar to gout. This is almost always averted if the patient is given an NSAID concomitantly. Therapy with NSAIDs should continue until 1 week after all symptoms have subsided. Once the aggravating factors have been eliminated, the patient seldom needs repeated injections. A recurrence of the bursitis within 7 days of the injection should raise a suspicion of septic bursitis, and reaspiration is indicated.

Patients with an infected bursa often have an elevated temperature. In addition, the overlying tissues may be hot, red, and exquisitely tender. Optimal treatment includes aspiration with culture and sensitivities. Patients with multiple systemic features should have blood cultures. Septic bursitis is usually due to a penicillin-resistant *Staphylococcus aureus* and should always be considered if the patient is a diabetic, an intravenous drug user, or is otherwise immunocompromised. Septic bursitis always requires systemic antibiotic therapy. Patients with a more serious underlying condition need intravenous antibiotic therapy. At the initiation of therapy, the bursal contents should be drained through a 16 to 18 gauge needle. This drainage may need to be repeated two to three times over the course of the first week of treatment (1).

Olecranon Bursitis. Risk factors for olecranon bursitis include gout, rheumatoid arthritis, or calcium pyrophosphate deposition. Local erythema should always raise the suspicion of a septic bursitis.

Trochanteric Bursitis. Trochanteric bursitis typically has a gradual onset. Risk factors include aging, being overweight, having osteoarthritis of lumbar spine or hip, leg length discrepancy, and scoliosis. Treatment includes local injection of corticosteroid using a 22-gauge 3.5 inch needle, use of NSAIDs,

Table 1. Commonly involved areas of bursitis.

Bursa	Symptom	Physical Findings
Olecranon*	Elbow pain	Swelling, tender on pressure over olecranon, no loss of motion
Trochanteric*	Lateral hip and thigh pain	Point tenderness over trochanteric bursa
Iliopsoas	Painful groin and anterior thigh	Tender over inguinal triangle
Ischial (weavers bottom)*	Pain on sitting or lying, may radiate down back of thigh	Point tenderness over ischium
Anserine*	Painful knee, worse on stair climbing	Tenderness over medial aspect of knee
Prepatellar (housemaid)*	Painful knee	Swelling and tenderness over patella
Infrapatellar*	Painful knee	Swelling and tenderness below patella
Achilles (pump bump)*	Painful heel	Subcutaneous swelling at back of Achilles tendon
Calcaneal	Painful plantar surface of heel	Tenderness over calcaneum

* Location specific considerations (see text).

weight loss, stretching and strength training, correcting biomechanical disruption, and use of a cane when indicated.

Ischial Bursitis. Use of cushions and injection of corticosteroids are indicated in the presence of ischial bursitis.

Anserine Bursitis. The preferred therapies for anserine bursitis are rest, weight loss (if indicated), corticosteroid injection, and stretching and strengthening of the quadriceps muscles.

Pre- and Infra-patellar Bursitis. Pre- and infra-patellar bursitis result from knee trauma such as frequent kneeling. A history of trauma with disruption of skin over the knee in addition to findings of swelling and heat should raise the suspicion of sepsis.

Subcutaneous Achilles Bursitis. Subcutaneous Achilles bursitis results from the pressure of shoes; the only treatment is relief of this pressure. Due to the risk of Achilles tendon rupture, the area should not be injected.

TENDINITIS

The term *tendinitis* refers to an inflammation of the peritendinous tissues or synovial sheaths (tenosynovitis). Most instances of tendinitis result from overuse or unaccustomed activity. Rest of the affected area is important in treatment (2). Commonly involved tendons and the accompanying findings are noted in Table 2. An accurately placed injection of corticosteroids provides the quickest symptomatic relief. Tendons themselves are never injected; it is the small space between the exterior surface of the tendon and the peritendinous sheath that is infiltrated with a mixture of corticosteroids and local anesthetic. To avoid snagging the tendon, it is important to have the bevel of the needle facing downward and parallel to the long axis of the tendon.

Supraspinatus. Supraspinatus tendinitis is often associated with calcific deposits. Risk factors include repetitive overhead

motion and the presence of an inflammatory process. There is often an osteophyte on the underside of the acromion-clavicular joint that irritates this tendon; in recurrent cases it should be removed via arthroscopy. Chronic involvement of the supraspinatus tendon predisposes to a partial or complete tear of the rotator cuff.

Finger Flexors. Alcoholism, epilepsy, diabetes, and heredity are risk factors for Dupuytren's tendinitis. Corticosteroid injections given intralesionally usually provide relief. However, surgery is indicated if contracture occurs.

Patellar. Local corticosteroids are contraindicated in patellar tendinitis.

Achilles. Risk factors for Achilles tendinitis include overuse, improper shoes, and inflammatory rheumatic conditions such as anklyosing spondylitis and Reiter's syndrome. Local injections should not be used with the Achilles tendon because of its propensity to rupture.

CARPAL TUNNEL SYNDROME

Pain or tingling in the hands is commonly caused by entrapment of the median nerve where it passes, along with the flexor tendons of the fingers, through a tunnel at the wrist. Symptoms include median paresthesias that may affect the index finger, middle fingers, and radial side of the ring fingers. Nocturnal paresthesias are common and may wake the patient. Any condition resulting in edema—including pregnancy, weight gain, inflammatory arthritis, or hypothyroidism—may precipitate carpal tunnel syndrome. Repetitive use of the hands is another common precipitating factor.

The physical examination should include Phalen's test, which is performed by holding the flexed fingers against each other for 60 seconds, or Tinel's test, which is performed by percussing over the median nerve on the volar aspect of the

Table 2. Commonly involved sites of tendinitis.

Tendon	Symptom	Physical Findings
Supraspinatus*	Pain in shoulder, especially lateral deltoid	Painful arc especially 60° to 120°; active abduction > passive
Bicipital	Pain anterior shoulder	Point tenderness over bicipital groove
Lateral epicondyle muscle attachment (tennis elbow)	Pain on motion such as lifting	Point tenderness just below lateral epicondyle
Extensor pollicis brevis and abductor pollis brevis (de Quervain's)	Wrist pain	Pain increases when thumb folded into palm and fingers flexed around thumb and wrist deviates toward ulnar side
Finger flexors (Dupuytren's)*	Trigger finger	Catching on extension of finger
Patellar*	Knee pain	Tenderness over patellar tendon
Achilles*	Anterior ankle pain	Tenderness over and proximal to attachment; increased pain on dorsiflexion

* Location specific considerations (see text).

wrist. While these tests lack a high degree of sensitivity, either test may be used for gross screening and is considered positive if paresthesia occurs. If symptoms persist despite conservative treatment, surgery should be considered. In this setting, the diagnosis may be aided by electrodiagnostic testing.

Treatment

The first line of treatment includes correction of any underlying disorder and avoidance of the aggravating factors. In milder cases, splinting of the wrists in the neutral positions, use of NSAIDs in doses sufficient for anti-inflammatory effect, and local steroid injections using a 25-gauge needle may produce relief. In more severe or recurrent cases, surgical intervention to decompress the tunnel is indicated. The patient should be warned that surgery does not guarantee against recurrence of the symptoms (3).

MYOFASCIAL PAIN

Myofascial pain has been reported as the most frequent cause of chronic pain syndromes. It presents as regional pain characterized by palpation of a tender spot in a taut band of muscle. The pain usually includes a "zone of reference," thus the irritative focus is commonly called a *trigger point*. Diagnosis and treatment of myofascial pain is dependent on the concept that the pain, restricted motion, taut bands, and zone of reference are caused by the trigger point within the muscle (4). Researchers have identified 147 trigger points and their zones of reference (5,6).

Many patients with myofascial pain are misdiagnosed as having bursitis, tendinitis, or nerve entrapment syndrome. Misdiagnosis, inappropriate testing, and inadequate treatment result in treatment failure and a labeling of the patient as having a "functional syndrome." In order to diagnose and adequately treat this syndrome, the examiner must first identify the proper trigger point. The contributing and perpetuating factors that cause increased tension in the muscles must be identified. These factors may include improper posture, especially forward head thrusting, repetitive overload, and emotional stress. Failure to identify and correct the underlying cause and treating only the zone of reference will result in treatment failure.

Therapy consists mainly of physical modalities. Aggravating factors should be identified and eliminated. Spray and stretch therapy may be used, consisting of the application of anesthetic spray (such as Fluori-Methane®) or a brief ice massage followed immediately by passive stretching of the muscle, as described below. Trigger point injections should be considered for highly irritable trigger points or for patients in whom the stretching does not resolve the pain (4–6).

Spray and Stretch

This type of therapy consists of an application of a vapocoolant spray over the muscle with simultaneous passive stretching. The cool spray is used as a distractionary technique based on the gate theory of pain; actual cooling of the muscle should be avoided. A fine stream of the spray is aimed at the skin directly overlying the muscle with the trigger point. A few sweeps of the spray are made over the trigger point and zone of reference.

This is followed by a progressively increasing passive stretch of the muscle. Frosting the skin and excessive sweeps tend to lower the temperature of the muscle and may aggravate the trigger point.

Trigger Point Injections

Before injecting trigger points, the patient should be educated that determining the exact location will depend on patient reports of increased pain felt at the moment of entering the trigger point. The exact trigger point should be palpated and marked. Once located, active or latent trigger points should be sought in the antagonist muscle, which may also need injecting in order to avoid recurrence.

Trigger points are usually injected with 3–5 ml of 1% procaine. Prior to injection, inquire whether the patient is allergic to local anesthetics. A 22- to 24-gauge needle is inserted into the trigger point, guided by the patients' report of pain. Signs that the trigger point has been entered include: 1) patients experience sudden pain; 2) there is increased resistance to the tip of the needle; and 3) a transient "twitch response" of the muscle is noted. Approximately 0.5 ml is injected, then the needle is partially withdrawn so that movement in and out of the muscle band but not the skin occurs. The needle is then reinserted into an adjacent area of the muscle. This peppering procedure is repeated until no further pain in the area is experienced (7).

Pain relief should occur within a few minutes in the zone of reference. After pain relief, the muscle should be stretched for 1 to 2 minutes to the fullest range of motion, followed by 30 minutes of heat application. A mild increase in pain may be felt 2 to 5 hours after the injection but should subside within 3 days. Instruct the patient to minimize the use of involved muscle groups for 5 to 7 days after the injection.

There are often several trigger points responsible for the pain, and more than one may need to be injected to receive total relief. Due to the increased risk of light-headedness, bradycardia, and hypotension from large volumes of anesthetic, the number of injected trigger points at one time should not exceed three. Repeat visits can be scheduled at 1 to 2 week intervals. Anaphylaxis is a rare complication of trigger point injections. Clinicians doing these procedures should have the appropriate emergency equipment for treating an anaphylatic reaction. Caution must be used when treating trigger points in the upper back and thorax, because a pneumothorax will occur if the needle penetrates the pleura of the lung. Entering trigger points at an oblique angle to the surface of the chest wall minimizes the likelihood of this complication. Contraindications to the use of trigger point injections include severe acute muscle injury, allergies to the specific anesthetics, bleeding difficulties or anticoagulant therapy, and infection in the area.

Other Treatment

An aggressive physical therapy program is crucial to the long-term success of the above techniques. It should consist of graded active and passive stretching and strengthening of the muscles and total body endurance (aerobic) training. Lack of exercise and improper use of muscles or poor posture are often correctable contributing factors to the development of trigger

Table 3. Diagnostic fibromyalgia paired tender points.

Name	Location
Occiput	Insertion of occipital muscles into base of skull
Low cervical	Cleido-mastoid over anterior part of C5–C7 intertransverse process
Trapezius	Midpoint upper border of muscle
Supraspinatus	Above scapular spine at medial border
Costo-chondral	Lateral to second costo-chondral junction; pectoralis major muscle
Epicondyle	Extensor origin; 2 cm distal to lateral epicondyle
Gluteal	Upper outer quadrant of buttocks; gluteal muscle
Greater trochanter	Gluteal muscle; just posterior to trochanteric prominence
Knee	Vastus medialis proximal to the joint line

points. Patients should be taught that the stretching, strength, and endurance program is lifelong (8).

There is little evidence that inflammation exists in myofascial pain. The use of NSAIDs may be beneficial only as analgesics; other analgesics with less gastrointestinal risk may be more appropriate. Analgesic medication is indicated especially during the first few days after trigger point injections when the patient may experience an increase in pain before receiving pain relief.

FIBROMYALGIA

Fibromyalgia is a syndrome of widespread body pain that has been present for at least 3 months and includes the physical finding of multiple tender points. The typical patient with fibromyalgia is a woman between 25 and 45 years of age. A recent prevalence study indicated that fibromyalgia affects 3.4% of women and 0.5% of men (9); it has been reported worldwide.

Although the etiology remains unknown, it is unlikely that a single etiologic mechanism results in the complexity of symptoms. The pain most likely arises from the muscle (10). The persistent muscle pain leads to changes in the central nervous system such that pain is perceived from stimuli not previously perceived as painful (11). Symptoms may wax and wane, but they are likely to persist over the course of the patient's life (12). There is no evidence that they necessarily progress in severity or that they are a prodrome to another illness.

In addition to diffuse generalized aching, most patients also feel exhausted even after a night of sleep. Typically, sleep is light and unrefreshing with a disordered sleep physiology characterized by alpha intrusion on non-REM sleep (13). Other commonly associated symptoms present in about one-third of patients with fibromyalgia include irritable bowel syndrome, tension headaches, sicca symptoms, and Raynaud's phenomenon.

A physical examination may be unrevealing unless the clinician pays attention to the characteristic tender points. In 1990 the American College of Rheumatology published diagnostic criteria that include the presence of at least 11 of 18 specified tender points (Table 3) (14). Presence of widespread pain for at least 3 months, the typical tender points, and unrefreshing sleep should suggest the diagnosis of fibromyalgia, whether or not the patient has additional concomitant disorders. There are no diagnostic laboratory tests.

The multiplicity of patient complaints along with normal laboratory testing has led many practitioners unfamiliar with fibromyalgia to label patients as psychologically dysfunctional. However, there is no evidence that these patients differ psychologically from other patients with a chronic pain disorder (15). The most frequently reported *Diagnostic and Statistical Manual of Mental Disorders (Fourth edition)* psychiatric disorder is depression, which has a lifetime prevalence of 30% in patients with fibromyalgia.

Treatment

Successful treatment of fibromyalgia must be individualized, holistic, comprehensive, and goal-oriented. Unlike medical conditions in which cure is the expected outcome, management of fibromyalgia must focus on functional goals and should place the patient in the role of the primary worker. One useful tool for monitoring progress in treatment is the Fibromyalgia Impact Questionnaire (16).

Currently there are no treatments available to eliminate the pain associated with fibromyalgia. However, management strategies can provide significant benefit, and most patients remain productive members of society. Treatment programs that include education, exercise, cognitive restructuring, and relaxation techniques have had greater success than traditional rheumatic disease management strategies (17). This approach has reported subjective improvements of 60% to 64%, and improvements in tender points of 46% (18).

Patients rarely respond to treatment with NSAIDs, and corticosteroids are never indicated as they have been shown to have no benefit. Fibromyalgia patients frequently have concomitant myofascial trigger points, which must be treated appropriately. If concomitant medical disorders, depression, or other psychological problems are present, they too must be appropriately treated.

Sleep

Almost all patients with fibromyalgia have a history of nonrefreshing sleep; therefore, any causes of the sleep disturbance (e.g., sleep apnea, bruxism, reflux) must be identified and treated. An often overlooked problem is periodic limb movement or nocturnal myoclonus; the bed partner may help verify this problem. These patients can also be identified by daytime restless leg syndrome characterized by extremity dysthesiae (feelings of numbness, tingling, insect crawling, etc.) and the need to constantly move legs. Sinemet® (carbidopa-levodopa; 10–100) or Klonopin® (clonazepam; 0.5 mg) taken with the evening meal can help this disorder (19). Sleep disturbance in fibromyalgia patients is improved by use of a tricyclic antidepressant. In general the dose is low, not more than one-fifth of the antidepressant dose. Effectiveness is thought to depend on the ability of tricyclic antidepressants to block the uptake of serotonin and antihistaminic activity.

Patients should be taught the basic principles of good sleep hygiene (see Chapter 21, Sleep Disturbance). While regular aerobic exercise aids in delta sleep, this exercise should not be undertaken within 4 hours of bedtime. Gentle stretching and relaxation exercise prior to bedtime may aid in refreshing sleep.

Exercise

The majority of patients with fibromyalgia also have deconditioning, which perpetuates problems of fatigue, pain, and makes the muscles more susceptible to damage. Thus, muscle conditioning plays an important role in the management of fibromyalgia. Patients may be reluctant to exercise, because attempts usually result in pain and a flare of symptoms often occurring 2-3 days after exertion. When prescribing exercise, it is important to note that eccentric work may exacerbate pain in fibromyalgia. This exacerbation of pain typically does not respond to eccentric training, which may be due to low levels of growth hormone found in many fibromyalgia patients (20). If a patient reports that vacuuming, overhead movements, walking downhill or downstairs causes flares, the patient probably has a problem with eccentric work. In this setting, the exercise prescription should minimize eccentric work. Attempts at eccentric training should be done very gently and slowly progress in intensity.

Initially, patients should undertake a program of gentle, progressive stretching. Stretching aids in the release of the often tightened muscle bands and, when properly performed, will provide pain relief. Prior to stretching, muscles should be warmed either actively by gentle exercise or passively by warm bath or hot tub. The amount of the stretch is important. Stretching to the point of resistance and then holding the stretch will allow the Golgi tendon apparatus to signal the muscle fibers to relax. Stretching to the point of increased pain, however, will precipitate a contraction of additional fibers and have the opposite effect. The stretch should be gentle and should be sustained for 60 seconds. Often patients must work up to this amount of time and start with 10–15 seconds on and 10–15 seconds off the stretch. No bouncing movements should be performed during stretching.

Successfully engaging in a stretching program will provide reinforcement for the patient to continue with exercise. Learning not to maintain sustained contractions may also aid in pain relief. For activities requiring repetitive contractions, a stretch break every 20 minutes will be of benefit.

Strength training should focus on functional strength and muscle toning, and should not be undertaken until the patient is engaging in a regular program of stretching. Use of bands, soft weights, or equipment such as Nautilus or Universal machines can provide resistance while not requiring a tightened grip and sustained contractions. Start with small sets of three to five repetitions and add sets as tolerated.

Concomitant with stretching and strength training, fibromyalgia patients should engage in activities that promote aerobic conditioning. The prescription should emphasize non-impact loading exercise such as pool exercise with aqua-belts, walking, and stationary cycling. One caution is that stationary bicycles may aggravate gluteal trigger points and produce symptoms resembling sciatica. Walking has the advantage of being easy to accomplish and does not require additional equipment. While most patients cannot initially complete 30 minutes of daily aerobic activity, they can start with two or three daily exercise bouts of 3–5 minutes duration. These bouts can be increased until patients are doing two 15-minute, three 10-minute, or one 30-minute bout daily. On bad days, patients can decrease the duration but should continue to exercise. Conversely, on good days patients should not try to make up for missed sessions.

Cognitive behavioral techniques are important for improving coping strategies for control over pain and less pain behavior (see Chapter 10, Cognitive Behavioral Interventions). Programs that include meditation to trigger the relaxation response and teaching mindfulness have been shown to be effective in the treatment of fibromyalgia (17). Mindfulness teaches patients to pay attention to "automatic thoughts" and to view them objectively.

Managing time and planning activities is crucial to the successful management of fibromyalgia. Patients should be encouraged to continue activities that are considered to be pleasurable. Achieving a better night's sleep, becoming physically fit, and using cognitive restructuring techniques are equally important components of the treatment plan.

REFERENCES

1. Canoso JJ: Bursitis, tenosynovitis, ganglions, and painful lesions of the wrist, elbow, and hand. Curr Opin Rheumatol 2:276–281, 1990
2. Stern P: Tendinitis, and overuse syndromes, tendon injuries. Hand Clin 6:467–476, 1990
3. Nakano KK: Entrapment neuropathies and related disorders. In, Textbook of Rheumatology. Edited by WN Kelley, ED Harris Jr, S Ruddy, CB Sledge. Philadelphia, WB Saunders, 1993, p. 1712
4. Fricton J: Clinical care for myofascial pain. Dent Clin North Am 35:1–28, 1991
5. Travell JG, Simons DG: Myofascial Pain and Dysfunction: The Trigger Point Manual. Baltimore, Williams & Wilkins, 1983
6. Travell J, Simons D: Myofascial Pain and Dysfunction: The Trigger Point Manual. Vol. 2. Baltimore, Williams & Wilkins, 1992
7. Hong C: Considerations and recommendations regarding myofascial trigger point injection. J Musculoskeletal Pain 2:29–59, 1994
8. Rosen N: The myofascial pain syndromes. Phys Med Rehabil Clin North Am 4:41–63, 1993
9. Wolfe F, Ross K, Anderson J, Russell IJ, Hebert L: The prevalence and characteristics of fibromyalgia in the general population. Arthritis Rheum 38:19–28, 1995
10. Bennett RM, Jacobsen S: Muscle function and origin of pain in fibromyalgia. Baillieres Clin Rheumatol 8:721–746, 1994
11. Mense S: Nociception from skeletal muscle in relation to clinical muscle pain. Pain 54:241–289, 1993
12. Bengtsson A, Backman E, Lindblom B, Skogh T: Long term follow-up of fibromyalgia patients: clinical symptoms, muscular function, laboratory tests—an eight year comparison study. J Musculoskeletal Pain 2:67–80, 1994
13. Moldofsky H, Scarisbrick P, England R, Smythe H: Musculosketal symptoms and non-REM sleep disturbance in patients with "fibrositis syndrome" and healthy subjects. Psychosom Med 37:341–351, 1975
14. Wolfe F, Smythe HA, Yunus MB, Bennett RM, Bombardier C, Goldenberg DL, Tugwell P, Campbell SM, Abeles M, Clark P, Fam AG, Farber SJ, Fiechtner JJ, Franklin CM, Gatter RA, Hamaty D, Lessard J, Lichtbroun AS, Masi AT, McCain GA, Reynolds WJ, Romano TJ, Russell IJ, Sheon RP: The American College of Rheumatology 1990 criteria for the classification of fibromyalgia: report of the Multicenter Criteria Committee. Arthritis Rheum 33:160–172, 1990
15. Ahles TA, Khan SA, Yunus MB, Spiegel DA, Masi AT: Psychiatric status of patients with primary fibromyalgia, patients with rheumatoid arthritis, and subjects without pain: a blind comparison of DSM-III diagnoses. Am J Psychiatry 148:1721–1726, 1991
16. Burckhardt CS, Clark SR, Bennett RM: The Fibromyalgia Impact Questionnaire: development and validation. J Rheumatol 18:728–733, 1991
17. Goldenberg DL, Kaplan KH, Nadeau MG, Brodeur C, Smith S, Schmid CH: A controlled study of a stress-reduction, cognitive-behavioral treatment program in fibromyalgia. J Musculoskeletal Pain 2:53–66, 1994
18. Bennett RM, Campbell S, Burckhardt C, Clark SR, O'Reilly C, Wiens A: A multidisciplinary approach to fibromyalgia treatment. J Musculoskeletal Med 8:21–32, 1991
19. Montplaisir J, Lapierre O, Warnes H, Pelletier G: The treatment of the restless leg syndrome with or without periodic leg movements in the sleep. Sleep 15:391–395, 1992
20. Bennett RM, Clark SR, Campbell SM, Burckhardt CS: Low levels of somatomedin C in patients with the fibromyalgia syndrome: a possible link between sleep and muscle pain. Arthritis Rheum 35:1113–1116, 1992

Additional Recommended Reading

1. Bennett RM: Fibromyalgia: the commonest cause of widespread pain. Compr Ther 21:269–275, 1995
2. Boissevain MD, McCain GA: Toward an integrated understanding of fibromyalgia syndrome. II. Psychological and phenomenological aspects. Pain 45:239–248, 1991
3. Clark SR: Prescribing exercise for fibromyalgia patients. Arthritis Care Res 7:221–225, 1994
4. King JC, Goddard MJ: Pain rehabilitation. 2. Chronic pain syndrome and myofascial pain. Arch Phys Med Rehabil 75:S9–S14, 1994
5. McClaflin RR: Myofascial pain syndrome: primary care strategies for early intervention. Postgrad Med 96:56–59,63–66,69–70, 1994
6. Myofascial pain syndrome, and the fibromyalgia syndrome, Second World Congress on Myofascial Pain and Fibromyalgia, Copenhagen. J Musculoskeletal Pain 1:1993
7. Masi AT, editor: Fibromyalgia and myofascial pain syndromes. Baillieres Clin Rheumatol, 1994

Regional Illness:
Managing Musculoskeletal Predicaments

NORTIN M. HADLER, MD, FACP, FACR

Coping with musculoskeletal symptomatology is one of life's challenges (1). Seldom is there a discrete or violent precipitant. Instead we become aware that using a musculoskeletal region, even in a fashion that is customary, causes discomfort. The symptoms rarely reflect a systemic musculoskeletal disease. Far more often, the pain and restriction of motion, even when severe, reflect a minor disorder of the tissue involved—a "regional musculoskeletal disorder."

REGIONAL MUSCULOSKELETAL SYMPTOMS

Approximately one-half of all individuals will be faced with an episode of regional musculoskeletal symptoms within the next 2 months. The majority of episodes involve some degree of low back pain that lasts about a week. Upper extremity and neck discomfort, including discomfort that interferes with customary function, is not quite as common. However, within the next 3 years nearly everyone will experience an episode of neck/upper extremity regional symptoms lasting about 1 month. No one is able to totally ignore these episodes; they instantly become a predicament of life. We are forced to consider their implications in terms of our healthfulness and to choose a course of action. Often the symptoms are familiar in that we have dealt successfully with similar experiences.

Most people rely on "common sense", the general understanding as to the cause of, implications of, and recourse for such an experience. However, common sense varies from place to place and from time to time. Health care providers should be cognizant of the common sense in their community so that they can disabuse patients of the more counterproductive precepts. For example, "common wisdom" often holds that usage which causes the pain to worsen is the usage that caused the pain in the first place. Such thinking underlies terms like tennis elbow or housemaid's knee. It may be that these regional disorders come and go without relationship to use; however, it is because of use that we become aware. Many more of us might be aware of our "tennis elbow" if we played tennis. The cause is not so important, but realization of the *pattern of usage* that exacerbates the symptom can prove palliative.

Nearly all regional musculoskeletal symptoms are self-limited, although their natural history can encompass months, and their severity can be daunting. Patients need to know that patience in coping will almost always be rewarded by healing and return to prior usage.

Many people will turn to over-the-counter medicines for pain. Prescription medications are often proffered, even if they are not sought. In terms of analgesic and anti-inflammatory effectiveness, there is little data to suggest that one agent is better than another. More importantly, there is little if any data to suggest that any anti-inflammatory agent or opiate offers more benefit to the patient than acetaminophen for these regional musculoskeletal disorders. Other agents offer a far greater potential for toxicity, particularly in the elderly, and most are far more costly.

Other people might turn to physical interventions. It is important to realize that any physical interventions must be comfortable, that none are mandatory or "indicated", and that nearly all are empirical. In the mind of the patient, benefits should clearly outweigh discomfort, inconvenience, stigmatization, or enforced disability. One should feel in control of all empirical decisions.

LESSONS OF CLINICAL EPIDEMIOLOGY

For centuries, nearly all clinical textbooks and papers were written by "expert" clinicians drawing inferences from personal experiences in the context of their institutional base. Many advances in diagnosis and therapy have resulted. So, too, have many false starts if not false steps. Today we know better than to assume that personal experience is not blinded by personal conviction or that the experience in one setting will generalize to any other setting.

The Fallacy of Generalization

There are dramatic examples of regional musculoskeletal disorders of the upper extremity. For example, there are examples of *tenosynovitis*, wherein the synovial tissue that normally ensheaths a moving tendon is inflamed (*-itis*) meaning painful, swollen, warm, and red. Moving such an inflamed tendon against resistance is painful. Such a finding is often a sign of a systemic rheumatic disease. Very occasionally, there is no systemic disorder to account for this obvious pathology, and none will develop over time. This is what de Quervain described at the abductor tendons at the base of the thumb, for example. However, great license has been taken with such terms as tendinitis, epicondylitis, fibrositis, and so on. Local tenderness or discomfort when the tendon is moved against resistance without any certain signs of redness, swelling, or warmth is also labeled tendinitis with an assumption that pain alone is a *forme fruste* of the classical disease. There is little justification for such an assumption. If all that is apparent is focal pain, then "focal pain" or "localized soreness" are the only meaningful labels available. Using clinical diagnoses that suggest greater disease than is demonstrable will distort the patient's perception of the problem in a way that is neither palliative nor defensible. Uncertainty as to the etiology of the

Table 1. Cardinal features that distinguish regional from systemic musculoskeletal disorders.

CHARACTERISTICS OF THE REGIONAL MUSCULOSKELETAL DISORDERS

1. The patient would feel well if it were not for the musculoskeletal region that hurts. There are no systemic symptoms such as fever or weight or appetite loss.
2. Night pain is not prominent. Resting the part that hurts is palliative.
3. There is a prominent biomechanical component to the symptomatology. Usage exacerbates pain.
4. Aside from restricted motion, there are few if any objective findings. In particular, overt inflammation (redness, swelling, warmth) affecting the symptomatic part is not present.

"RED FLAGS" FOR THE POSSIBILITY OF SYSTEMIC ILLNESS

1. Even without the musculoskeletal symptoms, the patient would feel ill. Symptoms may include fever, weight loss, loss of appetite, and pathologic fatigue.
2. Beware of night pain. Resting may palliate regional pain, but not systemic pain. Night pain that causes the patient to pace or fidget often indicates bone pain and may suggest metastatic neoplasms or infection.
3. Beware of pain that causes any motion, particularly writhing, which may indicate a vascular or visceral catastrophe.
4. Any patient who has findings of overt, objective inflammation should be evaluated for systemic diseases. Any redness or swelling should exclude regional disorders as presumptive diagnoses.
5. There should be no suggestion of atrophy, dystrophy or infarction of muscles or skin.
6. Beware of joints that do not have a normal range of motion. If articular motion is compromised, systemic disease becomes a possibility.

"focal pain" is reassuring; nearly all such presentations are self-limited and benign.

The False Positive Test

The standard literature urges us to elicit a Tinel's or Phalen's sign because of its specificity for carpal tunnel syndrome, to palpate the lateral epicondyle for the tenderness that is tennis elbow, to quantify spinal mobility, and to yank and crunch the knee. However, such urgings reflect the accrual biases of generations of prominent "experts" who described and applied the tests. In order to assess the utility of a particular test, the population must be appropriate to the setting in which the test is to be applied. In actuality, the predictive values of most classic signs of the regional disorders, when applied to any but the "classic" populations of yesteryear, is so low as to render them useless.

DISTINGUISHING REGIONAL DISORDERS

Several clues are useful in discriminating systemic disease from all the regional disorders. First, systemic illness presenting with musculoskeletal symptoms is relatively uncommon in persons between the ages of 18 and 50. These illnesses also are uncommon in youth, but the young seldom complain of regional illness, so any complaint should be reviewed. They are more common in the elderly who are so accustomed to coping with regional illnesses that any verbalized complaint bears perspicacity. But for the vast majority of the working age population, musculoskeletal symptoms are likely to be regional, lacking the "red flags" for systemic illness (Table 1).

OSTEOARTHRITIS

Osteoarthritis (OA), also called degenerative joint disease, describes the progressive loss of cartilage accompanied by bony reactions including sclerosis and osteophyte (spur) formation that affects many joints in the body (see Chapter 30, Osteoarthritis). Osteoarthritis is highly prevalent; in fact, no axial skeleton is spared by mid-life. The tradition in medicine is to ascribe regional musculoskeletal symptoms to radiographic OA of associated joints. That tradition must be reexamined (2). Although joints undergo pathologic changes and consequently lose range of motion, the patient may experience no pain. Regions suffering the pathology of OA often are painful. However, the pain is usually intermittent while the pathology is relentless. Therefore, a diagnosis of OA does not diagnose the cause of the pain, nor does it have prognostic significance. Too many patients are led to believe that their spurs, or disc disease, or "bad joints" account for their pain and seal their fate. Spurs, "ruptured discs", and the like are largely irrelevant. As a corollary, radiographs should not be obtained with the goal of seeking OA; rather, imaging studies are useful to help exclude systemic diseases in the appropriate setting.

HAND AND WRIST PAIN

Hand and wrist pain with motion and soreness to the touch will affect some 15% of us for 1 week each year. Almost all discomfort and tenderness is self-limited and bodes no evil. Until recently, most people coped without seeking medical assistance. However, the current wisdom is that people with hand/wrist pain should not cope on their own. The population seeking care for hand/wrist complaints is larger than and unlike any before.

Osteoarthritis of the Hand and Wrist

Most hand/wrist discomfort relates to the soft tissues. However, there are symptoms at the hand and wrist that are associated with OA. These become nearly ubiquitous by late life. They can be recognized by their two principle manifestations.

Deformity. Osteoarthritis of the hands has a readily recognizable pattern of involvement (Figure 1), with both cosmetic and functional implications. The precision and power of pinch are most at risk.

Discomfort. Persons with OA of the hands experience intermittent discomfort in a distinctive fashion. The involved joints are intermittently inflamed, although to a modest degree at worst. Slight swelling, aching pain, and morning stiffness can come and go, usually lasting no more than days, seldom interfering with function, and usually responding to conservative treatment.

A more persistent and compromising problem relates to power pinch with the thumb. Power pinch at the thumb pivots at the first carpometacarpal (CMC) joint. In the normal hand, the CMC slides laterally before stabilizing against its ligaments. With OA of the CMC, power is compromised. Often, pinch causes pain in the region of the joint. Pain at this location is often misinterpreted as a soft tissue illness, more particularly as de Quervain's tenosynovitis, which deprives the patient of the insights that follow from the correct diagnosis (Figure 2).

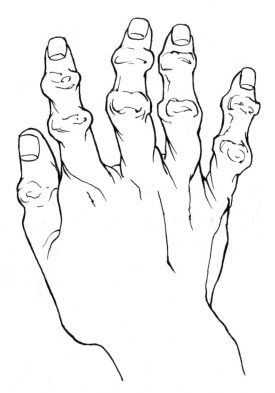

Figure 1. Osteoarthritis affects the majority of postmenopausal women. Men are affected as well, though later in life and with lesser severity. The pattern of involvement is distinctive. The distal interphalangeal joints (DIP) undergo loss of joint space and mobility. Efforts at repair lead to the growth of cartilagenous excrescences at the dorsolateral joint margins, Heberden's nodes, and malalignment. The first carpometacarpal joint (CMC) at the base of the thumb is similarly involved (see Figure 2). The proximal interphalangeal joints are also involved, leading to the formation of Bouchard's nodes and further malalignment.

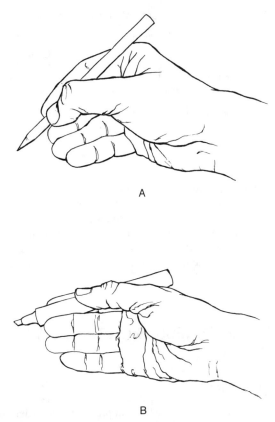

Figure 2. The first carpometacarpal joint (CMC) at the base of the thumb is frequently involved in osteoarthritis. Ability to abduct the thumb is compromised; progressively the thumb is forced into adduction. The typical symptom, however, is pain with power pinch. Power pinch **(A)** can be circumvented by employing an implement of larger diameter, thus permitting grasp in the length of the opposing digits **(B)**.

Soft Tissue Pain

Often, there is no good physical explanation for hand and wrist pain. Aside from focal tenderness and increased pain with motion of the painful region, little can be determined upon examination. We can demonstrate no reproducible anatomic or pathophysiologic abnormality despite the marvels of modern diagnostics. The cause is subtle, indeterminate, and usually benign. Reassuring the patient as to outcome without exacerbating the uncertainties that confound any illness is paramount. Informing and educating the patient is mandatory; in fact, it is the first line of therapy.

Today the traditional language of diagnostics for regional musculoskeletal disorders is unsupportable and iatrogenic. We lose nothing in content if we talk about tenderness at the lateral wrist rather than tenosynovitis. Furthermore, we will not confuse our patient nor encourage unwarranted leaps as to pathogenesis or prognosis. Focal tenderness exacerbated by certain usages of the hand and wrist is a frequent predicament. These conditions are self limited and should not cause alarm. Appropriate alteration in hand usage is usually palliative. Little else is as reliably effective.

Ganglion

A ganglion is a subcutaneous cystic structure usually presenting at the dorsal wrist and occasionally at the volar wrist. The skin moves freely over this "bump", which is bound to the underlying hard tissues. There may be some tenderness and discomfort associated with wrist motion. The cause of ganglia has not been definitively established. Even their pathology is not straightforward; occasionally they are outpouchings of the synovial cavity but more often they are self-contained cystic structures filled with mucinous debris, suggesting embryologic rests. Management is based on informing and reassuring the patient. Surgery is a cosmetic option.

Neuropathic Pain

The three major nerves to the upper extremity emanating from the brachial plexus are at risk for localized, isolated pathology. Fortunately, such processes rarely occur without overt trauma. By far the most common peripheral neuropathy of the upper extremity is a median neuropathy (see Chapter 33, Soft Tissue Rheumatic Diseases). Even idiopathic carpal tunnel syndrome has a frequency of only one diagnosed case in 2,000 adults followed for 1 year; a frequency that is not increased in any population regardless of the quality of hand or arm usage (3).

Irritation of nerve roots as they exit the cervical spine is a far more common cause of arm/hand pain than any peripheral neuropathy. These radiculopathies are distinctive in the quality and distribution of pain. The discomfort is dysesthetic and is neither exacerbated nor relieved by hand motion. Table 2 offers a summary of the classical distribution of the cervical

Table 2. Signs and symptoms of cervical radiculopathies.

Root	Pain Numbness	Sensory Loss	Motor Loss	Reflex Loss
C3	Occipital region	Occiput	None	None
C4	Back of neck	Back of neck	None	None
C5	Neck to outer shoulder and arm	Over shoulder	Deltoid	Biceps Supinator
C6	Outer arm to thumb and index fingers	Thumb and index fingers	Biceps (triceps) and wrist extensors	Triceps Supinator Biceps
C7	Outer arm to middle finger	Index and middle fingers	Triceps	Triceps
C8	Inner arm to fourth and fifth fingers	Fourth and fifth fingers	Intrinsics, Extrinsics	None

radiculopathies. However, short of overt weakness or certain atrophy, there is no reason for alarm or surgical referral. Most cervical radiculopathies are self-limited. Reassurance, acetaminophen, and warm showers are palliative. Patients may be advised to avoid flexion or extension of the neck, which increase stress on the neural structures as they exit the cervical spine.

REGIONAL ILLNESSES OF THE LOW BACK AND NECK

It may be said that the choice to be a patient for a regional backache is, nearly always, just that—a choice. The volitional aspect of seeking care must be appreciated in order to do justice to the choice, which is often driven by confounding issues that must be addressed if therapy is to succeed (4). If the response is to prescribe analgesia and/or proscribe function, the result will be a costly compromise in patient satisfaction with care, in patient understanding of the illness, and in patient function (5). If the response is contingent on defining the cause of the pain, the search is almost always futile. If the response is to seek a cure, the only ally in the exercise is natural history. The only therapeutic contract that can be successfully enjoined relates to coping.

The data addressing issues related to the management of acute low back pain is rich and informative. It is also readily accessible (see additional recommended reading). The discussion of regional low back pain extrapolates to regional neck pain reasonably well. Table 3 summarizes the author's version of evidence-based management. This advice represents a radical departure from the tone and substance of precedent reviews, and will be discussed below.

Symptoms and Signs. Quantification of reproducibility (6), and of sensitivity and specificity (7), places the physical signs long held to be useful in the diagnosis of regional back pain into perspective. With the exception of cauda equina syndrome, none can offer substantial insights when it comes to the diagnosis or management of low back pain. Short of overt weakness, no finding—not even stretch signs or focal neurologic abnormalities—can alter the diagnostic synthesis or restructure therapeutic options for sciatica or other leg pain syndromes (8). Sciatica is no more ominous a presentation than regional low back pain alone (9).

Imaging Modalities. Pinpointing the cause of regional low back pain is difficult. The conundrum arises from the fact that pathoanatomy is so common in the adult as to be "normal". Only a minority of adults have the pristine lumbosacral anatomy they were born with (10). The clinically meaningful question is not whether there is pathoanatomy. Instead, it

should be "Which aberration accounts for this episode of regional low back pain or of regional sciatica?"

Surgery and Other Invasive Interventions. In spite of 50 years of zeal, which appears to know no bounds (11,12), the surgeon has little if anything to offer the patient with regional low back pain or regional sciatica. There are patients for whom elective surgery is sensible; but they are exceptional indeed. There is no substantive data to show that invasive procedures of any kind afford benefit beyond that of the natural history. For facet joint injections (13), benefit proved elusive in a well designed study with sufficient statistical power to detect even minor salutary effect. There have been two decades of conflicting results on epidural steroid injection for sciatica. Percutaneous discectomy proved more disappointing even than chemonucleolysis in a compellingly elegant study (14). Discectomy may help some patients with sciatica whose illness persists for a month or two (15). However, the information is from a single, barely interpretable trial that represents the underpinnings of one of the most frequently performed surgical procedures in the U.S. This putative minor benefit is not easily reproducible (16) nor readily justifiable (17,18).

SUMMARY

It is necessary to understand regional arm and axial syndromes in order to appropriately inform and advise patients. For the

Table 3. Evidence-based management of a patient with a regional backache.

1. When eliciting the history of the present illness, the clinician must probe for psychosocial confounders.
2. The elicitation of the history of the present illness is an instructional event for the patient as well as the physician. The patient should be disabused of any false inferences, including those regarding causation, pathophysiology, and prognosis.
3. The physical examination can assuage clinical uncertainty, to some degree, regarding the regional nature of the illness. However, it offers little in terms of pathophysiologic insight.
4. Imaging modalities offer the potential for great anatomic definition. However, even dramatic degenerative changes at the lumbosacral spine are common in the asymptomatic and persist in the patient long after symptoms have subsided.
5. Do not "invalid" your patient either by your attitude or by your prescription. Urge coping and advise neutral postures but do not prescribe bed rest.
6. Do not prescribe an analgesic for impaired coping; doing so clouds the issues further and promulgates prolonged illness. Seldom is any prescription analgesic mandatory; attention to posture and to psychosocial confounders are the front line of therapy.
7. Regional low back pain is not a surgical disease. There is no compelling evidence that any invasive, even "minimally invasive", technique can provide benefit.

vast majority of patients, specialized facilities are unnecessary, and more specialized insights are ephemeral. There are five tenets for management of these patients: 1) listen closely to the predicament without presuppositions; 2) provide explanations and reassurance regarding the natural history of the syndrome; 3) avoid unreliable diagnostic labeling; 4) explore alternative patterns of usage of the painful region, both on and off the job; and 5) prescribe acetaminophen as the first-line agent of choice if any analgesia is necessary.

REFERENCES

1. Verbrugge LM, Ascione FJ: Exploring the iceberg: common symptoms and how people care for them. Med Care 25:481–486, 1987
2. Hadler NM: Knee pain is the malady - not osteoarthritis. Ann Intern Med 116:598–599, 1992
3. Hadler NM: A keyboard for 'Daubert'. J Occup Environ Med 38:469–476, 1996
4. Hadler NM: The injured worker and the internist. Ann Intern Med 120:163–164, 1994
5. Von Korff M, Barlow W, Cherkin D, Deyo RA: Effects of practice style in managing back pain. Ann Intern Med 121:187–195, 1994
6. McCombe PF, Fairbank JCT, Cockersole BC, Pynsent PB: Reproducibility of physical signs in low-back pain. Spine 14:908–918, 1989
7. Deyo RA, Rainville J, Kent DL: What can the history and physical examination tell us about low back pain? JAMA 268:760–765, 1992
8. Van den Hoogen HMM, Koes BW, van Eijk JTM, Bouter LM: On the accuracy of history, physical examination, and erythrocyte sedimentation rate in diagnosing low back pain in general practice: a criteria-based review of the literature. Spine 20:318–327, 1995
9. Weber H: The natural history of disc herniation and the influence of intervention. Spine 19:2234–2238, 1994
10. Jensen MC, Brant-Zawadski MN, Obuchowski N, Modic MT, Malkasian D, Ross JS: Magnetic resonance imaging of the lumbar spine in people without back pain. N Engl J Med 331:69–73, 1994
11. Davis H: Increasing rates of cervical and lumbar spine surgery in the United States, 1979–1990. Spine 19:1117–1124, 1994
12. McGuire SM, Phillips KT, Weinstein JN: Factors that affect surgical rates in Iowa. Spine 19:1117–1124, 1994
13. Carette S, Marcoux S, Truchon R, Grondin C, Gagnon J, Allard Y, Latulippe M: A controlled trial of corticosteroid injections into facet joints for chronic low back pain. N Engl J Med 325:1002–1007, 1991
14. Revel M, Payan C, Vallee C, et al: Automated percutaneous lumbar discectomy versus chemonucleolysis in the treatment of sciatica: a randomized multicenter trial. Spine 18:1–7, 1993
15. Hoffman RM, Wheeler KJ, Deyo RA: Surgery for herniated lumbar discs: a literature synthesis. J Gen Intern Med 8:487–498, 1993
16. Alaranta H, Hurme M, Einola S, et al: A prospective study of patients with sciatica: a comparison between conservatively treated patients and patients who have undergone operation. Part II: results after one year follow-up. Spine 15:1345–1349, 1990
17. Shvartzman L, Wengerten E, Sherry H, Levin S, Persaud A: Cost-effectiveness analysis of extended conservative therapy versus surgical intervention in the management of herniated lumbar intervertebral disc. Spine 17:176–182, 1992
18. Weber H: The natural history of disc herniation and the influence of intervention. Spine 19:2234–2238, 1994

Additional Recommended Reading

1. Hadler NM: Occupational Musculoskeletal Disorders. New York, Raven Press, 1993
2. Bigos S, Bowyer O, Braen G, et al: Acute Low Back Problems in Adults. Clinical Practice Guideline No. 14. AHCPR Publication No. 95–0642. Rockville, MD, Agency for Health Care Policy and Research, Public Health Service, U.S. Department of Health and Human Services, December 1994

<table>
<tr><td>CHAPTER

35</td><td># Impact of Rheumatic Disease
on Society</td></tr>
</table>

CHAPTER

35

Impact of Rheumatic Disease on Society

LEIGH F. CALLAHAN, PhD

Rheumatic disease and musculoskeletal conditions are the most prevalent chronic conditions in the U.S. and are projected to remain prevalent in the future. In 1990, an estimated 37 million individuals in the United States population (15.0%) reported having rheumatic diseases, including 22.8 million women (18.0%) and 14.2 million men (11.7%) (1). In addition to being the most prevalent chronic condition, rheumatic disease is one of the leading causes of disability (1,2). It is also associated with significant work disability and limitations in performing activities (3–5).

The economic, social, and psychological impact associated with rheumatic diseases is enormous (6). While some of the effects are easily translated into economic terms such as medical care costs and lost wages, others are not easily determined, such as the inability to enjoy leisure activity, a reduction in housekeeping activities, or pain. The impact of rheumatic disease is underestimated because of difficulties in quantifying many of the consequences and the high prevalence among older persons and women (7).

Despite its prevalence and impact, the public health importance of rheumatic disease has not been emphasized previously (8). Public health agencies, health care providers, and researchers often focus resources and prevention efforts on diseases associated with acute mortality, rather than on conditions contributing to reduced quality of life, activity limitations, and increased health care utilization (8). Although there are no cures for chronic arthritis, there are a number of strategies for primary, secondary, and tertiary prevention that should be considered.

PREVALENCE

In a report using data from the National Health Interview Survey (NHIS), prevalence estimates were derived from self-reported arthritis in the United States for 1990. Survey respondents were asked about the presence of any of a variety of musculoskeletal conditions during the preceding twelve months and for details of these conditions. Each condition was assigned an *International Classification of Diseases, Ninth Revision, Clinical Modification* (ICD-9-CM) code. "Arthritis" was classified as a condition that matched ICD-9-CM codes selected by the National Arthritis Data Workgroup (1). Data were weighted to provide average annual prevalence estimates;

synthetic state estimates were developed by applying respective regional arthritis rates that were stratified by age, sex, race, and ethnicity to the stratum-specific population rates.

An estimated 37 million persons (15.0%) of the U.S. population reported arthritis during 1990 (1). The estimated prevalence rate increased directly with age, with rates of 1.3% for individuals age 24 years or less, 6.6% aged 25–34 years, 12.7% aged 35–44 years, 22.6% aged 45–54 years, 36.5% aged 55–64 years, 45.4% aged 65–74 years, 55.2% aged 75–84 years, and 57.1% for individuals aged 85 years or older (Figure 1). Age-adjusted rates were higher in women (17.1%) than in men (12.5%). Age-adjusted rates were also higher in individuals with 11 years or less of formal education, and in those who resided in households with an annual income less than $20,000. Rates were similar for blacks and whites.

When the average rank and prevalence of chronic medical conditions (minus mental conditions) in the U.S. in 1983 to 1985 were compared by age and gender, arthritis was the sixth ranked condition in women aged 18–44 years, with a rate of 63.6 per 1,000 women, and the tenth ranked condition in men 18–44 years, with a rate of 40.7 per 1,000 (8). In men and women 65 years and older, arthritis was the first ranked condition, with rates of 382.6 and 544.1 per 1,000 in men and women, respectively. Arthritis was the pre-eminent chronic condition in older men and women, followed by high blood pressure and hearing impairment (8).

As the average age of the U.S. population increases, an estimated 59.4 million individuals (18.2% of the estimated population) may be affected by rheumatic diseases by the year 2020 (1). This represents an increase of 57% in the estimated number of persons with arthritis, largely attributable to the high prevalence of these diseases among older persons and the increasing age of the U.S. population.

IMPACT OF DISEASE

Disability and Activity Limitations

The symptoms and consequences of rheumatic disease often result in limitations in functional capacity and the ability to perform activities of daily living. An estimated 6.9 million (2.8%) individuals in the U.S. reported arthritis as a major or contributing cause of activity limitation during 1990 (1). Re-

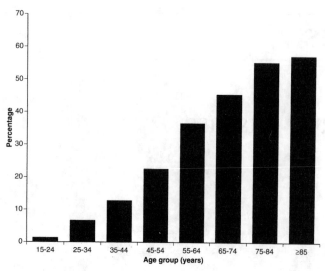

Figure 1. Estimated average annual prevalence of self-reported arthritis in the U.S. in 1990, by age category. Data from *Morbidity and Mortality Weekly Report*, June 24, 1994.

spondents were asked whether they were limited in working, housekeeping, or performing other activities as a result of health condition(s) and were asked what condition(s) they considered to be responsible for these activity limitations. Activity limitation associated with rheumatic disease increased directly with age. Age-adjusted rates of activity limitation were significantly higher for blacks (4.0%) and American Indians/Alaskan natives (4.2%) than for whites (2.6%). Rates of activity limitation attributed to arthritis were higher in individuals with fewer years of formal education and a lower annual income (1).

When the rank and prevalence of chronic conditions causing disability in the U.S. in 1991–1992 were analyzed in the Survey of Income and Program Participation (SIPP), arthritis was the leading cause of disability (Figure 2) (2). Measures of disability used in the SIPP were derived from D- and I-codes in the *International Classification of Impairments, Disabilities, and Handicaps*. Disability was assessed using five measures:

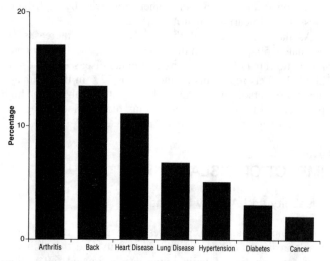

Figure 2. Prevalence of chronic conditions causing disability in the U.S. in 1991 to 1992. Data from *Morbidity and Mortality Weekly Report*, 1994.

1) ability to perform functional activities; 2) activities of daily living; 3) instrumental activities of daily living; 4) presence of selected impairments; and 5) use of assistive aids. Results from the SIPP estimated that 42 million persons in the U.S. reported one or more conditions they believed to be associated with their disability. Of those individuals, 17.1% reported arthritis or rheumatism, 13.5% reported back or spine problems, and 11.1% reported heart trouble as being associated with their disability (2).

Work Disability and Role Limitations

The capacity of individuals with rheumatic diseases to work is significantly affected (3–5). In fact, rheumatic disease is the leading cause of work loss. Approximately one-half of the patients with rheumatoid arthritis (RA) who are working at the onset of disease become work disabled (3), and substantial earnings losses and work disability have been noted in individuals younger than age 65 with asymmetric oligoarthritis, surrogate for osteoarthritis (OA) (5). Work autonomy, social factors, and disease factors are significant predictors of work disability in individuals with arthritis (3,4). However, it has also been demonstrated that the risk of becoming work disabled in 5 years in a cohort of individuals with RA was predicted more by clinical status at study entry than by work structure (9). A more extensive discussion of the rates of work disability in arthritis, as well as the individual and societal factors influencing disability, is presented in Chapter 25, Work Disability.

Economic Consequences

In 1992 terms, the total costs of arthritis and musculoskeletal conditions were $149.4 billion dollars, or the equivalent of 2.5% of the 1992 Gross National Product (Table 1) (6). Just under one-half of the total costs were due to direct costs of medical care. Of these direct costs, 41.5% of the costs reflect hospital and physician inpatient costs, 15.8% are outpatient costs, 20.3% represent nursing home care, and the remainder is attributed to drugs, nonphysician health care professional visits, administration, and other costs (6). Indirect costs, primarily due to lost wages, account for $77.1 billion of the costs associated with arthritis and musculoskeletal conditions (6). For all types of arthritis, the total costs were $64.8 billion. The direct costs of medical care account for an even smaller proportion (23.5%) of the total costs. The magnitude of work loss costs due to arthritis is $49.6 billion; this estimate would be

Table 1. Total costs of musculoskeletal and associated conditions in billions of 1992 dollars, by condition* (6).

Condition	Direct Costs %	Indirect Costs %	Total
Musculoskeletal conditions, except injuries	45.7 (38.6)	72.8 (61.4)	118.5
All forms of arthritis	15.2 (23.5)	49.6 (76.5)	64.8
Musculoskeletal injuries	26.7 (86.1)	4.3 (13.8)	31.0
Fractures	19.6 (82.0)	4.3 (18.0)	23.9
Total-all musculoskeletal conditions	72.3 (48.4)	77.1 (51.6)	149.4

* Values are the cost in billions of dollars (% of total).

even larger if the costs attributed to loss of homemaking functions could be more easily determined (6).

The economic costs associated with RA approximate those of coronary heart disease (10–12). In the U.S., the direct costs of RA are, on average, three times the costs of medical care for persons of the same age and gender who do not have RA (10). The per-person annual medical care costs have been estimated at approximately $5,400 (in 1994 terms) (12). Physician-visit costs comprised over $1,500 of this annual cost, and hospital admissions accounted for over $3,500 despite the relatively infrequent occurrence of hospitalizations. However, as demonstrated for all rheumatic diseases, the indirect costs of RA, primarily from lost wages, exceed direct medical care costs by a wide margin. These indirect costs are three to four times higher than direct costs (11,12).

Psychological and Social Consequences

In addition to the significant economic costs associated with rheumatic disease, the psychological and social impact has been documented. The impact of arthritis on psychological status has been measured in terms of depression, coping strategies, anxiety, cognitive changes, self-efficacy, and learned helplessness (6). Most reports indicate higher levels of psychological distress in individuals with rheumatic disease than in the general population, comparable to levels noted in clinical samples of individuals with other chronic conditions (13). Higher levels of psychological distress in individuals with arthritis have also been noted to be associated with poorer status on clinical outcome variables, as well as with increased health services utilization (14).

Research efforts on depressive symptoms and disorders have focused on RA, OA, systemic lupus erythematosus, and fibromyalgia (13). Depressive symptoms and disorders are more common among clinical samples of individuals with arthritis than in the general population (13); however, the majority of individuals with rheumatic disease do not report increased depression. Among persons with RA, the loss of valued activities and the self-perception of the ability to do activities also are strongly correlated with psychological status (15).

PUBLIC HEALTH STRATEGIES

Disability and prevention in rheumatic diseases can be discussed in terms of the World Health Organization (WHO) classification of impairment, disability, and handicap (16). *Impairment* is defined by WHO as any loss or abnormality of psychological, physiologic, or anatomic structure or function. *Disability* refers to any restriction or lack of ability (resulting from impairment) to perform an activity in the manner or within the standard range for a human being. Disabilities reflect the consequences of impairment in terms of activity and functional performance. *Handicap* is defined as a disadvantage for a given individual, resulting from an impairment or disability. Thus, diagnosis of a rheumatic condition is an impairment that can lead to disability and handicap.

Although there is no cure for arthritis, there are interventions targeting primary, secondary, and tertiary prevention (Table 2). The aim of primary prevention is to reduce the incidence of symptomatic disease (impairment); however, in order for primary prevention to be successful or even feasible, the risk factors for disease must be known. The risk factors for many rheumatic diseases are not known, but data from cross-sectional and longitudinal studies reveal that obesity and occupational and sports-related injuries are risk factors for OA (17–19). The Framingham Osteoarthritis Study demonstrated that weight change significantly affected the risk for development of OA of the knee in women; a weight reduction of 5.1 kg (11.2 lbs) over a 10-year period reduced the risk of symptomatic knee OA by more than 50% (19). In addition, the physical demands of occupation as a risk factor for OA of the knee have been observed in several studies (17,18,20). Data from Framingham and the first National Health and Nutrition Examination Survey (NHANES I) indicate jobs that require knee bending and have at least medium physical demands are associated with increased rates of radiographic and clinical OA of the knee (18,20). Risk factor modification such as weight reduction and avoidance of occupational and other injuries may prevent the development of OA of the knee.

Another target for primary prevention is exposure to ticks that carry the spirochete *Borrelia burgdorferi*. The spirochete is a known risk factor for Lyme disease, an infectious arthritis that may have chronic manifestations. Avoiding tick-infested areas, checking the skin regularly for ticks, and using anti-tick pesticides are primary preventive measures for Lyme disease.

Secondary prevention is aimed at early detection and treatment of a disease so that its course may be controlled or favorably altered. Secondary prevention seeks to reduce disability and generally involves screening for disease. Currently, the most appropriate screening test for rheumatic disease is a complete history and physical examination (21). There are a wide variety of clinical presentations, which may or may not

Table 2. Examples of prevention strategies for persons with arthritis.

	Primary Prevention	Secondary Prevention	Tertiary Prevention
Goals	Reduce incidence of disease	Detect disease at early, treatable stage	Reduce disease complications
Target population	Susceptible	Asymptomatic	Symptomatic
Examples	Weight reduction Avoiding sports- & occupational-associated injuries Avoiding tick exposure, checking self and pets for ticks (Lyme)	History and physical Improved education of health professionals Public education to encourage early diagnosis & treatment HLA/genetic testing (potential)	Improved education of health professionals Medication Physical therapy Exercise Occupational therapy Assistive devices Education Use of effective coping strategies Joint replacement surgery

involve the musculoskeletal system; thus, a complete history and physical examination allow the clinician to develop a differential diagnosis, order the appropriate laboratory studies, and formulate a diagnosis and treatment plan. Because early, aggressive therapy may be associated with improved outcomes, it is imperative that the clinician consider these diagnoses when evaluating individuals with musculoskeletal or ill-defined systemic complaints. In order for secondary prevention to be successful in improving outcomes, it will be necessary to increase efforts to educate health professionals about the rheumatic diseases. It is also imperative to increase public awareness about the value of early diagnosis and treatment of rheumatic conditions.

Tertiary prevention is aimed at reducing the complications and handicap resulting from the impairment or disease in symptomatic persons. Most research efforts in the rheumatic diseases have focused on tertiary prevention. Treating individuals with arthritis is often a multidisciplinary effort, involving medications to reduce pain and inflammation; physical therapy, exercise, and occupational therapy to maintain functional status and prevent disability; and education to develop coping and health management skills.

Despite its importance in reducing disability, exercise is a frequently neglected part of the treatment plan. In contrast to the traditional belief that those with rheumatic disease should avoid vigorous physical activity, recent studies have demonstrated that people with arthritis can benefit from appropriate aerobic exercise without exacerbating disease (22,23). Compared to their non-involved peers, people with arthritis are often deconditioned, which may worsen disability. This deconditioning may be reinforced by physicians' recommendations to reduce physical activity. Prolonged inactivity can produce muscle weakness, decreased flexibility, poor endurance, osteoporosis, cardiovascular deficit, fatigue, depression, and other problems that historically have been accepted as either the natural progression of arthritis or the consequences of therapy (22). (See also Chapter 23, Deconditioning.)

In a trial of supervised fitness walking, people with OA of the knee had significant improvement in walking distance and functional status and a decrease in pain and medication usage compared to the control group (23). Similarly, in a trial of people with RA and OA of weight-bearing joints, those randomized to aerobic exercises had a significant improvement over controls in aerobic capacity, 50-foot walking time, depression, anxiety, and physical activity (24). In a 5-year follow-up study of a conditioning program for people with RA, participants who reported more than 5 hours of exercise per week showed less radiographic progression of joint damage, less hospitalization, and less work disability (25). Thus, the benefits of regular aerobic exercise in persons with arthritis may extend beyond improved physical functioning.

Patient education programs are another adjunct in the treatment of people with arthritis. A meta-analysis of 15 controlled evaluations of psychoeducational interventions for people with RA or OA showed improvements in pain, depression, and disability (26). There is an emphasis on educational processes that increase self-efficacy and empower the participants to make appropriate health decisions. In a 4-year follow-up study, participants in the Arthritis Self Management Course retained improvements in pain level and self-efficacy and had a 43% decrease in physician visits compared to nonparticipants (27). Based on reaching just 1% of the population with RA and OA, the projected cost-savings to society that would result from a broader implementation of the program would be $33 million (27). Effective self-management programs with similar content and self-efficacy enhancing processes are also available for people with other rheumatic diseases. For example, the Bone-Up on Arthritis program is a home-study intervention consisting of audiocassettes and print materials written at the fifth-grade reading level. Participants in this program experienced significantly positive changes in self-care behavior, helplessness, pain, disability, and depression compared to nonparticipants (28).

CONCLUSIONS AND POLICY IMPLICATIONS

Given the high prevalence and the significant functional, economic, social and psychological consequences of rheumatic diseases, they should receive considerable attention. This will require changes in policy discussions that currently place more priority on conditions with high mortality rates (8). The research and program funds devoted to rheumatic conditions need to be more commensurate with the frequency and impact of these diseases. Messages regarding primary, secondary, and tertiary prevention must be disseminated more broadly in the public health, research, medical, and lay communities. Public education efforts must be intensified to increase awareness of the value of early diagnosis and appropriate treatment.

According to a recent report by the Centers for Disease Control and Prevention, 6 million individuals believe they have arthritis but have never consulted a physician (1). The high incidence of self-diagnosis and/or delay in seeking medical attention have been observed in other surveys as well (29,30). These high rates may be at least partly attributable to misconceptions about the value of treatment. In interviews with 1,000 adults in two diverse communities, about 40% of people with musculoskeletal conditions thought that nothing could be done for their arthritis (29,30). Clearly, the message that there are effective treatments for arthritis is not reaching the public.

Implementation of strategies to decrease the incidence of rheumatic disease should be incorporated into public health agendas. Individuals should be informed through public and patient education activities of ways to reduce the risk of contracting forms of arthritis with identifiable risk factors. An obvious example is teaching people about the relationship between obesity and knee OA. However, it is also important to incorporate information about the benefits of weight control for arthritis, in addition to cardiovascular and other chronic diseases, into general public health messages. Policies should provide incentives for assessment of and intervention in work-site activities involving repetitive motion and other potentially harmful activities.

Public and professional education efforts should be aimed at changing misconceptions about rheumatic disease and physical activity. Educational messages should focus on the impact of inactivity and how low-intensity aerobic exercises can improve fitness, functional ability, and psychosocial status. Physicians should be encouraged to include conditioning exercise as an important part of their treatment recommendations and to refer their patients to physical therapists or other rehabilitation specialists for detailed exercise instruction. Health professionals should also be encouraged to refer their patients to community-based programs such as the Arthritis Foundation's self-management and exercise classes, which have demonstrated the ability to improve participant outcomes. Greater awareness by health professionals and persons with rheumatic disease of the relevancy of the Americans with Disabilities Act (ADA) for employment accommodation, public access, and housing is necessary to prevent handicap (31).

Rheumatic diseases have complex etiologies that involve interactions among genetic, immunologic, environmental, and behavioral factors. The degree to which an individual remains independent or becomes disabled is also multideterminant. Further studies are needed to identify biopsychosocial risk factors that contribute to the development of the various forms of rheumatic disease and to the progression of disability. Where risk factors have been identified, there is still a need for multidisciplinary intervention studies and population-based longitudinal studies. Because morbidity is higher in some underserved populations like African-Americans, intervention studies are needed to determine how best to deliver and/or modify interventions. There are currently no national, community-based longitudinal studies of working age adults with sufficient sample sizes to estimate the prognosis for persons with arthritis in terms of function and work capacity. Creating a longitudinal version of the National Health Interview Survey would improve understanding of how working-age persons with arthritis withdraw from the labor force. The probable underestimation of the impact of arthritis in women raises questions about the adequacy of current methods of counting impacts and costs that reflect a strong masculine bias.

Recognition of rheumatic disease as a disease of public health importance is necessary for the condition to receive appropriate attention when policymakers are setting their health agendas. More resources should be committed to arthritis research and programs. Concomitantly, the burden of rheumatic disease in society could be reduced by broader dissemination and implementation of known prevention strategies and interventions.

REFERENCES

1. Centers for Disease Control and Prevention: Arthritis prevalence and activity limitations-United States, 1990. MMWR Morb Mortal Wkly Rep 43:433–438, 1994
2. Centers for Disease Control and Prevention: Prevalence of disabilities and associated health conditions-United States, 1991–1992. MMWR Morb Mortal Wkly Rep 43:730–739, 1994
3. Yelin EH: Work disability and rheumatoid arthritis. In, Rheumatoid Arthritis: Pathogenesis, Assessment, Outcome, and Treatment. Edited by F Wolfe, T Pincus. New York, Marcel Dekker, Inc., 1994, pp. 261–272
4. Yelin EH, Henke CJ, Epstein WV: Work disability among persons with musculoskeletal conditions. Arthritis Rheum 29:1322–1333, 1986
5. Pincus T, Mitchell JM, Burkhauser RV: Substantial work disability and earnings losses in individuals less than age 65 with osteoarthritis: comparisons with rheumatoid arthritis. J Clin Epidemiol 42:449–457, 1989
6. Yelin E, Callahan L, for the National Arthritis Data Work Group: The economic cost and social and psychological impact of musculosketetal conditions. Arthritis Rheum 38:1351–1362, 1995
7. Reisine S, Fifield J: Expanding the definition of disability: implications for planning, policy, and research. Milbank Q 70:491–508, 1995
8. Verbrugge L, Patrick D: Seven chronic conditions: their impact on US adults' activity levels and use of medical services. Am J Public Health 85:173–182, 1994
9. Reisine S, McQuillan J, Fifield J: Predictors of work disability in rheumatoid arthritis patients: a five-year followup. Arthritis Rheum 38:1630–1637, 1995
10. Allaire SH, Prashker M, Meenan RF: The costs of rheumatoid arthritis. Pharmacoeconomics 6:513–522, 1994
11. Lubeck DP: The economic impact of arthritis. Arthritis Care Res 8:304–310, 1995
12. Yelin E: The costs of rheumatoid arthritis: absolute, incremental, and marginal estimates. J Rheumatol 23 (Suppl 44):47–51, 1996
13. DeVellis B: Depression in rheumatological diseases. Baillieres Clin Rheumatol 7:241–257, 1993
14. Hawley DJ, Wolfe F: Anxiety and depression in patients with rheumatoid arthritis: a prospective study of 400 patients. J Rheumatol 15:932–941, 1988
15. Katz PP, Yelin EH: Life activities of persons with rheumatoid arthritis with and without depressive symptoms. Arthritis Care Res 7:69–77, 1994
16. Wood PHN: Appreciating the consequences of disease: the international classification of impairments, disabilities and handicaps. WHO Chron 34:376–380, 1980
17. Cooper C, McAlindon T, Coggon D, Eggger P, Dieppe P: Occupational activity and osteoarthritis of the knee. Ann Rheum Dis 53:90–93, 1994
18. Felson DT, Hannan MT, Naimark A, Berkeley J, Gordon G, Wilson PWF, Anderson J: Occupational physical demands, knee bending, and knee osteoarthritis: results from the Framingham Study. J Rheumatol 18:1587–1592, 1991
19. Felson DT, Zhang Y, Anthony JM, Naimark A, Anderson JJ: Weight loss reduces the risk for symptomatic knee osteoarthritis in women: the Framingham Study. Ann Intern Med 116:535–539, 1992
20. Anderson JJ, Felson DT: Factors associated with osteoarthritis of the knee in the first national health and nutrition examination survey (NHANES I): evidence for an association with overweight, race and physical demands of work. Am J Epidemiol 128:179–189, 1988
21. Pincus T: A pragmatic approach to cost-effective use of laboratory tests and imaging procedures in patients with musculoskeletal symptoms. Prim Care 20:795–814, 1993
22. Minor M: Physical activity and management of arthritis. Ann Behav Med 13:117–124, 1991
23. Kovar P, Allegrante J, MacKenzie C, Peterson M, Gutin B, Charleson M: Supervised fitness walking in patients with osteoarthritis of the knee: a randomized controlled trial. Ann Intern Med 116:529–534, 1992
24. Minor MA, Hewett JE, Webel RR, Anderson SK, Kay DR: Efficacy of physical conditioning exercise in patients with rheumatoid arthritis and osteoarthritis. Arthritis Rheum 32:1396–1405, 1989
25. Nordemar R, Ekblom B, Zachrisson L, Lundquist K: Physical training in rheumatoid arthritis: a long-term study I. Scand J Rheumatol 10:10–23, 1981
26. Mullen PD, Laville EA, Biddle AK, Lorig K: Efficacy of psychoeducational interventions on pain, depression, and disability in people with arthritis: a meta-analysis. J Rheumatol 14 (Suppl 15):33–39, 1987
27. Lorig KR, Mazonson PD, Holman HR: Evidence suggesting that health education for self-management in patients with chronic arthritis has sustained health benefits while reducing health care costs. Arthritis Rheum 36:439–446, 1993
28. Goeppinger J, Arthur MW, Baglioni A Jr, Brunk SE, Brunner CM: A reexamination of the effectiveness of self-care education for persons with arthritis. Arthritis Rheum 32:706–716, 1989
29. A Study of Help-Seeking Among Individuals with Musculoskeletal Conditions in San Mateo County, California: A Report to the San Mateo Arthritis Project. San Francisco, Communication Technologies, July 1, 1993
30. A Study of Help-Seeking Among Individuals with Musculoskeletal Conditions in the Greater Atlanta Area: a Report to the Arthritis Foundation. San Francisco, Communication Technologies, May 23, 1994
31. Greenwald S, Gerber L: The Americans with Disabilities Act. Bull Rheum Dis 41:5–7, 1992

Treatment Efficacy and Cost Effectiveness

CHRISTOPHER D. LORISH, PhD

Payers, providers, and consumers of health care services have an interest in delivering effective health care for less cost. The legislative, administrative, and research responses to this effort are already underway and will continue to affect not only the quantity and quality of care that patients receive but also health professionals' practice standards and working conditions. Well-designed studies are needed to inform legislative debate and administrative decisions. This might counterbalance the marketplace inclination to maximize cost reductions and profit, possibly at the patient's expense. Health professionals should participate in these studies and be critical consumers of the research literature in order to maintain credibility and influence in the debate (1–3).

TREATMENT COST AND EFFECTIVENESS STUDIES

The shift in health care from a focus on process quality standards to outcomes has found its research analogue in studies testing comparative treatment effectiveness and, more recently, cost-effectiveness. The differences in the purposes of these studies are important. Treatment effectiveness studies use clinical experiments to determine which of two or more treatments produces the most, best, or quickest return to health with the least harm. A drug study in which, for example, a new nonsteroidal anti-inflammatory drug (NSAID) is compared to aspirin or another NSAID in its relative ability to reduce pain, inflammation, and improve function is a model case. In physical therapy, comparing manual therapy treatment to electrical stimulation to reduce pain and increase function in patients with acute low back pain is another example. Such clinical experiments permit clinicians to develop and use scientifically verified or evidence-based treatments, rather than tradition or normative-based practices (4).

If resources to pay for health care were unlimited, clinical experiments testing cost effectiveness of treatments would be of little interest. However, resources *are* limited and payers of health care—business, taxpayers, and the consumer—are asking a more complicated question. Cost-effectiveness studies, which are grounded in the utilitarian precept of providing the greatest good for the greatest number, use a variety of methods to identify the most efficacious treatments for the least cost so that government or insurance officials can rationally distribute limited health care resources to the most people. When outcomes of treatment are translated from their natural units (such as years of remission or number of deaths) to an economic unit (such as dollars), the study is termed a cost-benefit analysis, a term revealing its economic lineage (5,6). Whether or not cost-effectiveness or cost-benefit analyses help accomplish the

utilitarian ideal will depend on an amalgam of science, politics, and a consensus of values regarding who should be treated or saved. As the values debate continues, health researchers can exert influence by providing answers to the prior question of comparative treatment effectiveness and costs, and practitioners can stimulate the treatment effectiveness research by a commitment to an evidence-based practice (4).

BECOMING A CRITICAL CONSUMER OF RESEARCH

The transition to empirically-based practice in which therapeutic decisions are based more on validated efficacy than on tradition has great promise for improving patient outcomes and reducing time and money spent on less effective treatments. In disciplines like physical and occupational therapy, progress is likely to be slow because the research traditions are young and have limited financial support. Treatment effectiveness research is presented regularly in the journals of these disciplines, and all the health professions must make judgements about the value of treatments on the basis of this often limited scientific evidence (7). While these judgements can be uncritically adopted from influential researchers and clinicians, another strategy is for each health professional to become a critical consumer of the treatment effectiveness research. Developing such a perspective requires that health professionals critically read studies of treatment effectiveness (1,8) and answer the following questions: 1) Is the research study being reported descriptive or experimental? 2) How credible is the causal relationship between the treatment and desired outcome (the study's internal validity)? 3) How clinically important are the results (the magnitude of the study's effects)? and 4) How applicable are the results to my practice (the study's generalizability to other patients)?

CLINICAL EXPERIMENTS VERSUS DESCRIPTIVE STUDIES

All research begins with questions. Clinical experiments assessing treatment effectiveness attempt to answer questions about the onset, duration, and degree of desired and harmful effects caused by one or more treatments (9). Effects can be focused on changes in tissues or organ system dysfunctions (impairments), functional limitations, and/or social, emotional, and role dysfunctions. Note the implicit causal sequence; that is, impairments cause functional limitations which cause role or other health status changes. Health professionals in the rheumatic diseases are the beneficiaries of years of work developing valid and reliable measures of outcomes at each of these levels (10). Measuring treatment impact on each level greatly increases a study's value, because it adds to our understanding of how impairments influence function.

Prior to conducting clinical experiments, descriptive data often need to be obtained. Clinical observation should be supplemented by systematic descriptive studies to identify characteristics of the condition and the range of desired and harmful treatment effects. Descriptive studies may be *laboratory studies* detailing the characteristics of normal and pathological tissues. They may be *epidemiologic studies* of the incidence and prevalence of rheumatologic conditions or correlational studies that identify potentially important causal relationships in the etiology or sequelae of a condition. They may be *case studies* or *surveys* soliciting patients' opinions or descriptions of a disease, its effects, and costs. They may be *qualitative studies,* which emphasize participant observation and copious description to provide insight into the meaning of a disease or treatment for patients. These kinds of descriptive studies lay the groundwork for both comparative treatment and cost-effectiveness studies by fully elaborating the characteristics of a condition and likely costs and benefits of the disease and treatments. For example, recent research in fibromyalgia consists of both descriptive and treatment efficacy studies, specifically tissue pathology, incidence and prevalence of the condition, functional limitations, and psychological, social, and role consequences to improve our understanding of the disease (11).

The key distinction between descriptive studies and experimental ones is that the latter attempt to demonstrate a causal relation between the application of a treatment and a desired outcome. For example, does a patient education program cause an improvement in patients' social and role functioning? Descriptive studies may *suggest* a causal connection, but their primary purpose is to help us know more about the object of interest. The task of an experimental study is to set up a test that unambiguously demonstrates the causal relationship between the treatment and effect.

DETERMINING CREDIBILITY OF CLINICAL EXPERIMENTAL RESULTS

Laboratory and clinical experiments follow rules of procedure and evidence to narrow the number of potential causes of an effect to the one of interest. This is no simple task when dealing with real people living in natural settings. Experimental researchers apply procedures to exert control over unwanted causes by eliminating them or exerting procedural and statistical controls. This increases the likelihood that the observed effect (e.g., reduced pain) is due to the treatment (the cause of interest). The number and success of control efforts determine a study's *internal validity.* Studies that successfully apply all the procedures are judged to have higher internal validity and the results are more likely to be judged credible by the scientific community. Thus, to answer the first question, "How credible is the causal relationship between the treatment and outcome?," the most important criterion is the amount of control exercised over other causes that threaten internal validity. Readers should examine research reports for the controls used in the study to minimize the influence of causes other than the treatment.

Numerous articles have been published detailing the procedural characteristics evidencing high internal validity (1). Rating schemes that give a summary score of a study's internal validity exist and have been used to evaluate the experimental literature in the allied health disciplines (12). Because no study with humans is ever able to rule out all possible competing causal explanations for the effect of interest, internal validity is achieved by degree, necessitating additional studies that overcome the uncontrolled causes of prior studies. The accumulation of similar findings from many studies with high internal validity gives that finding the highest credibility.

Inclusion–Exclusion Criteria

To control other causes (sometimes termed *biases*), researchers use a variety of procedures to eliminate, minimize, or make such causes explicit. The more control procedures used in an experiment, the more confidence the reader can have in the study's results. Clinical experiments consist of comparisons of two or more treatment (intervention) groups in which subjects in each group are selected, assigned, and compared after exposure to a treatment. Because people vary in many ways, some of which may affect the outcome of interest, the first control measure used by investigators is specific subject inclusion and exclusion criteria to try to obtain a more homogeneous pool of subjects. Persons with characteristics known to affect the outcome are usually excluded. For example, in a study on the efficacy of electrical stimulation versus NSAID therapy for controlling pain, persons with an aversion to electricity or with gastric problems would probably be excluded because of an increased likelihood that they would not comply with the treatment, thereby reducing the treatment's full effects. Careful examination of the study's inclusion–exclusion criteria alerts the reader to other causes that may have operated to either enhance or diminish the treatment's effects.

Random Assignment to Groups

Even with selection criteria that eliminate persons with characteristics known to affect the outcome, there will likely be causally important differences among subjects. A second control measure is *random assignment*. Random assignment of subjects to groups equilibrates groups at the study's outset, where the distribution and effects of other subject characteristics that can affect the outcome are more likely to be the same in both groups.

While randomization is the best method for equilibrating subject-related causal influences, it does not guarantee initial comparability. The likelihood that the distribution of subject characterisitics is similar in both groups is related to the number of study subjects. This is illustrated by the distribution of heads and tails when a coin is flipped 500 times versus 10 times. The former is most likely to achieve a 50–50 split, while the latter most likely would deviate from the 50–50 split. Thus, even with randomization a reader cannot be assured that groups were equilibrated at the outset if the group sizes were small (<10 per group). In a study with a small number of subjects per group, authors should provide additional evidence of group equivalency at the study's outset on characteristics most likely to influence the outcome.

Note that randomization at the outset does not guarantee that roups will remain comparable throughout the study. Unexpected events occur in studies, especially those occurring over months or years. Good research reports will discuss how the study was monitored and the responses to unexpected changes that add ambiguity to the causal connection between the treatment and outcome of interest.

Statistical Control

A third control method is *statistical control,* in which measures of variables known to be associated with the outcome are included in the statistical analysis. A study may examine the effects of two treatments but also include subgroups within each treatment (e.g., men and women). Differences between these subgroups within each treatment group can be tested by statistical procedures like analysis of variance (ANOVA) or multiple regression. Studies that purposely build in subgroups have the additional advantage of providing more definitive evidence of the efficacy of treatment on different types of patients. The most common use of statistics is to rule out whether chance variation is a possible explanation for the results. The usual statistical criterion sets a probability value (P value) equal to or less than 0.05, indicating this result would only occur 5 times out of 100 by chance alone. These three control procedures—inclusion-exclusion criteria, randomization, and statistical analyses—proactively reduce bias, but other events can occur during a study that threaten internal validity and require scrutiny by the reader of a research report.

The Missing Data Threat

Data not collected on subjects (missing data) or subjects who quit the study after its start (dropouts) pose a serious threat to the comparability of groups obtained by randomization. At the end of the study, it can no longer be assumed that groups are comparable. For example, in a study of two strengthening regimens, random assignment is the best way to ensure that differences in pre-study strength, exercise motivation, and other influences are equally distributed between the groups at the outset. Confidence in the results is greatly diminished if there is a significant number of dropouts or data not collected in any or all of the groups. The distribution of pre-study strength or other causes that could influence the outcome may have changed, and the effects of these causes can no longer be assumed to be comparable between the groups. Look for discussion of the amount of study dropouts and missing data and what the authors have done to identify its effects on the results. The results of a clinical experiment with dropouts that exceed 20% (15% is the FDA standard) should probably be viewed with healthy skepticism (13).

The Variable Treatment Implementation Threat

Poor control of the treatment implementation and measurement procedures can lead to ambiguous cause–effect relationships. The report should convince the reader that 1) treatments were clearly different and consistently applied and/or followed by subjects; 2) subjects were not exposed to other treatments, such as home remedies or other prescribed medications, outside of the study; and 3) measures were appropriate (measurement

validity) and consistently applied (reliability). Treatments and measures haphazardly applied or frequently modified result in a causal stew of unknown ingredients.

Control procedures should minimize unwanted treatment implementation influences. Data collectors may unknowingly encourage a treatment subject to respond in a desirable way or a treatment provider may do more or less to a comparison group patient out of a "sense of fairness." This treatment and measurement control is best accomplished by keeping study subjects, data collectors, and treatment staff ignorant ("blinded") of treatment group membership. Maintaining subjects' ignorance of the treatment received is especially important in order to minimize bias in self-report measures.

The careful reader should be aware of the steps taken to keep subjects and study personnel ignorant of study group membership and to ensure the consistent implementation of the treatment. For example, in a study comparing the efficacy of at-home exercise versus manual therapy techniques on low back pain patients, a stronger study will include the following: 1) evidence that the subjects in the exercise group did the same or at least similar exercises (within group treatment homogeneity) and that each person did them correctly and regularly during the study period (treatment adherence); 2) subjects received no other treatments, such as acupuncture, chiropracty, or any others, that were likely to affect the outcome measures during the study; and 3) personnel taking measures were ignorant of a subject's group assignment and that the measures were taken consistently in the same way (intra- and inter-rater reliability). Indications that patients did less or more of the specified treatment or other treatments, that opportunities were missed to keep study personnel and subjects ignorant of a subject's group assignment, and low (<80%) intra- and inter-rater measurement reliability (self-report measures are often lower) are significant threats to internal validity and weaken the inference that one treatment was superior, even if one group is statistically different from the other.

DETERMINING CLINICAL IMPORTANCE

Assume that an investigator has done a credible job of minimizing and identifying threats to internal validity and that the statistical analyses indicate that the differences between the groups were probably not due to chance variation in the population. The reader can more confidently believe that for the sample studied, one treatment was superior to another in producing a clinical effect. The reader must now ask whether the difference (effect size) is *clinically important.* This may be intuitively determined by examining the outcome data and its scale. For example, if one of the outcomes in the back pain study was pain measured by 10-cm visual analogue scale (10) and the difference between the two groups at the end of the study was a 1-cm reduction in pain favoring the exercise treatment, the advantage to exercise may be judged trivial given the reader's clinical experience. A small difference between treatments can be statistically significant if the sample is large and valid and reliable measurements are used. Both increase the sensitivity (statistical power) of the statistical test to detect a significant difference. Thus, the obtained probability level (e.g., $P < 0.05$) is a poor indicator of both the magnitude of a study's effect and its clinical importance.

Treatment Effect Size

An alternative indicator that is often not reported is the treatment's *effect size*. Effect size is an index of the magnitude of an effect independent of the scale on which it is measured. While the effect size can be calculated in different ways, one common way is to take the difference between the end-of-study means of two groups and divide that by the standard deviation of the mean of the control group. This provides a number that can be compared with effect sizes from other studies or used for planning future studies. If prior studies do not exist, Cohen (14) provides guidelines for classifying an effect as small, medium, or large.

If the study also collected data on all the direct and indirect costs associated with each treatment, a cost-effectiveness ratio can be calculated by dividing the benefit obtained (e.g., the effect size for a treatment) by its costs in dollars multiplied by $1,000 to give the number of benefit units per $1,000 of cost. These ratios can be directly compared to ascertain which treatments gave the most benefit per unit of cost. This simplistic example glosses over the necessity to quantify a benefit unit based on all benefits adjusted by all harmful effects of the treatment and dividing by the sum of all present and future costs. The conceptual simplicity of the cost-effective ratio belies complex methodological problems, the solutions to which are still emerging and controversial.

The use of effect sizes for computing cost-effective ratios of treatments may be beyond most clinical researchers now; however, its use in study planning is not. The author should indicate how the study's sample size was determined using an effect size estimate preferably obtained from the most recent, similar published study. If no published study exists, then the author may cite a pilot study effect size. This planning step is crucial in avoiding the unfortunate situation of reading a research report in which the internal validity was high, but there were not enough subjects to demonstrate statistical significance.

Meta-analysis

Another approach to determining a study's clinical significance is to place the obtained effect size in the context of other studies. *Meta-analysis*, a quantitative study of studies, aggregates the effect sizes of other similar studies to produce an average effect size for a treatment (15). This quantitative approach to synthesizing findings from numerous studies with similar treatments and outcomes provides a quantitative accounting of our knowledge. For example, a meta-analytic study of the effect of NSAID therapy in similar patients would produce an average effect size that could be directly compared with splinting to reduce inflammation. Analyses of the average effects of a treatment and comparisons of effect sizes with other treatments for the same condition will help answer the question of which treatments are most efficacious and should be considered first-line therapy. Extant meta-analyses of interest to rheumatic disease health professionals include patient education and psychoeducation interventions (16), multidisciplinary pain treatment (17), aerobic fitness (18), nursing interventions (19), and psychosocial treatments of depression (20). This approach to integrating findings is relatively new and requires a number of comparative experiments before it can be completed. Because of the relative youth of the allied health disciplines, there may not be enough comparative experiment to conduct a meta-analysis on a specific treatment, leaving the therapist to gauge the clinical importance and relevance to practice on a study-by-study basis.

DETERMINING APPLICABILITY TO PRACTICE

In addition to judging a study's clinical importance, the health professional must also assess the relevance of the study's results to his or her practice. The more similar the practice patients are to the study patients, the more applicable the study's results are. One guideline is to ask if the patients seen in practice fit the inclusion criteria of the study and would not be eliminated by the exclusion criteria. Some investigators apply a more liberal standard by suggesting that a practitioner should ask if there is a compelling reason why the result should not be applied, such as comorbidities, greater disease severity, or greater risks for harm (8). Ideally, clinical effectiveness research will be used to develop treatment guidelines in the form, "For patients with X, Y, and Z characteristics Treatment A is the best choice for producing the greatest change in Outcome C." Until the treatment effectiveness data exist to create such guides, clinicians must weigh scientific uncertainty, use caution, and rely on clinical judgement in treating their patients.

Health practitioners must become more involved in the collection of data that answers important clinical effectiveness questions. How can they become more involved in this effort when many feel overwhelmed by patient care activities, revenue generation, and paperwork? One promising model is the development of clinical data bases at practice sites. If set up carefully and fed with valid and reliable process and outcome data, these data bases can help answer treatment efficacy and cost questions. Another approach would be single subject protocols shared through the Internet that individual clinicians could implement. A study of one subject in which the study protocol is already developed is a much less daunting task than planning and implementing a clinical experiment. At the study's completion, the data would be returned to the originating site for aggregation, resulting in an "N=1" study replicated many times. A variation of this model is a research partnership between academic researchers and clinical sites that works together to develop and test treatment protocols. This latter model is more inclusive than the former and permits both partners to contribute their respective strengths to the effort. The clinician brings a source of subjects and insight into important treatment questions to be asked, while the academic brings a strong knowledge of the requirements for an internally valid clinical experiment and the possibility of obtaining financial support for the work. Through such collaborative efforts or "N=1" studies numerously replicated, it is more likely that busy practitioners can participate in and benefit from treatment effectiveness experiments.

REFERENCES

1. Guyatt GH, Sackett DL, Cook DJ, for the Evidence-Based Medicine Working Group: User's guide to the medical literature: II. How to use an article about therapy or prevention A. Are the results of the study valid JAMA 270:2598–2601, 1993

2. Bork CE: Research in Physical Therapy. Philadelphia, JB Lippincott, 1993
3. DePoy E, Gitlin L: Introduction to Research: Multiple Strategies For Health and Human Services. St. Louis, Mosby, 1994
4. Sackett DL, Haynes RB, Guyatt GH, Tugwell P: Clinical Epidemiology: A Basic Science For Clinical Medicine. Boston, MA, Little Brown, 1991
5. Eddy DM: Cost-effectiveness analysis: a conversation with my father. JAMA 267:1669–1675, 1992
6. Eddy DM: Applying cost-effectiveness analysis: the inside story. JAMA 268:2575–2582, 1992
7. Robertson VJ: A quantitative analysis of research in physical therapy. Phys Ther 75:69–83, 1995
8. Guyatt GH, Sackett DL, Cook DJ: Users' guide to the medical literature: II. How to use an article about therapy or prevention. B. What were the results and will they help me in caring for my patients? JAMA 271:59–63, 1994
9. Liang MH, Andersson G, Bombardier C, et al: Strategies for outcome research in spinal disorders: an introduction. Spine 185(S):2037–2040, 1994
10. Gall E, Gibofsky A: Rheumatoid Arthritis: Clinical Tools for Outcome Assessment. Atlanta, Arthritis Foundation, 1994
11. Freundlich B, Leventhal L: The fibromyalgia syndrome. In, Primer on the Rheumatic Diseases, Tenth edition. Edited by HR Schumacher, JH Klippel, WJ Koopman. Atlanta, GA, Arthritis Foundation, 1993, p. 247
12. Barr JT: Critical Literature Review: Clinical Effectiveness In Allied Health Practices. Pub No. 940029. Rockville, MD, Agency for Health Care Policy and Research, 1995
13. Shekelle PG, Andersson G, Bombardier C, et al: A brief introduction to the critical reading of the clinical literature. Spine 19(S):2028–2031, 1994
14. Cohen J: Statistical Power Analysis for the Behavioral Sciences. Second edition. New York, Academic Press, 1988
15. Mullen B: Advanced BASIC Meta-Analysis. Hillsdale, NJ, Lawrence Earlbaum Associates, 1989
16. Mullen PD, Laville EA, Biddle AK, Lorig K: Efficacy of psychoeducational interventions on pain, depression, and disability in people with arthritis: a meta-analysis. J Rheumatol 14:33–39, 1987
17. Flor H, Fydrich T, Turk D: Efficacy of multidisciplinary pain treatment centers: a meta-analytic review. Pain 49:221–230, 1992
18. Crews DJ, Landers DM: A meta-analytic review of aerobic fitness and reactivity to psychosocial stressors. Med Sci Sports Exerc 19:S114–S120, 1987
19. Heater BS, Becker AM, Olson RK: Nursing interventions and patient outcomes: a meta-analysis of studies. Nurs Res 37:303–307, 1988
20. Scogin F, McElreath L: Efficacy of psychosocial treatments for geriatric depression: a quantitative review. J Consult Clin Psychol 62:69–74, 1994

Subject Index